Head and Neck Ultrasonography

Head and Neck Ultrasonography

Edited by
Lisa A. Orloff, MD

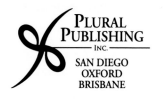

PLURAL
PUBLISHING
INC.

SAN DIEGO
OXFORD
BRISBANE

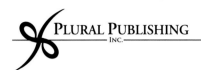

PLURAL PUBLISHING
INC.

5521 Ruffin Road
San Diego, CA 92123

e-mail: info@pluralpublishing.com
Web site: http://www.pluralpublishing.com

49 Bath Street
Abingdon, Oxfordshire OX14 1EA
United Kingdom

Library of Congress Cataloging-in-Publication Data:

Head and neck ultrasonography / [edited by] Lisa Orloff.
        p. ; cm.
  Includes bibliographical references.
  ISBN-13: 978-1-59756-075-7 (alk. paper)
  ISBN-10: 1-59756-075-8 (alk. paper)
  1. Head–Ultrasonic imaging. 2. Neck–Ultrasonic imaging.
  [DNLM: 1. Head–ultrasonography. 2. Neck–ultrasonography. 3. Ultrasonography–
methods. WE 705 H4313 2007] I. Orloff, Lisa.
  RC936.H436 2007
  617.5'107543–dc22

                                                                2007049396

CONTENTS

PREFACE

Head and Neck Ultrasonography is the first, and one hopes the definitive, English-language textbook of head and neck ultrasonography by and for clinicians, and particularly surgeons. Although the current reference literature includes a number of textbooks of head and neck ultrasonography written by and for diagnostic radiologists, there is no comprehensive textbook of office-based and intraoperative ultrasonography for the English-speaking surgeon who manages patients with head and neck disorders. This void exists at precisely the time when ultrasonography is experiencing an explosion in interest and application within nearly every medical subspecialty. No longer regarded as the sole domain of the radiologist who is not engaged in direct patient care, ultrasonography is being utilized at the bedside in fields ranging from emergency medicine to cardiology to breast oncology. The anatomy of the head and neck is particularly accessible and amenable to ultrasound examination, and otolaryngologists/head and neck surgeons and endocrine surgeons are increasingly incorporating ultrasonography into their clinical practices. There is a rapidly growing body of journal literature citing the utility and advantages of neck ultrasonography, especially in the management of thyroid disease, head and neck cancer, and benign neoplasms and masses in the head and neck. There are evolving applications to active processes such as swallowing, sleep dynamics, and speech. The publication of this complete textbook of head and neck ultrasonography is the ideal complement to this surge in appreciation and utilization of ultrasonography.

Head and Neck Ultrasonography covers the fundamentals of ultrasound physics, equipment, normal head and neck ultrasound anatomy, and technique. Individual chapters cover specific anatomy and pathology. Interventional ultrasonography and dynamic ultrasonography are included. New directions and techniques in ultrasonography are also presented.

This textbook is unique both in its thoroughness and in its relevance to the clinical setting, where ultrasonographic examination is a dynamic and interactive process between physician and patient. Although numerous examples of still ultrasound images are necessary and invaluable (and are the traditional format of ultrasound textbooks), this book also takes advantage of dynamic video clips that can be viewed on DVD to best illustrate both the process and the interpretation of specific examinations and procedures. Images (both still and video) are predominantly black and white, as in standard B-mode ultrasonography, but color Doppler sonography is included where pertinent.

Head and Neck Ultrasonography is organized into chapters written by individuals with particular expertise in the given topic. Contributors include surgeons predominantly, but also radiologists, gastroenterologists, neurologists, and research scientists whom I have had the privilege of learning from and collaborating with as experts in head and neck ultrasonography who are helping to move forward the applications of this powerful tool. To the clinician caring for head and neck disorders, one hopes that this book will be a useful resource for trainees and experienced practitioners alike, and will provide stimulation for new applications of ultrasonography within the region.

Lisa A. Orloff, MD

ACKNOWLEDGMENTS

Many people have contributed to bringing this textbook to fruition. However, I would like to give special thanks to the following individuals: my original ultrasonography instructors, especially Wolf Mann, Peter Jecker, and the HNO residents at the Uni-Klinikum Mainz and the University of Regensburg; all of my contributing authors for their hard work and commitment to educating the readers of this book about the infinite benefits of clinical ultrasonography; Dave Eisele for having the foresight and enthusiasm to support the integration of ultrasonography into our clinical practice of head and neck surgery; Carole Benson for her technical help with the DVD compilation; and Senator J. William Fulbright for having established a program that sponsors cultural and scientific exchange and mutual understanding, and enables those of us so fortunate to participate in this program to meet and learn about amazing people and ideas such as those represented by this book.

Lisa A. Orloff, MD

CONTRIBUTORS

Timothy J. Beale, FRCS, FRCR
Consultant Radiologist
The Royal National Throat Nose and Ear Hospital
London, England
Chapter 9

Jonas A. Castelijns, MD, PhD
Professor of Radiology, Vice-Chairman
Department of Radiology
VU Medical Center
Amsterdam, The Netherlands
Chapter 15

Marc D. Coltrera, MD
Professor and Vice Chairman
Department of Otolaryngology-Head and Neck
    Surgery
University of Washington
Seattle, Washington
Chapter 2

Kristin K. Egan, MD
Department of Otolaryngology-Head and Neck
    Surgery
University of California, San Francisco
San Francisco, California
Chapter 12

Christine G. Gourin MD, FACS
Associate Professor
Director of Clinical Research Program in Head
    and Neck Cancer
Department of Otolaryngology- Head and Neck
    Surgery
Johns Hopkins University
Baltimore, MD
Chapter 4

Peter Jecker, MD, PhD
Chief, Division of Otolaryngology, Head and
    Neck Surgery

Klinikum Bad Salzungen gGmbH
Bad Salzungen
Germany
Chapters 7 and 11

Theresa B. Kim, MD
Resident
Department of Otolaryngology, Head and Neck
    Surgery
University of California, San Francisco
San Francisco, California
Chapter 5

Wolf J. Mann, MD, PhD, FACS
Professor and Chairman
Department of Otolaryngology
Mainz, Germany
Chapter 1

Jeri L. Miller, PhD
Clinical Research Scientist
Rehabilitation Medicine Department
National Institutes of Health
Bethesda, Maryland
Chapter 14

Michael Moussouttas, MD
Postdoctoral Clinical Fellow
Vascular and Critical Care Neurology
Columbia University Medical Center
New York, New York
Chapter 13

V. Raman Muthusamy, MD
Assistant Clinical Professor of Medicine
Division of Gastroenterology
H.H. Chao Comprehensive Digestive Disease
    Center
University of California, Irvine
Chapter 10

Lisa A. Orloff, MD, FACS
Professor of Otolaryngology/Head and Neck
  Surgery
Chief, Division of Head and Neck and Endocrine
  Surgery
University of California, San Francisco
San Francisco, California
Chapters 4, 5, 7, and 12

John S. Rubin MD, FACS, FRCS
Consultant Ear Nose and Throat Surgeon
Clinical Director
Royal National Throat Nose and Ear Hospital
  Directorate
Royal Free Hampstead NHS Trust
London England
Chapter 9

Tatjana Rundek, MD, PhD
Associate Professor of Neurology
Department of Neurology
Miller School of Medicine, University of Miami
Miami, Florida
Chapter 13

Janak N. Shah, MD
Director of Endoscopy
San Francisco VA Medical Center
Assistant Clinical Professor of Medicine
University of California, San Francisco
San Francisco, California
Chapter 10

Barbara C. Sonies, PhD, CCC/slp
Board Recognized Specialist in Swallowing and
  Swallowing Disorders
Research Professor, Hearing and Speech
  Sciences, University of Maryland
College Park, MD
Adjunct Professor, George Washington
  University, Speech and Hearing Department
Washington, D.C.
Chapter 14

Antonia E. Stephen, MD
Assistant in Surgery

Division of Surgical Oncology
Massachusetts General Hospital
Boston, Massachusetts
Chapter 3

David L. Steward, MD
Associate Professor
Director of Thyroid and Parathyroid Surgery
Dept. of Otolaryngology
Head and Neck Surgery
University of Cincinnati Medical Center
Cincinnati, Ohio
Chapter 6

Samuel H. Trocio, Jr., MD, RVT
Technical Director
Non-Invasive Doppler Laboratory
Neurological Institute, Division of Stroke and
  Critical Care
Columbia University Medical Center
New York, New York
Chapter 13

Michiel W.M. van den Brekel, MD, PhD
Department of Otolaryngology
Head and Neck Surgeon
Netherlands Cancer Institute and Academic
  Medical Center
Amsterdam, The Netherlands
Chapter 15

Mikhail Vaysberg, DO
Assistant Professor
Department of Otolaryngology/Head & Neck
  Surgery
University of Florida
Gainesville, Florida
Chapter 6

Hans J. Welkoborsky, MD, DDS, PhD
Department of Otolaryngology
Head and Neck Surgery
Nordstadt Clinic
Academic Hospital
Hannover, Germany
Chapter 8

To my family: Paul, Stuart, and Eric
Who have lovingly shared, and endured, the many hours, adventures, and miles traveled in
the course of acquiring and passing on the knowledge contained herein

And my parents
Who have always taught by example and will forever be my mentors

Chapter 1

HISTORY OF HEAD AND NECK ULTRASONOGRAPHY

Wolf J. Mann

Historical Development of Medical Ultrasound

Ultrasound is based on the piezoelectric effect which was discovered by the brothers Pièrre and Jacques Curie in 1880[1] (Fig 1-1). Ultrasonography (US) experienced further development in 1912 by the physicist A. Behm[2] with the invention of maritime sonar, a development which was accelerated by the tragedy of the sinking of the Titanic. The first medical application of US was in the field of neurology, led by Dussik,[3] with the description of the so-called "hyperphonography" for evaluating the ventricular

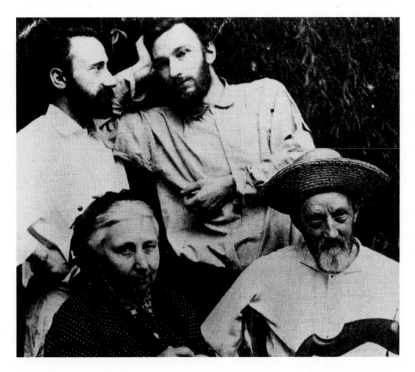

Fig 1-1. The brothers Pierre (*top right*) and Jacques Curie (*top left*) with their parents.

system of the brain. Ultrasound transducer and receiver were located on opposite sides of the patient's head. Shortly after this time Keidel[4] reported the use of US for diagnosis of paranasal sinus disease. Between 1950 and 1968, it was mostly echoencephalography that established the role of US in neurologic diagnosis for intracranial space occupying lesions.[5-7] Almost simultaneously, developments took place in perinatology[8-10] and in gynecology, allowing for the differentiation between cystic and solid tumors.[8,9,11] Other applications of US within the fields of ophthalmology,[12-14] cardiology,[15,16] oncology (diagnosis of the abdominal and the retroperitoneal space),[17,18] and dentistry[19] followed.

It was in 1963 that Holms and Howry[20] used ultrasonic scanners through water basins to examine the head and neck area in addition to the abdomen. US for head and neck pathology was initially applied to the evaluation of thyroid disease,[21,22] the diagnosis of head and neck tumors,[23] and for assessment of motion of the lateral pharyngeal wall.[24] Kitamura et al[23] used US for recording vocal fold motions and Abramson et al[25] used US for diagnosis of middle ear effusions. For sinus disease Kitamura and Kaneko,[26] Gilbricht and Heidelbach,[27] and Mann[28] based diagno-

sis mainly on A-scan (amplitude mode) US (Fig 1-2), but before long compound scanners were introduced for two-dimensional diagnosis of paranasal sinus disease[29,30] (Fig 1-3). Revonta soon introduced this method in northern Europe.[31]

In the mid-1970s Wiley et al,[32] Gooding et al,[33] Scheible,[34] and Leopold used B-mode US technology for the clinical evaluation of neoplastic neck masses. In the late 1970s and the early 1980s, US was increasingly described in the English, German, and French literature for examination of head and neck lesions including those of the salivary glands.[35-37] It is understandable that head and neck US was first validated for diagnosis of lesions in parenchymatous organs like the parotid gland and the thyroid because their homogeneous echotexture allowed for detection of tumors within their structure.[38,39]

It was in 1984 that Mann[40] published the first textbook of US in head and neck surgery in the German literature, summarizing the knowledge and the possible application of US by clinicians to a spectrum of diseases of the head and neck. Since then, several additional German textbooks on this topic have been published.[41,42] This adaptation was made possible through the evolution and application of

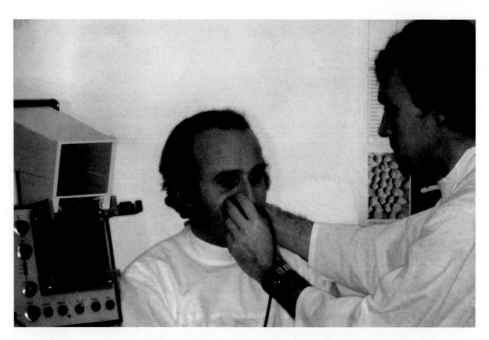

Fig 1-2. A-scan ultrasonography of the maxillary sinus in 1974.

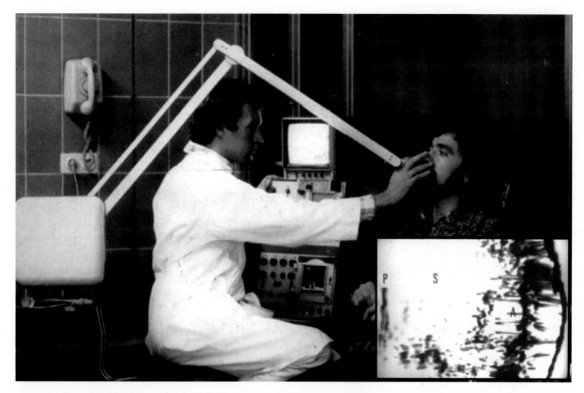

Fig 1–3. First compound scanner of the maxillary sinus in 1974 using the Combison® (Kretz, Zipf, Austria). Inset: gray-scale image of maxillary sinus in a vertical plane for a patient with acute maxillary sinusitis. A = anterior wall of the sinus; P = posterior wall; S = sinus lumen with secretion.

new technologies, beginning with A-scan US for sinus disease, followed by compound scanning, first routinely used in obstetrics and gynecology[11] and extrapolated to the head and neck. Subsequent development of the first real-time ultrasonic scanner Videoson® (Siemens, Germany) allowed for the generation of 16 black and white images per second, albeit in a form that was quite bulky for application in the head and neck (Fig 1–4). Tissue differentiation technology using gray scale imaging was developed in 1972 by the Australians Kossoff and Garrett[43] and was soon to be incorporated into medical technology. For the first time the advantages of A-scan sonography were combined with B-mode (brightness or gray scale) display of tissue differentiation and anatomic orientation in one image. Based on this development, many new machines were designed in the 1980s, which were characterized by progressive improvement in transducer technology, higher

resolution, and increased storage capacity. Still, US transducers remained cumbersome for examination of the head and neck. A 7.5-MHz transducer built in 1986 had a length of 5.1 cm, and a 5-MHz transducer measured 8.5 cm. Compared to this, modern small parts transducers with variable frequencies have a dimension of 4 cm or less, enabling improved contact with the surfaces of the head and neck region.

In the mid-1990s color-coded Doppler sonography was applied to the examination of head and neck lymph nodes with the aim of differentiating benign from malignant lymphadenopathy by analyzing vascular perfusion pattern.[44,45] Transcranial Doppler sonography was used for evaluating possible occlusion of the common carotid artery during surgery of N3 neck nodes[46] and ultrasound-guided needle aspiration for cytologic examination of diseases of the thyroid, the parotid gland, and the neck nodes became standard.

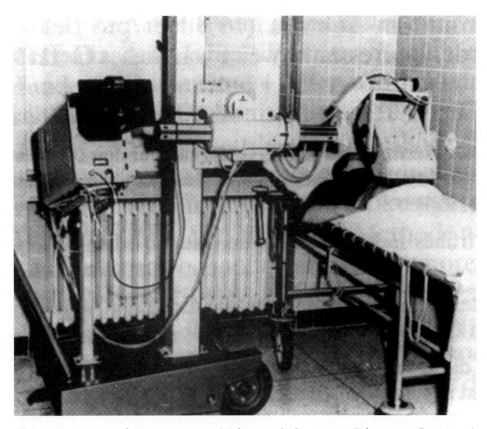

Fig 1–4. First real-time scanner (Videoson®, Siemens, Erlangen, Germany) with bulky transducer for B-mode ultrasound examination of the abdomen.

Modern Refinements

The introduction of color–coded duplex sonography created the possibility not only to demonstrate the vascularity of head and neck tumors and lymph nodes, but also to quantify vascularity and to define certain patterns of vascularization. Parallel to the advances in CT-scanning and MR-imaging, various groups attempted to classify lesions into malignant or benign entities depending on the vascularization pattern; however, without achieving sufficient sensitivity and specificity. Due to the prohibitive costs of these new US machines and the limited market, clinical head and neck US had to rely on technology which was adapted for broader indications in various specialties such as obstetrics and gynecology and gastroenterology.

During this time, so-called high-end US systems entered the market characterized by fast calculating capabilities and customized modules, which allowed for improved "small parts" application including head and neck examination. This led to the introduction of additional new technology for examination of head and neck structures such as panoramic imaging, which allows for serial images of an entire anatomic area to be composed into ultrasonic tomographic pictures. Harmonic imaging was developed which allowed for optimizing contrast and spatial resolution.[47] Three-dimensional (3D) US was adapted from obstetrics for lesions of the head and neck, and "daylight sonography" enabled examination of patients without dimming the light in the examining room. The introduction of "signal enhancers" combined with color-coded duplex sonography yielded additional information on the vascularity of certain neck masses, allowing for diagnoses such as glomus tumors including carotid body tumors without further need for angiographic examinations.[48]

The Incorporation of Ultrasound into the Clinician's Practice

Ultrasound technology, which found its first clinical application in the 1940s, was further developed in isolated centers in the mid-1960s and found broad application in the various medical fields in the early 1970s. Thanks to a rapid development from analogue to digital technology, this imaging modality became available at many centers throughout the world. By 1970, national ultrasound societies had been founded in the United States, Germany, Japan, the United Kingdom, Switzerland, and Austria, although representation by head and neck clinicians was limited to nonexistent. Umbrella organizations like the American Institute of Ultrasound in Medicine (AIUM), the European Federation for Ultrasound in Medicine (EFSUM), and the World Ultrasound Federation (WUFSUM) evolved. The AIUM, founded in the early 1950s, was initially focused on ultrasonics in research; in the later 1950s therapeutic applications for ultrasound energy were the main area of interest. By 1964 the AIUM had broadened its interests to include both diagnostic and therapeutic applications of ultrasound, and the focus on diagnostic ultrasound has grown and diversified ever since. Still, as an example, during the European trinational (Swiss, Austrian, and German) interdisciplinary ultrasound meeting in Davos in 1979, only one presentation focused on examination of the head and neck; whereas in 2001 on the same occasion, 30 oral presentations were given on various topics for head and neck examinations. The 1980s and 1990s saw a tremendous expansion in the application of ultrasound to head and neck imaging worldwide. In the mid-1990s, ultrasound examination of the head and neck also became part of the training requirement for board certification in otolaryngology in Germany, which made it mandatory for each training program to acquire appropriate expertise. The same is not yet the case in the United States, but the tide is turn-

ing. Simultaneously, this examination became reimbursed by health insurance companies, not only for radiologists but also for otolaryngologists and specialists in various disciplines of medicine, thus eliminating a long-standing obstacle to incorporation of ultrasound into clinical practice across medical subspecialties. In 1998, the American College of Surgeons released statement ST-31, supporting the use of ultrasound by appropriately trained surgeons. Similarly, in recognition of ultrasound as a tool to be utilized across medical specialties, the American Medical Association drafted a resolution in 2000 affirming that ultrasound imaging is within the scope of practice of appropriately trained physicians [Resolution H-230.960].

Indications for Head and Neck Ultrasonography

Many recent developments have led to broad acceptance of US as a diagnostic tool in the clinical evaluation of patients with head and neck diseases. The true value of US is maximized when it is incorporated into the clinical examination of patients during office visits. In this setting, imaging information is immediately obtained by the clinician caring for the patient regarding lesions that are palpable or nonpalpable, suspected or unsuspected, or known to reside deep within the structures of the head and neck beyond the reach of inspection and palpation. Anatomic detail is delineated without radiation exposure and with a minimum of cost relative to any other diagnostic imaging modality. Dynamic, interactive anatomic images are augmented by maneuvers that yield functional information regarding swallowing, mastication, and phonation. Thus, US enables real-time interpretation by the examiner, who is familiar with the clinical context. For this reason US is best performed by physicians caring for patients rather than by US assistants.

Specific indications for head and neck US are presented throughout the rest of this textbook. To summarize, indications include: to characterize neck masses; to detect adenopathy and to aid in TNM staging; to identify suspected *and* unsuspected pathology; to perform dynamic assessment of function; to monitor therapy; to enhance sensitivity of oncologic follow-up; to distinguish benign from malignant features of lesions; and to guide intervention (FNA, treatment, surgery).

On review of the literature of the last decade, it is clear that US has established its place in the evaluation of thyroid and parathyroid pathology, benign and malignant lymph nodes in the neck, congenital and cystic lesions, tumors of soft tissue, hematomas, foreign bodies, and glandular disorders. Ultrasound-guided needle biopsies and therapeutic procedures are commonplace, and for good reason. Ultrasound examination of the operated and radiated neck is far superior to palpation alone. Through US, information can be obtained about the relationship between neck nodes and vascular structures.

US is useful in the examination of lesions of the upper aerodigestive tract itself. US is now a standard examination for diseases of the major and minor salivary glands, providing information which rivals CT or MRI for tumors, acute and chronic sialadenitis, and sialolithiasis.

US has long been the standard for imaging of the thyroid and parathyroid glands, but has traditionally been done through radiology departments, often with review of images and reports outside the presence of the patient. Only in the last decade has the obvious advantage of office-based US been adopted by endocrinologists and surgeons in their initial consultation and follow-up management of patients with thyroid and parathyroid disease. US of the paranasal sinuses and the orbital contents have a similar tradition shared by ophthalmologists and otolaryngologists. More recently realized applications include evaluation in maxillofacial trauma, where US can detect fractures of the mandible, the nasal bones, the zygoma, the maxilla, and the frontal bone. Still newer uses include a spectrum of image-guided procedures, such as interstitial laser therapy in patients with facial vascular malformations. Other new developments include US for measuring depth of penetration of skin tumors, such as melanomas, using 20-MHz transducers[49]; updating preoperatively gained imaging for computer-assisted surgery to correct for soft tissue shift in skull base lesions[50]; and the intraoperative use of US to localize difficult to palpate lesions in situ during surgery to minimize surgical exposure.[51]

Advantages and Disadvantages of Ultrasonography

The advantages of US are self-evident as this is an imaging technology without radiation exposure that allows for real-time information acquisition by the examiner during evaluation and care of the patient. US is easily repeatable, reproducible, convenient, inexpensive, painless, quick, portable, and well-tolerated by patients of any age in just about any clinical situation. The main logistical disadvantage of US is the fact that it should be performed by the physician him- or herself, which can be relatively time consuming and not necessarily appropriately reimbursed. For the already busy practitioner it may take some creativity to incorporate US into one's clinical practice. Compared to interpreting CT and MRI, the US examiner must possess profound knowledge of variable anatomic planes in the neck to accurately interpret US images obtained through variable positions of the sound transducer in horizontal, oblique, or sagittal planes. In addition to anatomic knowledge, an understanding of US physics is required to maximize the yield of the US exam. Thus, there is a learning curve with US, and the yield from the examination is operator dependent. In general, only small windows on anatomy corresponding to the linear dimensions of the transducers are visualized at a given time, making the context of the field of view all important and encouraging the person performing the examination to be the one who interprets it. Furthermore, the cost of US equipment may be an initial obstacle to its incorporation into office practice, in spite of the fact that the long-term benefits to the patients and the physician offset the investment.

Ultrasound Training— Ongoing Evolution

Head and neck US has become an integral part of specialty training in German otolaryngology residency programs. Training in thyroid US has become quite common in American endocrinology fellowships. US training is beginning to become available in otolaryngology and surgery residency programs in the United States, but such training is not yet standard. For specialists who intend to bill for US examinations, a quality control process, including quality of image interpretation, must be guaranteed, and legal implications do exist. The American Medical Association policy on ultrasound imaging affirms that privileging of the physician to perform ultrasound imaging procedures in a hospital setting should be a function of hospital medical staffs and should be specifically delineated on the Department's Delineation of Privileges form. The AMA further states that hospital medical staffs should review and approve criteria for granting ultrasound privileges that are in accordance with recommended training and education standards developed by each physician's respective specialty. As medical specialty boards range from having developed US standards to having no defined standards at all, this process can be nebulous and may require pioneering efforts by some clinicians aiming to begin practicing US. It is helpful that physician groups such as the American College of Surgeons (ACS) and the American Association of Clinical Endocrinologists (AACE) have developed US certification courses with standardized curricula and criteria for completion. The opportunities for US training and education can only be expected to grow with time, and it is the hope of the contributing authors that this textbook will be a foundation, a stimulus, and a reflection of that growth.

References

1. Curie J, Curie P. (quoted in Jecker P, Frentzel-Beyme B). Zur Geschichte der Kopf/Hals-Sonographie. *Laryngo-Rhino-Otol.* 2002;81:900–905.

2. Behm A. (quoted in Frentzel-Beyme B). Als die Bilder laufen lernten. *Ultraschall Klin Prax.* 1994; 8:265–287.

3. Dussik K. Über die Möglichkeit hochfrequente mechanische Schwingungen als diagnostisches Hilfsmittel zu verwerten. *Z ges Neurol Psychiat.* 1942;174:153–156.

4. Keidel W. Über die Verwendung des Ultraschalls in der klinischen Diagnostik. *Ärztl Forsch Z Forschungsergebn Med.* 1947;1:349–355.

5. French LA, Wild J, Neal D. Detection of cerebral tumors by ultrasonic pulses: pilot studies on post mortem material. *Cancer.* 1950;3:705–709.

6. Leksell L. Echoencephalography, I. Detection of intracranial complications following head injury. *Acta Chir Scand.* 1955;110:301–304.

7. Kazner E, Kunze S, Schiefer E. Die Bedeutung der Echoenzephalographie für die Erkennung epiduraler Hämatome. *Langenbecks Arch klin Chir.* 1965;310:267–270.

8. Willocks J, Donald I, Duggan TC, Day N. Fetal cephalometry by ultrasound. *J Obstet. Gynaec Cwlth.* 1964;171:11–16.

9. Kratochwil A. *Ultraschalldiagnostik in Geburtshilfe und Gynäkologie.* Stuttgart; Thieme: 1968.

10. Hoffbauer H. Die Bedeutung der Ultraschalldiagnostik in der Frühschwangerschaft. *Elektromedica.* 1970;3:227–231.

11. Donald J, Brown TG. Demonstration of tissue interfaces within the body by ultrasonic echo sounding. *Br J Radiol.* 1961;34:539–542.

12. Mundt GH, Hughes WF. Ultrasonics in ocular diagnosis. *Amer J Ophthal.* 1956;41:488–493.

13. Baum G, Greenwood J. The application of ultrasonic locating techniques to ophthalmology. *Amer Arch Ophth.* 1958;60:263–267.

14. Ossoinig K. Zur Ultraschalldiagnostik der Tumoren des Auges. *Mbl Augenheilk.* 1965;146:321–326.

15. Edler J. The diagnostic use of ultrasound in heart diseases. *Acta Med Scand Suppl.* 1955;308:32–37.

16. Effert S. Diagnostic value of ultrasonic cardiography. *Br J Radiol.* 1963;36:302–305.

17. Kikuchi Y, Uckida R, Tanaka K, Wagai T. Early cancer diagnoses through ultrasonics. *J Acoust Soc Amer.* 1957;29:824–828.

18. Bannaski H, Fischer KH. Neue diagnostische Möglichkeiten des Ultraschall-Impulsechoverfahrens. *Med Klin.* 1958;53:51–57.

19. Spranger H. Sofortdiagnose des marginalen Knochenabbaues anhand der eindimensionalen Ultraschallechodarstellung des Limbus alveolaris. *Dtsch Zahnärtzl Z.* 1970;25:501–506.

20. Holms JH, Howry DH. Ultrasonic diagnosis of abdominal disease. *Amer J Digest Dis.* 1963;8:12–16.

21. Fujimoto Y, Oka A, Omoto R. Ultrasound scanning of the thyroid gland as a new diagnostic approach. *Ultrasonics.* 1967;5:177–181.

22. Damascelli B, Cascinelli N, Kivraghi T. Preoperative approach to thyroid tumors by two-dimensional pulsed echo technique. *Ultrasonics.* 1968;6: 242–246.

23. Kitamura T, Kaneko T, Asano H, Muira T. Ultrasonic diagnosis in otorhinolaryngology. *Eye Ear Nose Throat Mon*. 1969;48:329–337.

24. Kelsey CA, Crummy AB, Sulman E. Comparison of ultrasonic and radiographic determination of lateral pharyngeal wall displacement. *Phys Med Biol*. 1969;14:332–334.

25. Abramson DH, Abramson AL, Coleman DJ. Ultrasonics in Otolaryngology. *Arch Otolaryngol*. 1972; 96:146–148.

26. Kitamura TA, Kanecko T. Le diagnostic des affections du sinus maxillaire par ultrasons impulsifs. *Ann Oto-Laryngol (Paris)*. 1965;82:711–714.

27. Gilbricht E, Heidelbach JG. Ultraschall in der Medizin und ihre Anwendungsmöglichkeiten im HNO-Bereich. *Z Laryngol Rhinol Otol*. 1968;47:737–746.

28. Mann W. Die Ultraschalldiagnostik der Nasennebenhöhlen und ihre Anwendung in der Freiburger HNO-Klinik. *Arch Oto-Rhino-Laryngol*. 1975;211: 154–155.

29. Mann W. Die Ultraschalldiagnostik der NNH-Erkrankungen mit A- und B-Scan. *Laryng Rhinol*. 1976;55:48–53.

30. Mann W. Diagnostic ultrasonography in paranasal sinus diseases—A 5-year review. *ORL, Oto-Rhino-Laryngology*. 1979;41:168–171.

31. Revonta M. Ultrasound in the diagnosis of maxillary and frontal sinusitis. *Acta Otolaryngol (Stockholm)*. 1980;(suppl. 370):1–34.

32. Wiley AL, Zagzebski JA, Tolbert DD, Baujavic RA. Ultrasound B-scans for clinical evaluation of neoplastic neck nodes. *Arch Otolaryngol*. 1975;101: 509–513.

33. Gooding GAW, Herzog KA, Lang FC. Ultrasonographic assessment of neck masses. *J Clin Ultrasound*. 1976;5:248–252.

34. Scheible FW, Leopold GR. Diagnostic imaging in head and neck disease: current application of ultrasound. *Head Neck Surg*. 1978;1:1–7.

35. Macridis CA, Kouloulas LA, Koutsimbelas B, Yannoulis G. Zur Diagnose von Speicheldrüsentumoren mit Ultraschall. *Elektromedica*. 1975;4:130–136.

36. Bruneton JN, Fenart D, Vallicioni J, Demard F. Séméiologie, échographique des tumeurs de la parotide. A propos de 40 observations. *J Radiol*. 1980;61:151–155.

37. Chodosh PL, Silbey R, Oen KT. Diagnostic use of ultrasound in diseases of the head and neck. *Laryngoscope*. 1980;90:814–817.

38. Blum M, Goldman AB, Hershovic A, Hernsberg J. Clinical application of thyroid echography. *N Engl J Med*. 1972;287:1164–1165.

39. Crocker EF, McLanghlin AF, Kossoff G, Jellins J. The grey-scale echographic appearance of thyroid malignancy. *J Clin Ultrasound*. 1974;2:305–309.

40. Mann W. *Ultraschall im Kopf/Hals-Bereich*. Tokyo, Berlin, Heidelberg, New York: Springer; 1984.

41. Hell B. *Atlas der Ultraschalldiagnostik im Kopf-Hals-Bereich*. New York, NY: Georg Thieme-Verlag; 1990.

42. Mann W, Welkoborsky HJ, Maurer J. *Kompendium Ultraschall im Kopf-Hals-Bereich*. New York, NY: Thieme-Stuttgart; 1997.

43. Kossoff G, Garrett W. 1972; quoted in Frentzel-Beyme, 1994 (see ref. 2).

44. Mann W, Beck A, Schreiber J, Maurer J, Amedee RG, Gluckman J. Ultrasonography for evaluation of the carotid artery in head and neck cancer. *Laryngoscope*. 1994;104:885–888.

45. Schreiber J, Mann W, Lieb W. Farbduplexsonographische Messung der Lymphknotenperfusion. Ein Beitrag zur Diagnostik der zervikalen Metastasierung. *Laryngo-Rhino-Otol*. 1993;72:187–192.

46. Maurer J, Ungersböck K, Amedee RG, Mann WJ, Perneczky A. Transcranial Doppler ultrasound recording with compression tests in patients with tumors involving the carotid artery. *Skull Base Surg*. 1993;3:11–15.

47. Jecker P, Maurer J, Mann WJ. Verbesserte Orts- und Kontrastauflösung in der Ultraschalldiagnostik durch Nutzung harmonischer Frequenzen. *Laryngo-Rhino-Otol*. 2001;80:203–208.

48. Jecker P, Engelke JC, Westhofen M. Über die Einsatzmöglichkeit eines Signalverstärkers für die Duplexsonographie in der Hals-, Nasen-, Ohrenheilkunde. *Laryngo-Rhino-Otol*. 1998;77:289–293.

49. Dummer W, Blaheta HJ, Bastian BC, Schenk T, Bropcker EV, Remy W. Preoperative characterization of pigmented skin lesions by epiluminescence microscopy and high-frequency ultrasound. *Arch Dermatol*. 1995;131(3):279–285.

50. Ecke U, Gosepath J, Mann WJ. Initial experience with intraoperative ultrasound in navigated soft tissue operations of the neck and below the base of the skull. *Ultraschall Med*. 2006;27:49–54.

51. Stetter S, Jecker P, Mann WJ. Einsatz des intraoperativen Ultraschalls in der Speicheldrüsenchirurgie. *Ultraschall in Med*. 2006;27:159–163.

Chapter 2

ESSENTIAL PHYSICS OF ULTRASOUND

Marc D. Coltrera

Although fascinating the underlying physics of many medical imaging technologies can be considered optional for nonradiologists. Not so for ultrasound. The generation of ultrasound images relies on sound reflection from interfaces between tissues with different acoustical characteristics. What the observer sees is affected as much by the characteristics associated with the target of interest as by the surrounding tissues. Artifacts abound and can be confounding factors or diagnostic attributes depending on the setting. The ultrasonographer/ultrasonologist needs to have a solid understanding of sound wave physics to properly perform the study and interpret the results.

This chapter aims to impart the essential physics required to perform head and neck ultrasound. For in-depth explanations of ultrasound physics the reader is directed elsewhere; several good sources for additional reading are listed at the end of this chapter.

The Sound Wave

Virtually all physical materials be they gas, liquid, or solid allow for propagation of mass vibrational energy. Just like billiard balls hitting each other in turn, vibrations are passed between molecules. To an observer sitting in one place mass movements of molecules are experienced as pressure waves alternating between compression and rarefaction as the vibrations pass by (Fig 2-1). Plotted on a graph of pressure versus time the repetitious nature of the pressure wave is self-evident. Each repetition of the wave is called a cycle. All waves can be characterized by their two fundamental properties: **wavelength** and **frequency**.

Wavelength (λ) is the distance between repeating points on the wave which occur once per cycle. In Figure 2-1 the wavelength is being measured peak-to-peak. For a stationary observer the time it takes for a complete pressure wave to pass completing a full cycle is called the wave's **period** (**T**), for example, the time period of passage. By convention the time scale most often used is seconds so T is expressed in units of sec/cycle. For convenient comparison of different waves it is easier to use the inverse of the wave's period, its **frequency** (f). For a wave with $T = 0.01$ sec/cycle, $f = 1/T = 1/0.01 = 100$ cycles/sec. The common unit used for frequency is the hertz (Hz) where 1 Hz = 1 cycle/sec. To simplify the expression of higher frequencies, kilohertz (kHz = 1000 Hz) and megahertz (MHz = 1,000,000 Hz) are also employed.

Under optimal conditions, the human ear is capable of detecting sound waves in the range of 20 Hz to 20,000 Hz (20 kHz). This is referred to as the audible or sonic range. Although some animals such as bats can detect sound waves in the range of

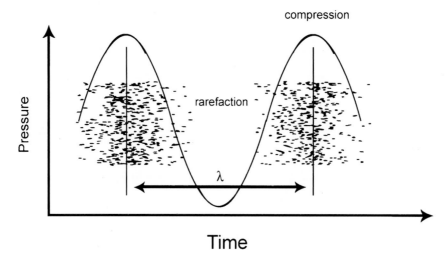

Fig 2–1. Sound waves propagate through a medium as varying pressure waves which alternately compress and rarefy the molecules of the medium. For a stationary observer, the time it takes for a complete pressure wave to pass completing a full cycle is called the wave's period (*T*). The distance between similar points on the time-pressure curve is the wavelength (λ).

80 kHz to 100 kHz, frequencies above the range of human hearing are defined as ultrasonic. The most common frequencies used for diagnostic head and neck ultrasound fall in the range from 7.5 MHz to 15 MHz.

The Speed of Sound

Clinical ultrasonography is fundamentally different from all other imaging modalities including magnetic resonance imaging (MRI), computed tomography (CT) scans, and positron emission tomography (PET) scans. It alone is based on measurement of reflected energy. Although transmission ultrasonography is possible, it is much more limited in its capabilities. Sound wave reflectance is fundamentally based on alterations in the speed of sound. Understand the speed of sound and you hold the key to ultrasonography.

Energy waves travel at a speed called the **propagation velocity**. In the case of gamma radiation used in CT scans, the waves travel at the speed of light. In a vacuum pure electromagnetic radiation such as light or gamma rays travels at 299,792,458 m/sec. In denser media the apparent speed of light slows down because of a conversion of the propagating wave into a hybrid of electromagnetic radiation and subatomic particle oscillations. Furthermore, the quantum nature of the subatomic interactions means that the frequency of the energy wave affects the propagation velocity through the medium.

Sound waves are limited to actions at the molecular level. Frequency has no effect on propagation velocity. The density of the medium still matters along with a measure of the interaction between molecules referred to as the elasticity or stiffness of the medium. The stiffness of the medium can be thought of as the springs interconnecting the molecules. The propagation velocity of sound depends on the stiffness and density of the medium in the following manner:

$$c = \sqrt{C/\rho}$$

where c is the propagation velocity, C is the coefficient of stiffness, and ρ is the density of the medium.

Figure 2–2 lists the propagation velocity of typical media encountered in the body. It makes intu-

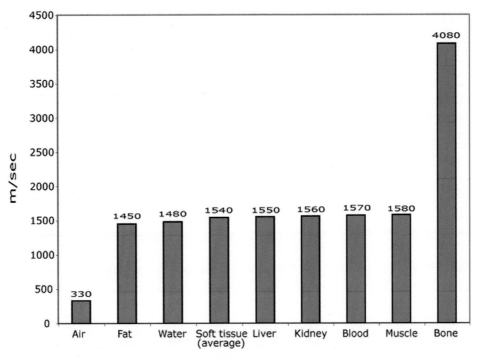

Fig 2–2. Propagation velocity varies depending on the medium's stiffness and density. For the purposes of calculating distance measurements, an average propagation velocity of 1540 m/sec is assumed.

itive sense that a stiffer medium transmits a pressure wave faster just like pulling on a tense spring transmits the impulse faster than pulling on a slack one. Looking at the graph in Figure 2-2, at first glance it appears counterintuitive that increasing density decreases the speed of sound as the propagation velocities increase in the denser media (air velocity < soft tissue velocity < bone velocity). The explanation lies in the fact that the stiffness of these media increases much faster than their density does. In general, the speed of sound increases when going from a gas to a liquid to a solid.

Knowing the speed of sound in a medium is critical for two reasons. The first reason is measuring distances with a reflected sound wave requires precise timing and knowing the speed of the wave (Fig 2-3). As there is no way of knowing what actual tissues are being imaged, designers of ultrasound machines have to base their calculations of distance on an average speed for the tissues involved. The standard value is 1540 m/sec which is derived from averaging the classic abdominal soft tissue set of fat, liver, kidney, blood, and muscle.[1] This value corre-

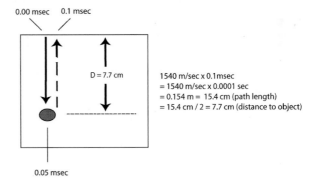

Fig 2–3. Ultrasound distances are calculated by precisely measuring the elapsed time between the pulse and the returned echo. The average propagation velocity 1540 m/sec is used to calculate the distance. If a large percentage of the tissues are fat, actual distances can be significantly different from the calculated distances.

sponds closely to the propagation velocities for the majority of the soft tissues in the neck which include muscles, blood-filled vessels, and parenchymal structures including the thyroid, lymph nodes, and salivary glands. However, if a large percentage of the neck tissues is composed of fat tissue (eg, in an obese individual) actual and measured distances can be significantly different: 1450 (speed in fat)/1540 (speed in average tissue) = 6% differential (Fig 2–4).

The second reason why the speed of sound in a given medium is critical is that the propagation velocity is related to frequency and wavelength:

$$c = f\lambda$$

The necessity for utilizing ultrasonic sound waves in medical quality imaging can be derived from this equation. The ability to distinguish between two closely spaced points requires the use of a wavelength of the same size or smaller than the distance between the two points. This means that the minimal resolving power for a 7.5-MHz sound wave would be:

$$\lambda = c/f = 1540 \text{ m sec}^{-1} / 7{,}500{,}000 \text{ cycles sec}^{-1}$$
$$= 0.205 \text{ mm}$$

In the head and neck region, common structures we are interested in resolving can be as small as 3 to 4 mm, for example, parathyroids and lymph nodes. Wavelengths in the range of 7.5 Mhz should be adequate for head and neck structures if a single cycle of sound energy is used, but as will be shown there are other considerations that can make the use of single cycle detection impractical in reality.

Acoustic Impedance: The Basis for Medical Ultrasound

Standard medical sonography equipment relies on reflected sound measurements. If sound waves flowed unimpeded through the tissues there would be no reflected waves to measure. Sound wave reflection occurs at interfaces between materials with different acoustic properties. The amount of energy reflected at the interface depends on the difference in acoustic impedances between the two media. The larger the difference in impedances the larger the reflection.

The acoustic impedance (Z) of a medium is the product of its density and the propagation velocity in the medium:

$$Z = \rho c$$

When an interface between two media is smooth and relatively large compared to the wavelength of the sound wave, it acts like a mirror. Such interfaces are referred to as specular reflectors. The diaphragm is a good example of a **specular reflector**. In the head and neck region, the carotid artery and fluid-filled cysts can also act as specular reflectors. Like a mirror a specular reflector that is perpendicular to the propagation path of the sound wave will reflect back to the transducer. Specular reflectors that are angled will reflect the sound energy away from the tranducer resulting in a loss of signal (Fig 2–5).

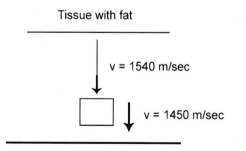

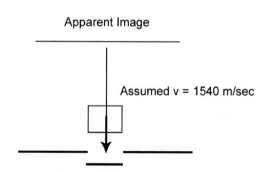

Fig 2–4. Distances are calculated based on precise timing of the reflected wave and the average propagation velocity of 1540 m/sec. When media such as fat make up a significant proportion of intervening tissues, the measured distance to deeper objects can be affected.

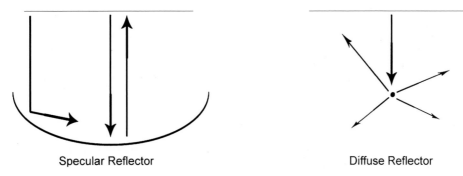

Specular Reflector   Diffuse Reflector

Fig 2–5. Objects in the body act as specular or diffuse reflectors based on the wavelength of the sound energy being reflected. Smooth acoustic interfaces which are significantly larger than the incident wavelength act as mirrors reflecting the energy directly back to the transducer or angling it obliquely away. Acoustic interfaces which are small in comparison to the incident wavelength scatter the energy wave in all directions.

The amount of energy reflected by a specular reflector expressed as a fraction of the energy delivered is called the reflection coefficient (*R*). In the special case of a specular reflector oriented in a plane perpendicular to the propagation path of the sound wave the reflection coefficient depends solely on the differential between the acoustic impedances of the media on each side of the interface:

$$R = (Z_2 - Z_1)^2 / (Z_2 + Z_1)^2$$

As impedance depends on density and the propagation velocity in the medium, the greatest reflectance in the head and neck region would be expected at air–soft tissue interfaces and bone-soft tissue interfaces (Fig 2-6). The minimal reflectance at an interface occurs when the impedances of the two media closely match. Gels created for use between the ultrasound transducer and the soft tissue are an example of a material with a good impedance match allowing transmission of most of the sound energy through to the soft tissue with minimal reflection.

When the size of a reflector is smaller than the wavelength of the sound wave, the sound energy is scattered rather than reflected in a coherent manner. These small reflectors are referred to as **diffuse reflectors** (see Fig 2-5). Diffuse reflectors are found throughout most soft tissues and account for the speckled patterns seen on ultrasound images.

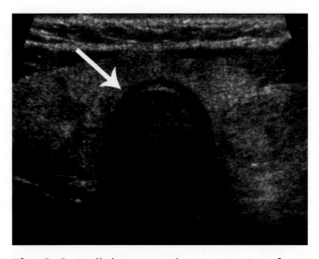

Fig 2–6. Well-demarcated acoustic interfaces occur where there are significant differences in acoustic impedances between tissues. In this transverse ultrasound view of the neck, the white arrow points to the interface between the soft tissue of the thyroid gland and the partially calcified tracheal cartilage ring.

Attenuation

As the basis of diagnostic ultrasound is the detection of reflected sound energy, anything which decreases or attenuates the energy of the returned pressure wave limits the potential depth of penetration. As noted previously, sound energy can be reflected obliquely by specular reflectors or scattered by diffuse reflectors leading to a loss of energy along the original path of propagation (see Fig 2-5). A third source of energy loss is absorbance by the medium. This occurs through the conversion of sound energy into heat. The conversion of sound energy into heat increases with the frequency of the sound wave and becomes the predominant factor in limiting the depth of tissue penetration for higher ultrasonic frequencies.

Attenuation of the sound wave is measured in relative units. Comparisons are made between the intensity levels of the sound energy at two points in the medium. Intensity is a measure of the spatial distribution of power:

$$\text{Power (in milliwatts [mW])/Area (in cm}^2) = I \text{ (Intensity in mW/cm}^2).$$

The relative unit employed to express the degree of attenuation is the decibel (dB), wherein the decibel is defined as $10 \times \log_{10}(I_2 / I_1)$. For example, if the intensity measured at $I_1 = 100$ mW/cm^2 and at $I_2 = 0.01$ mW/cm^2 the attenuation between the two points is:

$$10 \times \log_{10}(0.01 / 100) = 10 \times \log_{10}(0.0001) = -40 \text{ dB}$$

Figure 2-7 lists the attenuation in dB/cm/MHz for typical media encountered in the body. Air has a very high attenuation coefficient because carbon dioxide has a high-absorbance cross-section for ultrasonic sound waves. The attenuation values for soft tissues, although much better than air, significantly limit the depth of penetration for higher frequency ultrasound used in visualizing small structures. To visualize the thyroid in the neck, typical depths of beam penetration range up to 5 cm. At 7.5 MHz the average attenuation of an ultrasound beam at 5 cm is greater than 25 dB. Adequate resolution for visualization of the parathyroids can require 12 MHz or higher leading to attenuation values greater than 45 dB at the same depth. These figures are based on the "average" soft tissue attenuation value of 0.70 dB/cm/MHz. Depending on the cross-section of the head and neck region being evaluated, the actual

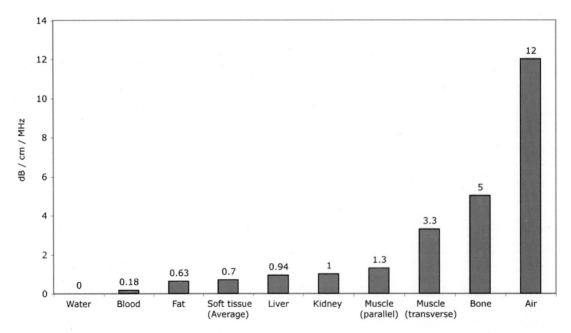

Fig 2–7. Attenuation of the sound wave occurs through reflection, scattering, and absorbance with conversion of sound energy to heat. Unlike propagation velocity, attenuation is affected by the frequency of the ultrasonic wave. Attenuation increases proportionally with the frequency.

attenuation values may be significantly higher. It should also be kept in mind that the reflected wave is subject to the same attenuation as it passes back through the overlying tissues effectively doubling the tissue effects.

The major effect of attenuation is ever decreasing energy delivered to deeper tissues which, in turn, results in weaker reflections from similar strength reflectors at different depths. To compensate for the weakened reflections, amplification of signals based on their distance can be employed. The greater the distance, the greater the attenuation and, hence, the greater the amplification required. Distance is inferred by the time for the reflection to return to the transducer so the amplification is referred to as **time-gain compensation** (**TGC**; Fig 2–8). The major limitation to TGC is the signal-to-noise ratio which approaches 1.0 at greater depths.

Doppler

Reflected sound waves contain three informational components which can be analyzed for different purposes: amplitude, phase, and frequency. B-scale ultrasonography rely on the amplitude of the re-

flected wave. The greater the amplitude of the reflected wave the brighter the image on the gray scale monitor. Doppler sonography analyzes the frequency of the reflected wave for the purpose of motion detection. Phase changes can also be used for motion detection.

The Doppler effect, frequency shifting based on the relative speed of the source and the observer, is a very well-known phenomenon (Fig 2–9). The classic example of the Doppler shift is a train whistle which goes from high to low pitch as the train approaches, passes, and then recedes from the observer. The basic formula describing the Doppler effect is the one for the Doppler (frequency) shift:

$$f_D = f_e - f_0$$

where f_D = Doppler shift, f_e = emitted frequency, f_0 = source frequency

In the train whistle example, the train is a moving transmitter and the observer is a stationary receiver.

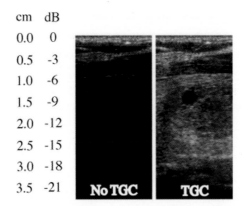

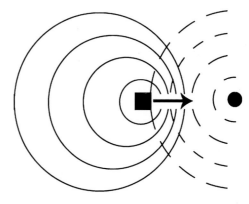

Fig 2–9. The Doppler shift is a frequency shift caused by the relative speeds of the emitter and receiver. Relative to a base frequency, an approaching object appears to be emitting a higher frequency whereas a receding object appears to emit a lower frequency. In Doppler ultrasonography the sound wave emitter and receiver, the transducer (*black circle*), is stationary whereas the reflector (eg, blood; *black square*) is moving. The reflector first "receives" a Doppler shifted sound wave and then "re-emits" a frequency which the stationary receiver detects as twice the Doppler shift expected for a simple moving emitter.

cm	dB
0.0	0
0.5	-3
1.0	-6
1.5	-9
2.0	-12
2.5	-15
3.0	-18
3.5	-21

No TGC   TGC

Fig 2–8. Time-gain compensation (TGC) is a graded amplification scheme meant to compensate for the weakened reflections due to attenuation at increased depths. For an 8.5-Mhz ultrasonic wave the average attenuation is 6 dB/cm. In the area of the thyroid the average attenuation of the neck cross-section may actually be higher.

The same shift in pitch is found if the transmitter remains stationary and the receiver moves, but the formulas must be rearranged.

The formula for a moving receiver and a stationary transmitter is:

$$f_r = f_0 ((c + v_r)/c)$$
where f_r = received frequency,
f_0 = source frequency, c = propagation velocity,
v_r = receiver speed

The formula for a moving transmitter and a stationary receiver is:

$$f_e = f_0 (c / (c - v_s))$$
where f_e = emitted frequency,
f_0 = source frequency, c = propagation velocity,
v_s = source speed

As Doppler sonography relies on reflected sound, both of these formulas need to be employed when analyzing moving objects such as blood. The reflector particle within the blood is first acting as a moving receiver for the ultrasonic sound wave (the first formula) and then as a moving transmitter of the reflected wave (the second formula). In other words, the source frequency for the moving transmitter is the received frequency for the moving receiver. Substituting the formulas derives a new formula for a moving reflector:

$$f_e = f_0 ((c + v) / (c - v))$$
where f_e = emitted frequency,
f_0 = source frequency, c = propagation velocity,
v = reflector speed

Returning to the Doppler shift formula and substituting for f_e obtains the formula for Doppler shift used in clinical ultrasonography:

$$f_D = f_0 (2v / (c - v)) \approx f_0 (2v / c)$$
where f_D = Doppler shift, f_0 = source frequency,
c = propagation velocity, v = reflector speed

The denominator can be simplified because the typical velocities (v) associated with blood flow are at most a few percent of the average propagation velocity of 1540 m/sec (c). The factor of two in the equation comes from the two Doppler shifts associated with the moving reflector.

Sonographic Doppler shift only occurs if the reflector's motion has a component of velocity in the direction of the ultrasound probe. If quantitative velocity analysis of blood is needed, the Doppler shift must be corrected for the angle formed between the direction of flow and the ultrasound beam (Fig 2-10):

$$f_D = f_0 (2v/c) \cos \theta$$

The angle θ is referred to as the Doppler angle. Two practical results come from this formula. At 90 degrees to the direction of flow, the cosine (cos) of θ is zero and no Doppler shift is seen. At angles between 60 degrees and 90 degrees the cosine of θ varies rapidly which amplifies a small error in measuring the Doppler angle into a large error in estimating Doppler shift (Fig 2-11).

Classical Doppler sonography is infrequently used in the head and neck region by practitioners

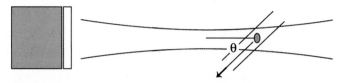

Fig 2–10. Doppler shift varies based on the cosine of θ, the angle between the insonation beam and the direction of flow. When the ultrasonic beam is perpendicular to the direction of flow, the cos of θ = 0 and there is no Doppler shift.

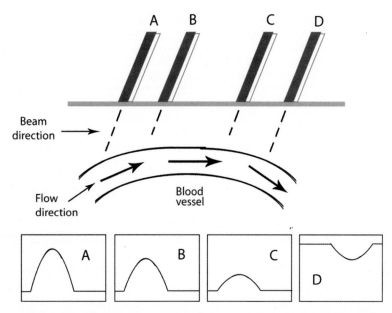

Fig 2–11. Changing angles affects the measured Doppler shift and the calculated flow based on the Doppler signal. The Doppler shift depends on the cosine of θ, the angle between the insonation beam and the direction of flow. The cosine of angles between 60 and 90 degrees varies rapidly leading to large potential errors in estimating flow rates.

other than vascular specialists. The most common presentation of Doppler sonography is an amalgam of Doppler frequency information and B-mode ultra-sonography called **color-flow Doppler** imaging (Fig 2-12). The stationary B-mode structures are overlaid on a Doppler frequency map. Relative velocity and direction is conveyed through the use of a Doppler frequency color map ranging from red hues (flow direction toward the transducer) to blue hues (flow direction away from the transducer).

Color-flow Doppler imaging is subject to sig-nal-to-noise problems which lead to incorrect repre-sentations of flow or completely spurious signals. Noise arises from many sources including pulsating vessel wall expansion and operator-induced move-ments. To minimize these problems, signal filtering is employed to exclude low-rate movements. The downside is that low-flow vessels such as small veins are excluded in color-flow Doppler images. An alternative to standard Doppler frequency mapping is an integrated power map of the Doppler signal

(Fig 2-13). This method, called **power-mode Doppler**, has the advantage of increasing signal-to-noise ratios allowing for more gain and the detec-tion of lower flow rates in smaller vessels. The limitations of power-mode Doppler are the loss of direction and velocity information.

Practical Issues in Transducer Design

Modern transducer designs combine the functions of the transmitter and the receiver for the produc-tion and detection of ultrasonic sound waves. The heart of the transducer is the piezoelectric ele-ment. Piezoelectricity is a phenomenon originally discovered by Pierre Curie in 1880. Certain crystals and ceramic materials generate a voltage when placed under mechanical stress. Conversely, when an external voltage is applied to them they undergo

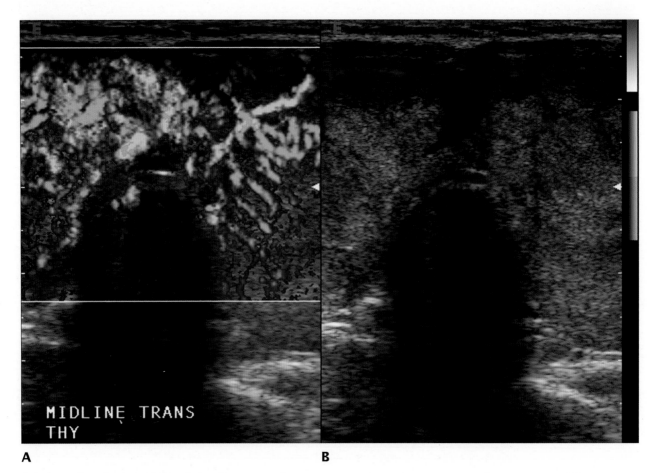

A   **B**

Figs 2–12A and 2–12B. Color-flow Doppler imaging. The stationary B-mode structures (B) are overlaid on a Doppler frequency map (Figure 12-A). This example shows relatively increased vascularity in the thyroid gland of a patient with Graves' disease. Relative velocity and direction is conveyed through the use of a Doppler frequency color map ranging from red hues (flow direction toward the transducer) to blue hues (flow direction away from the transducer).

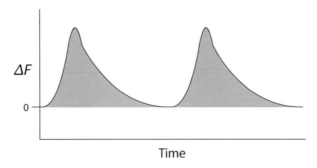

Fig 2–13. Doppler frequency mapping used in color-flow Doppler measures the change in the Doppler shift and calculates flow direction and rates based on the shift. The higher the peak, the stronger the implied flow rate. Low-level Doppler shifts must be filtered out to avoid problems with noise. Power-mode Doppler uses the integrated wave form (*the shaded area under the curve*) allowing for more sensitivity in detecting flow, but losing direction and rate information.

mechanical deformation to a small degree (Fig 2–14). The first practical use of the piezoelectric effect was the development of sonar during World War I for the detection of submarines. Application of varying voltages to quartz sheets placed between steel plates would cause expansion and contraction leading to the generation of a sharp ping. Hydrophones were then used to detect the reflected sound off the submarine's hull. Modern ultrasonic transducers use the same piezoelectric element to first produce the sound energy and then to detect the reflected sound waves.

The quality of an image is based on the maximum resolution of the imaging system. In ultrasonography resolution is measured in three dimensions with respect to the transducer beam and named accordingly: **axial**, **lateral**, and **elevation** (or azimuth) (Fig 2–15). The generation of an ultrasonic

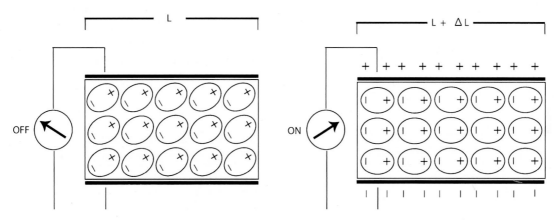

Fig 2–14. The piezoelectric effect was originally described in crystalline structures such as quartz. Application of a voltage causes dipolar elements in the crystal to align changing the shape of the crystal (ΔL). Alternating or pulsating voltages by producing expansion and contraction of the crystal can be harnessed to produce sound waves.

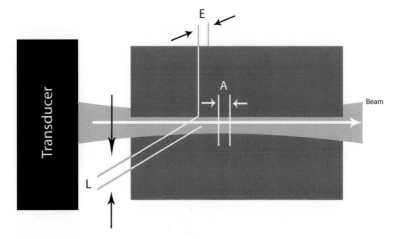

Fig 2–15. Beam resolution is measured in three planes: (*A*)xial, (*L*)ateral, and (*E*)levation (or azimuth). Axial resolution is measured along the beam axis. Lateral resolution is measured in a plane which is perpendicular to the beam and parallel to the transducer. Elevation resolution is a function of the thickness of the beam measured in the plane perpendicular to the beam axis and the transducer axis.

pulse by a piezoelectric element is subject to physical limitations which affect the achievable resolution in all three dimensions.

Axial resolution is measured along the beam axis. As previously mentioned, the closest two points in space can be, while still resolvable as two separate objects, is the length of the wavelength being employed to image them (Fig 2–16). For a 7.5-MHz sound wave the wavelength is equal to 0.205 mm. The problem is that it is virtually impossible to generate a single cycle pulse. Like a bell being struck with a hammer, a piezoelectric element will ring for 1 or 2 additional cycles after an applied voltage is discontinued. The length of the entire pulse determines the achievable axial resolution. For a 7.5-MHz stimulus this would be 0.615 mm. When trying to visualize small objects such as a parathyroid with a cross-sectional dimension of 2 to 3 mm, it is clear that higher resolutions are required such as can only be obtained with higher frequency beams.

Lateral resolution and elevation resolution are typically less than the achievable axial resolution. Both are a function of the design dimensions of the piezoelectric element. Lateral resolution is measured in a plane which is perpendicular to the beam and parallel to the transducer. Lateral resolution is governed to a first approximation by the width of the piezoelectric elements making up the transducer. Although the pressure wave generated by the piezoelectric element starts out the same size as the element's interface, it spreads out with increasing

depth leading to loss of resolution (Fig 2–17). This can be partially compensated for by focusing the ultrasonic beam at the depth of interest. Focusing of ultrasonic beams is achieved by timing the firing of the piezoelectric elements (Fig 2–18). The changes in timing compensate for the varying path lengths followed by the sound waves.

Elevation resolution is a function of the thickness of the beam measured in the plane perpendicular to the beam axis and the transducer axis. The beam "thickness" is due to more than just the finite size of the piezoelectric element's face. Because the piezoelectric element has edges, the primary pressure wave is generated by the center whereas less

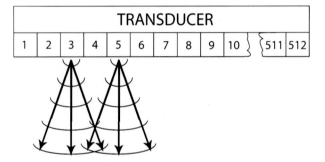

Fig 2–17. The shape and size of the piezoelectric elements define the initial shape and size of the generated sound wave. But as the depth increases diffusion of the sound waves generated by different piezoelectric elements causes them to overlap leading to a loss of resolution.

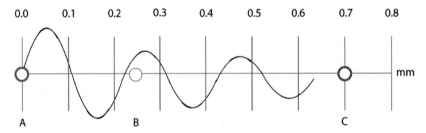

Fig 2–16. In theory axial resolution is limited only by the wavelength of the sound energy. For a 7.5-MHz ultrasonic wave the wave length is 0.205 mm. Point B would be resolvable under optimal circumstances. Because of design limitations for the piezoelectric element, 2 to 3 cycles are typically the minimum pulse which can be generated by the transducer. The pulse length, as long as 0.615 mm for a 7.5-MHz beam, becomes the limiting factor for axial resolution.

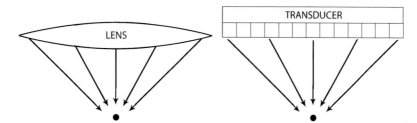

Fig 2–18. Lateral resolution can be improved by focusing the transducer beam electronically. Electronic ultrasound beam focusing is achieved by firing the piezoelectric elements at different times. The elements with longer path lengths (elements at the edge of the transducer in this example) are fired sooner than the elements with the shorter path lengths.

intense energy waves are given off at the margins (Fig 2-19), These marginal waves are called side lobes. Although the side lobes are of lesser energy they can interact with strong reflectors which are out of the primary beam plane creating artifacts. Proper piezoelectric element design can minimize the side lobes, but cannot eliminate them.

After generation of the ultrasonic pulse, sufficient time must be allowed for reflections to return to the transducer. The speed of sound in the tissues limits the rate that pulses can be generated by the transducer to obtain unambiguous reflection data. The rate at which pulses can be fired off by the transducer is called the **pulse repetition frequency (PRF)**. In the neck, maximal depths are on the order of 7.5 cm resulting in a total path length of 15 cm. The maximal PRF would be:

$$1540 \text{ m sec}^{-1} / 0.15 \text{ m } = 10 \text{ kHz.}$$

Attenuation of the sound wave by the tissues actually helps by minimizing the reflectance of deeper objects allowing for higher frequency PRFs.

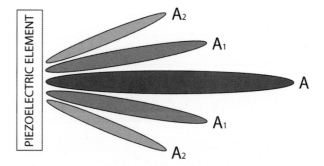

Fig 2–19. Piezoelectric elements have a finite shape and size with definite edges. Like a xylophone key being struck with a mallet, the primary energy wave (*the beam*) is emitted by a piezoelectric element in line with its central axis (*A*). Some of the vibrational energy is emitted toward the edges of the piezoelectric element. These additional side beams are called side lobes and are of lower intensity than the primary beam.

Artifacts as a Consequence of Physics

While a study is being performed, most artifacts are easily uncovered by rotating the transducer or varying its angle a small amount. The most common

artifacts seen in B-mode head and neck ultrasound include reverberation, multipath, shadowing, enhancement, side lobe, and refraction. An understanding of the first five simply requires applying the principles of physics already outlined. Refraction introduces one final concept embodied in Snell's law.

Reverberation artifacts occur when the ultrasonic sound waves repeatedly reflect between two interfaces. Optimal conditions for reverberations to occur typically include interfaces with high acoustic impedance mismatches, and relative proximity to the transducer to minimize attenuation of the signal through other tissues. In the head and neck region the most commonly encountered reverberation artifact occurs at a tracheal ring (Fig 2-20). In older individuals, cartilage rings are calcified to varying degrees approximating the acoustic impedance of bone. The anterior border is a soft tissue-to-cartilage interface and the posterior border is a cartilage-to-air interface. The apparent path length for the sound wave is increased by the serial reflections. Changing the angle of the incident beam helps reduce or eliminate this artifact.

Multipath artifacts arise from specular reflectors and can alter the position as well as the shape of objects (Fig 2-21). In these situations two objects will be perceived when there is only one. As the head and neck region has relatively small specular reflectors such as the carotid artery wall, multipath

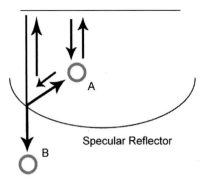

Fig 2–21. Multipath artifacts arise from reflections off specular reflectors. Object A acts as a reflector for ultrasound waves following the direct path length as well as the indirect path. The indirect path being longer is interpreted as a spurious object B at a greater depth.

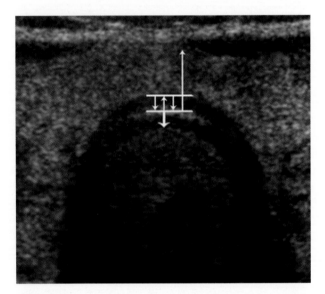

Fig 2–20. Reverberation artifacts occur at closely spaced interfaces with significantly mismatched acoustic impedances. Akin to light reflecting between two mirrors, the ultrasound wave repeatedly reflects between the interfaces delaying the return to the transducer. The increased interval for subsequent echos is interpreted as additional reflectors at greater depths than the first reflector. In the head and neck region the tracheal rings shown in this picture are a prime example of this phenomenon.

artifacts are not as much of a problem compared with other regions of the body.

Shadowing artifacts result from the attenuation of sound energy along the beam axis deep to a superficial object. Little or no reflections are returned from deeper objects because there is a lack of sound energy. Attenuation can occur through energy absorbance (eg, thick muscles or fat) as well as through reflectance off an object such as calcifications within a thyroid or the side wall of the carotid (Fig 2-22A). Shadowing can also occur because of operator error. Loss of beam penetration, poor scanning angles, and inadequate adjustment of time gain compensation can all contribute.

Enhancement artifacts occur when the attenuation of overlying tissues vary (Fig 2-22B). Fluid-filled cysts and blood within blood vessels have significantly lower attenuation values than surrounding soft tissues. In Figure 2-7, the attenuation of blood is given as 0.18 dB/cm/MHz which compares to an average attenuation for soft tissue of 0.70 dB/cm/MHz. Beams passing through the carotid have more of their sound energy available for reflection off of deeper structures when compared with similar beams passing through the thyroid. With more energy reflected, the tissues deep to the carotid appear brighter than those at the same level in the thyroid (see Fig 2-22B).

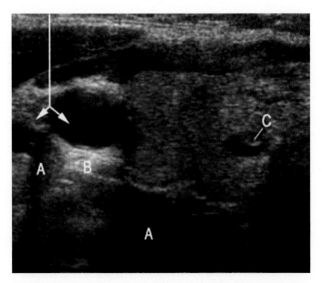

Fig 2–22. Transverse cross-section of the neck at the level of the thyroid. Examples of shadowing artifacts (**A**) are due to two mechanisms in this sonogram: On the left side of the sonogram a linear shadowing artifact is seen in line with the carotid sidewall due to reflectance and/or refraction at the sidewall (*bent arrows*). At the bottom center, the shadowing artifact is due to attenuation from the overlying tissues. **B** is an example of an enhancement artifact deep to the carotid because of a lack of attenuation of the beam through the blood. **C** is an example of a side lobe artifact. The side lobe beam is glancing off the wall of the cyst just out of the plane of the primary ultrasound beam.

Side lobe artifacts arise when there are strong reflectors adjacent to the primary ultrasonic energy beam. Reflection off a cyst wall just outside the sonographic plane can make it appear that there is a mass within the cyst (Fig 2–22C). Changing the angle or plane of the transducer can identify these artifacts.

Refraction artifacts like multipath artifacts move the position of objects resulting in spurious duplicates. Refraction is a change in the direction of propagation which can occur when a sound wave passes between two media with differing propagation velocities (Fig 2–23). The change in angle is described by Snell's law:

$$\sin \theta_1 / \sin \theta_2 = c_1 / c_2$$

where θ_1 is the angle of incidence approaching the interface, θ_2 is the angle of refraction leaving the interface, c_1 is the propagation velocity in Medium 1, and c_2 is the propagation velocity in Medium 2.

Significant refraction artifacts are rare in the head and neck region, but can occur at the edge of muscles (See Fig 2–23). Changing the angle of the incident beam can uncover this artifact.

Ultrasound Safety Issues

Ultrasound is one of the safest forms of imaging available. The American Institute of Ultrasound Official Statement on Clinical Safety, last revised in 1997, states that there are no confirmed reports of adverse biological effects on patients or ultrasonographers using machines which meet the current diagnostic equipment standards. However, there are potential concerns which the ultrasonographer needs to be aware of.

Ultrasound tissue effects can be broadly characterized as thermal or nonthermal. Thermal effects are due to energy absorption and conversion into heat. Nonthermal effects chiefly center on gaseous cavitation within fluid-filled areas. In the head and neck region nonthermal effects are a relatively small issue and are not discussed further. More information can be found in the recommended readings.

Thermal side effects due to ultrasound absorption are the same as for any mode of tissue heating. In general, the effects of heat depend on the rate of rise, the absolute temperature, and the duration. Common sense will lead the reader to realize that temperature variations of up to 2°C (eg, a low-grade fever) are well tolerated for extended periods of time. Experimentally temperature changes on this order have been maintained for over 50 hours without adverse effect.[2] On that basis, the general concept was born that a temperature rise of 1°C in an afebrile individual was acceptable for ultrasound exams. Temperature rises above 1°C might require consideration of the relative risk and benefit.

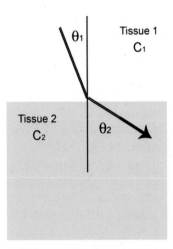
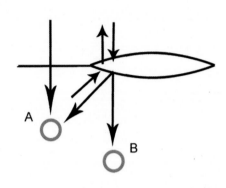

Fig 2–23. Refraction is a change in the direction of propagation which can occur when a sound wave passes between two media with differing propagation velocities. The change in angle is described by Snell's law: $\sin \theta_1 / \sin \theta_2 = c_1 / c_2$. An example of refraction at the edge of a muscle is shown on the right. Object A acts as a reflector for ultrasound waves following the direct path length as well as the indirect path. The indirect path being longer is interpreted as a spurious object B at a greater depth.

As previously discussed, tissue absorption is one of three components contributing to ultrasound attenuation. The greatest tissue attenuation, hence the greatest heating effects, are seen in bone (see Fig 2-7). Bone attenuation is up to seven times that of the average soft tissue. Bone heating can be a potential issue in obstetrical ultrasound where the partially calcified fetal calvarium is a target of interest. In the head and neck region the calcified tissues include the spine and incompletely calcified cartilage (eg, thyroid and cricoid cartilage) found in older individuals. For the typical frequencies used in head and neck ultrasound, the majority of absorption occurs within the soft tissues superficial to the spine (see Fig 2-22). Soft tissue absorption is the only significant consideration in most of these ultrasound studies.

Many factors affect the potential temperature rise in tissues including pulse power, pulse duration, beam shape, and beam frequency. Actual temperature rise in tissues is difficult to measure and can vary between subjects. In order to give some guidance to an ultrasonographer during an examination, equipment manufacturers will typically display a value called the Thermal Index (TI):

$$TI = W_0 / W_{deg}$$

where W_0 is the ultrasonic power output for the current exam and W_{deg} is the ultrasonic power output capable of creating a 1°C increase in temperature under specified conditions

The TI is meant to be a measure of the relative risk of a temperature rise rather than a measure of the actual temperature rise. Using this formula, a TI of 1 would be expected to limit the temperature rise in the tissue to 1°C or less; a TI of 2 would be expected to limit the temperature rise in the tissue to 2°C or less.

Following the safety guidelines outlined above, ultrasound exams with a TI of 1 or less would be considered safe and a TI of 2 or less would be considered generally acceptable, but might require consideration of the relative risk and benefit. In general, the amount of energy used in Doppler studies is significantly higher than for B-mode ultrasound. For example, in a series of obstetrical fetal exams where the B-mode portion lasted an average of 17 minutes and the Doppler portion took an average of 0.9 minutes, the B-mode TI averaged 0.3 whereas the color mode Doppler TI averaged 0.8 and the pulsed wave

Doppler TI averaged 1.5.[3] Extrapolating these findings to the average head and neck ultrasound exam, the typical exam should have a good safety margin.

References

1. Chivers RC, Parry RJ. Ultrasonic velocity and attenuation in mammalian tissues. *J Acoust Soc Am.* 1978;63:940-953.
2. Miller MW, Ziskin MC. Biological consequences of hyperthermia. *Ultrasound Med Biol.* 1989;15: 707-722.
3. Sheiner E, Shoham-Vardi I, Pombar X, Hussey MJ, Strassner HT, Abramowicz JS. An increased thermal index can be achieved when performing doppler studies in obstetric sonography. *J Ultrasound Med.* 2007;26:71-76.

Recommended Readings

The Core Curriculum: Ultrasound. William E. Brant. Philadelphia, Pa: Lippincott Williams & Wilkins; 2001.

Diagnostic Ultrasound. Carol M. Rumack, Stephanie R. Wilson, J. William Charboneau, Jo-Ann M. Johnson, eds. Philadelphia, Pa: Elsevier Mosby; 2005.

Chapter 3

ULTRASOUND EQUIPMENT, TECHNIQUES, AND ADVANCES

Antonia E. Stephen

Introduction

In recent years, the number of clinicians who care for patients with head and neck disorders who use ultrasound as an office-based tool has increased dramatically.[1] Both surgeons and nonsurgeon clinicians are using ultrasonography (US) to augment the physical examination,[2] and recent literature has documented its impact on patient management.[3,4] For head and neck and endocrine surgeons as well as endocrinologists experienced in US, performing these examinations and guided biopsies and interventions is an essential component of their clinical practice and adds an enormous amount of information and versatility to the traditional office-based history and physical examination. After obtaining fundamental US training, the first step to introducing US into a clinical practice is the selection and acquisition of the appropriate equipment and the setup of the office space to facilitate the efficient performance of ultrasound examinations and ultrasound-guided biopsies and procedures. If the US system and transducers are purchased without forethought, or if the office space is not organized in an appropriate fashion, performing US in the office can be uncomfortable for the patient and quite frustrating for the physician, not to mention misleading and inaccurate. On the other hand, when done under the appropriate conditions, US can be extremely informative while being quite painless and simple for all involved.

Options and Criteria for Selecting Equipment

There are a number of manufacturers of ultrasound equipment in the current era of office-based and clinician-performed US. Each manufacturer offers a variety of ultrasound machines and transducers, at a wide range of cost. The sheer volume of equipment to choose from can be overwhelming, especially to the US novice. The challenge of selecting the right ultrasound equipment is compounded by the fact that many, if not most, nonradiologist physicians are not sufficiently exposed to US during residency training, and thus lack knowledge of and familiarity with the equipment.

Before purchasing equipment, it is helpful to carefully review the logistical factors listed in Table 3–1. Once these practical considerations have been taken into account, the next step is to contact manufacturers or distributors and begin to test specific ultrasound equipment on a trial basis (Table 3–2). It is essential to decide what the ultrasound machine will be used for, that is, for neck ultrasound only, versus neck and

Table 3–1. Practical Considerations in Selecting an Ultrasound Machine for Office Use

1. Users and usage
2. Ability to perform biopsies
3. Office space and portability
4. Cost and billing
5. Politics

Table 3–2. Steps to Purchasing an Ultrasound Machine for Office Use

1. Consider the factors listed in Table 3–1
2. Discuss with other clinicians their recent experiences with ultrasound equipment
3. Determine the compatibility of prospective systems with your institution's digitized imaging systems or databases
4. Test ultrasound machines and probes in other departments or offices if possible
5. Contact manufacturers and trial specific machines and transducers in your own office

additional regions such as breast and/or abdominal ultrasound, and with or without vascular ultrasound capability. The intended applications are an especially important consideration when a group of individual specialists will be sharing usage of the ultrasound machine. Simple localization of blood vessels for performing US-guided vascular access procedures can be performed on relatively low-resolution, low-cost machines such as those available in emergency departments and anesthesiology environments. For higher resolution diagnostic imaging, higher end, higher resolution but still economical and even portable units are available. A single ultrasound machine can usually accommodate a variety of transducers for a wide array of purposes. If the ultrasound machine will be used exclusively for head and neck US, one transducer will usually suffice; the same transducer can also be used for neck US and for breast US. However, in order to use the same machine for abdominal US (gallbladder, adrenal,

etc), a transducer of a different (larger) size and (lower) frequency range is required. Deciding for whom and for what the machine will be used will help determine the best system and transducers to purchase. Depending on the individual vendor and machine, additional transducers can usually be purchased later, if and when usage of the machine is expanded to other purposes; this type of flexibility should be assessed when considering a purchase. Different transducers are better designed for biopsies; smaller sized, less bulky transducers that are easily maneuvered in one hand over the contours of the head and neck and that are not in the way of a biopsy needle work better for this purpose than the larger sized transducers. Another important consideration is the amount of space available for the machine and whether it needs to be portable or not. Some clinicians designate a specific room, often with ample space, for performance of ultrasound examinations and biopsies. In such circumstances space may also be desirable for a desktop microscope for a cytopathologist to use on site (Fig 3–1). With this type of arrangement the machine is not moved around regularly, and does not need to be particularly small or lightweight. On the other hand, if space is limited, or if the machine needs to be moved to different rooms or buildings on a regular basis, size and portability become more important. It is essential to test the machine, ideally for several days or weeks and under different clinical circumstances, before committing to a purchase.

Most modern ultrasound machines utilize computer technology for data storage, annotation, editing, and transferring images to other storage media. Therefore, it is important to determine the compatibility of a given system's software with other office-based computers and with the need to transfer stored images into files for presentations, or to share files with a hospital-based digital imaging system as is used by many radiology departments. In addition to storing data, most ultrasound systems also come with a black-and-white or color printer for immediate documentation of an examination by hard copy that can be filed in a patient's chart, sent to referring physicians, or given to the patient.

When considering the technical aspects and embarking on trials of various machines, the economics of purchasing a system naturally come into

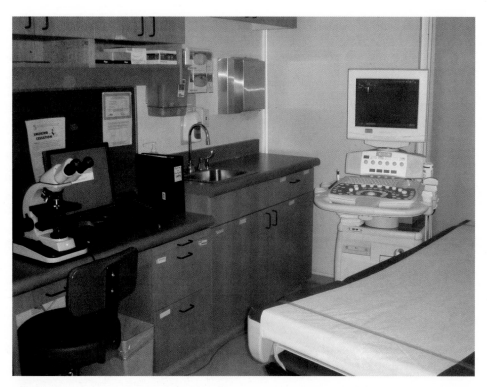

Fig 3–1. Examination room setup for ultrasonography, with on-site cyto-pathology setup as well.

play. A group of clinicians may decide to share an ultrasound machine, maximizing its usage and curtailing the cost for any one individual. Each practice group, hospital, and state have widely different policies regarding the billing of US by nonradiologists, and even within one practice, different insurance companies reimburse at different rates for diagnostic ultrasound examinations and ultrasound-guided procedures. A careful investigation of these policies is essential before any assumptions are made regarding reimbursement for US. Finally, the influence of politics on purchasing an ultrasound machine and using it in an office based setting cannot be ignored. In recent years there has been an enormous increase in the use of ultrasound by nonradiologists, including trauma surgeons, emergency room physicians, endocrinologists, breast and abdominal surgeons, urologists, obstetricians, and many others. The fact that there may be overlap in a particular hospital or institution with regard to which type of physician performs, and expects to bill for, head and neck ultrasound examinations, should be carefully taken

into account before purchase of the machine. With the respectful notification of all interested parties, and negotiation and compromise when necessary, in most circumstances the details can be worked out to everyone's satisfaction, and most importantly, to the benefit of patients.

Performing US of the Head and Neck

Office Setup

The successful performance of any procedure requires the appropriate setup. Office-based US and ultrasound-guided biopsies are no exception. Table 3–3 lists simple but essential equipment and supplies for performing US and US-guided biopsies in the office and supplies required for biopsies are listed in Table 3-4. By the time an ultrasound machine has been purchased, a space in which to

Table 3–3. List of Essential Equipment and Supplies for Performing US in the Office

1. Ultrasound machine and transducer(s)

2. Adjustable examination table or chair

3. Two separate lights: an overhead light and a desk or table light

4. Ultrasound gel

5. Medium sized towels, tissues, or absorbent pads to protect and clean patient

6. Printer paper

Table 3–4. Detailed List of Essential Supplies for Performing US-Guided Biopsies in the Office

Gloves

Needles (22–25g, 1.5-inch) (longer [eg, spinal]) needles for rare use in biopsying deep masses; finer [eg, 27g] if local anesthesia is to be used)

5 to 10-cc syringes (slip-tip often preferred)

Plastic wrap

Gauze

(Syringe holder)

Alcohol wipes or bottle of alcohol

Band-Aids

Local anesthetic (eg, lidocaine)

Cytology lab slips

Glass tubes for collecting samples for PTH, Thyroglobulin, Calcitonin, and so forth.

If preparing your own slides for cytologic evaluation:
    Paper clips (used to separate slides)
    Pencil
    Frost-ended microscope slides
    Hemostat for grasping needle shaft to "flick" material out of needle hub onto slide
    Slide fixative in glass jar (95% ethanol, Cytolyte, or similar)
    Cytology solution and saline for rinsing needle for thin prep slides and chemistry

use the machine should have been identified. There must be enough space in the room for the machine, an examination table or reclining chair, and a table or surface with the equipment needed for biopsies. The examination table should allow the examiner to have access to the patient from both sides; this is particularly important during biopsies, when the examiner may need to stand opposite the ultrasound machine to easily view the monitor while performing the procedure. The table with equipment and supplies needed for biopsies should be close enough to the physician who does his or her own slide preparation so that he or she can smear slides rapidly to avoid drying artifact and minimize nondiagnostic results. Also helpful is having a separate small desk light for the biopsy table as the overhead lights are typically dimmed or turned off during the ultrasound exam. For rooms with windows, adequate window shades are also necessary to provide sufficient darkness during examinations. Additional counter space and a microscope are necessary if microscopy is to be performed on site. The position of the ultrasound machine in relation to the examination table may depend somewhat on examiner preference, but for a right-handed examiner, it is generally most comfortable to place the ultrasound machine to the left of the head of the examination table (to the patient's right when lying supine, which is the examiner's left when facing the patient on the exam table) (Fig 3–2).

Patient Positioning

After the history and physical examination have been performed, the patient is asked to lie down on the examination table with the back of the table flat or elevated up to 45 degrees. A small pillow or shoulder roll can be placed underneath the patient's shoulders to gently hyperextend the neck; the neck position should be essentially the same as when performing thyroid or parathyroid surgery. If a patient cannot lie down or is in a wheelchair, the patient's chin is lifted and the neck slightly extended while the patient is sitting or only semireclined. Similarly, if the patient is unable to extend the neck, US can be performed without the neck extended; in such

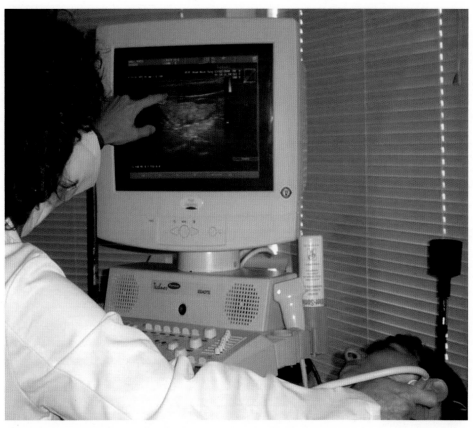

Fig 3–2. Example of examination table and ultrasound machine position for a right-handed examiner who is standing during the procedure.

patients US provides important preoperative information regarding accessibility of the thyroid and parathyroid glands during anticipated surgery, and the examination still provides useful if not maximal imaging information. In general, the examiner stands or sits to the right of the patient, facing the ultrasound monitor. The transducer is used in the right-handed examiner's right hand to examine the neck, and the ultrasound machine controls are manipulated with the left hand. A left-handed examiner may choose to adapt to this positioning, or to arrange the entire setup in a mirror image configuration to what has been described. It is essential that both the patient and the examiner be sufficiently comfortable to maintain their positions long enough for the examination to be completed—from 5 to 15 minutes or so—or else the exam will be rushed, and potentially useful information will be lost. It is worth

taking the few seconds to adjust the table height, bend the patient's knees, or move the pillow under the patient's shoulders to maximize comfort. A towel or absorbent pad is then tucked around the collar of the patient's shirt or the shirt is removed to protect the clothing from the ultrasound gel (which is water-soluble), and a generous amount of gel is applied to the patient's neck for sound transduction. Gel can be warmed although warming is not necessary.

General Principles of Ultrasound Transducers

The thyroid gland and surrounding area are best imaged using a "small parts" transducer at a frequency of 7.5 to 12 MHz or greater; this range is referred to as high frequency.[5-7] High-frequency US results in greater resolution than low-frequency US, at the expense of depth of penetration of the sound waves. However, as the majority of anatomic structures of interest in the neck are within 4 cm of the skin surface, loss of penetration is usually of little concern. Neck US is best conducted with a small parts transducer so that the probe can be easily maneuvered around the contoured and curved anatomy while still maintaining contact with the skin over the full length of the transducer. Most transducers used for head and neck US are linear array transducers that scan the rectangular section of tissue to which the transducer is directly applied. The curvilinear array transducers examine a convex shape of tissue, such that a wider area of tissue is imaged beneath the area of transducer contact. Curvilinear transducers are often used for intraoperative scanning, where very small contact areas are available for probe placement. Either type of transducer can be used for office US of the head and neck (Fig 3–3).

Ultrasound System Controls— Adjusting Settings to Optimize the Exam

Before starting an examination, patient identification is entered into the ultrasound system for documentation and data storage. Appropriate setup of the ultrasound machine for a neck examination is confirmed. The latter is particularly relevant when the ultrasound machine is used for a variety of purposes or by different examiners. Most ultrasound machines have preset parameters for different anatomic areas (ie, breast, thyroid, abdominal) that can be set with assistance from the vendor at the time of purchase, and need not be changed on a regular basis. Preset parameters limit the amount of control adjustment necessary during a patient examination, and reduce the effort required to reset the machine after each use. The parameters that are most often varied during an individual examination

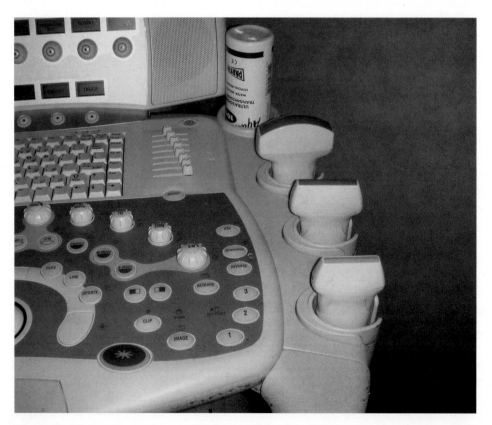

Fig 3–3. Various transducers can be used for head and neck ultrasonography.

are thus minimized, and typically include frequency, gain, depth of the focal zone, and zoom or depth of the field. Also used intermittently but frequently during an examination are calipers for measurement, color flow or power Doppler, and annotation controls. Although the number of knobs and buttons on any particular machine may initially seem daunting, the examiner can quickly become facile with those that are most useful for specific purposes during individual examinations. The ability to manually adjust specific settings does however, enable optimization of each exam.

Frequency

Most transducers have a range of frequencies that can be adjusted during an examination to optimize evaluation of individual anatomic structures at a variety of depths within the head and neck. With increased frequency, the detail resolution of the ultrasound image increases, but the tissue penetration decreases.[8] Because the thyroid is a relatively superficial and solid organ, it is well evaluated with high-frequency ultrasound. For patients with thin necks, 10 to 12 MHz or even higher frequencies provide exceptionally clear images, whereas in larger patients or those with deeper lesions, lower frequencies help to achieve better tissue penetration. The thyroid gland is a common starting point for ultrasound examination of the neck, and frequency is adjusted as the exam proceeds, to higher frequencies for superficial structures (thyroid isthmus, superficial lymph nodes), and lower frequencies for deeper structures (superior parathyroid glands, deep muscles and lymph nodes, deep parotid, tongue).

Gain

Gain refers to the overall brightness of the image on the screen. The gain can and should be adjusted and fine tuned throughout the exam, according to the area being examined and the eyesight of the examiner. For example, adjusting the gain while scrutinizing a thyroid nodule may help in defining the area of pathology in relation to surrounding tissues and parenchyma of varying echogenicity.

Focal Zones

The depth at which the ultrasound image is best focused can also be changed during an exam, depending on the depth of the object that is of greatest interest. Adjustment of focal zone is particularly useful when examining deep and superficial structures within the same patient, such as superior and inferior parathyroid glands, respectively, or thyroid nodules and associated cervical lymph nodes.

Planes of Imaging

When starting an examination, the orientation of the transducer is confirmed in relation to the image displayed on the ultrasound monitor. A simple method of doing so is to hold the probe (away from the patient) in the transverse orientation and press one's finger on one side of the probe to confirm that the motion is detected on the correct side of the monitor. Once the orientation is confirmed, examination of the neck is typically initiated in the transverse plane. One's personal algorithm for examining all structures may vary, but one basic sequence is to start in the low anterior midline over the trachea, and after identifying the airway and the thyroid isthmus, to slowly move laterally over each thyroid lobe. After completing the examination of both thyroid lobes in the transverse plane, the transducer is rotated 90 degrees and each thyroid lobe is examined in the longitudinal (or sagittal) plane. Measurements of thyroid lobes and nodules or masses should be done in three dimensions—longitudinal (height), transverse (width), and anteroposterior (depth).[9] Once the thyroid lobes are measured, overall thyroid volume can then be calculated manually using the standard formula, Volume = $(H \times W \times D) \times \pi/6$, or computed automatically by software within the ultrasound system. After the thyroid gland examination is complete, the ultrasound transducer is moved laterally over the carotid artery and jugular vein on either side to examine for cervical lymph nodes and other masses. Comprehensive nodal examination (levels I–VI) is best done with the transducer in the transverse orientation. However, preliminary examination of the parotid glands is often easier with the transducer in a longitudinal orientation. All nodular structures, including thyroid, parathyroid, and salivary gland tumors, as well as lymph nodes, should be examined in at least two planes; what may appear suspect as a mass in the transverse plane may prove to be muscle or blood vessel when it is examined in the perpendicular longitudinal plane. Examination of the midline structures superior to the thyroid (larynx, suprahyoid region, tongue, and floor of mouth) should also be carried out in two planes, usually starting with the transverse plane. Once a full survey of the thyroid gland and surrounding areas is completed, the examination can be further focused and directed toward any areas of particular interest or concern.

Interactive Ultrasound

Several physical maneuvers can be used during neck US to enhance information acquired. The transducer itself can be used to palpate and even move lesions or structures in the neck. Parathyroid adenomas tend to lie adjacent to, but separate from, the thyroid gland. It is often difficult to distinguish a closely situated parathyroid gland resting alongside the thyroid from a hypoechoic thyroid nodule. By pressing the probe firmly onto the thyroid gland, a parathyroid adenoma will move separately from the thyroid gland, whereas a thyroid nodule will move with it. Asking the patient to swallow during the exam achieves a similar effect, with mobile lesions within the thyroid gland sliding underneath the strap muscles along with the thyroid. Swallowing by the patient also helps delineate the esophagus and distinguish it from paratracheal pathology. Pharyngeal or esophageal pathologies (such as Zenker's diverticula) can be recognized by their appearance during rest and swallowing. "Sonopalpation" of masses (manual palpation of a neck mass with one hand while holding the transducer with the other hand) can demonstrate whether there is adherence or invasion of that mass with respect to surrounding structures such as the carotid artery (Videos 3A and 3B). Voluntary tongue movement helps delineate the base of tongue as well as the symmetry of tongue musculature (Video 3C), and respiration and phonation can be observed in the assessment of gross vocal fold mobility (Video 3D). These are but some of the maneuvers that make neck US a dynamic, interactive, and more informative study.

Color-Flow Doppler

Ultrasound systems equipped with color Doppler are able to measure the direction and velocity of blood flow. Doppler is useful both in identifying blood vessels and for assessing the vascularity of structures in the neck. Structures that appear round in the transverse plane, such as parathyroid adenomas or lymph nodes, can be easily distinguished from major blood vessels that are also round by the presence of luminal blood flow in the latter but not the former on color Doppler sonography. The combination of Doppler US and examination of structures in at least two perpendicular planes should prevent the mistaken interpretation of any blood vessel as a mass lesion, and helps distinguish vessels from ductal structures (Fig 3–4). The amount and architecture of blood flow in thyroid nodules, lymph nodes, and other lesions can be measured directly and has been shown to be useful in predicting risk of malignancy.[10] The vascularity of the thyroid gland itself, often increased in Graves' disease, can be assessed. Conversely, diminished blood flow, such as in chronic lymphocytic thyroiditis, can also be demonstrated. Both the gain and the velocity can be adjusted when using color Doppler to detect blood flow; fine tuning the flow gain decreases the background speckling that can occur with color Doppler and changing the velocity will detect flow in lower velocity vessels or tissues with low vascularity. Very low flow can be detected with the power Doppler mode, which increases the sensitivity of detection of low velocity blood flow at the expense of directional information.

Ultrasound-Guided Biopsy and Other Procedures

A detailed discussion of ultrasound-guided biopsies and interventions is found in Chapter 12. Briefly, the examination room should be organized to facilitate

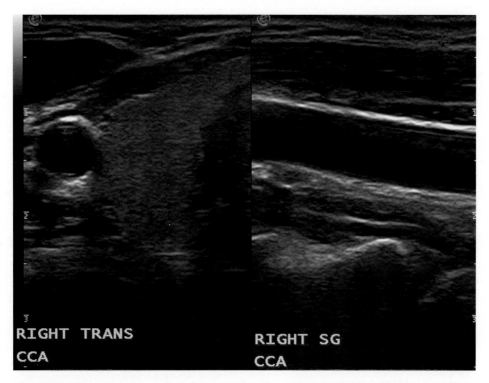

Fig 3-4. Examination of structures in two perpendicular planes, such as the transverse (*left*) and sagittal (*right*) views of the common carotid artery shown here, helps to distinguish nodular structures from tubular ones. Doppler sonography further helps to distinguish vascular structures (with moving blood) from ductal ones.

the performance of ultrasound-guided procedures. All equipment and supplies should be completely set up before beginning the procedure, and should be positioned at arm's length from the examiner and operator. Such thoughtful organization prevents fumbling with the equipment during the procedure and avoids unnecessary delays in preparing the aspirates obtained for evaluation, as well as unwanted turning of attention away from the patient. Some operators find it helpful to use a biopsy holder for the syringe, making it is easier to stabilize the syringe and needle with respect to the transducer, or to aspirate and apply suction with one hand. However, free-hand performance of ultrasound-guided biopsies yields maximum flexibility to the operator. Ultrasound-guided biopsy of thyroid nodules,[11] lymph nodes,[12] and other hard-to-palpate masses, and, in select circumstances, suspected parathyroid lesions,[13] has been shown to be highly accurate when performed as an office-based procedure. Table 3–4 lists the essential supplies for performing ultrasound-guided biopsies in the office.

Advanced and Emerging Ultrasound Techniques

The introduction of high resolution US in the late 1980s and early 1990s led to a dramatic increase in its widespread use. Truly excellent and affordable ultrasound technology is available to the independent practitioner. Still, new innovations are being developed to improve ultrasound imaging even further.[14]

Power Doppler can be used to objectively measure blood flow in tumors and lymph nodes using a power Doppler index (PDI) that quantifies the number of pixels in a defined region of interest. The PDI has been applied to selected frames of B-mode US images of tumors with power Doppler overlay, and found to have high diagnostic value in discriminating between certain benign and malignant masses.[15]

The use of intravenous contrast is routine for computed tomography and magnetic resonance imaging, and is currently being used with US in Europe. In the United States, the use of ultrasound contrast is still considered experimental and has been primarily used for vascular and cardiac imaging.[16] Ultrasound contrast agents contain microscopic air bubbles; the microbubbles reflect ultrasound waves and increase the contrast between adjacent structures to create more detailed images, especially with respect to perfusion mapping.[8,17] Contrast-enhanced Doppler US has been studied in the context of cervical lymphadenopathy and found to show some differences between vessel size and vessel density in malignant versus benign inflammatory nodes, but definitive differentiation has remained difficult.[18]

Three-dimensional (3D) reconstructions of ultrasound images are another advancement under current investigation. 3D reconstruction has become quite commonplace for computed tomography and magnetic resonance imaging, and has been used for fetal US as well.[19] The 3D images are typically reconstructed after the imaging and data collection is completed, not in real time. Prenatal two-dimensional (2D) US has for many years enabled measurement of fetal neck translucency that has increased the detection of aneuploidies and heart malformations. The addition of three-dimensional (3D), and even four-dimensional (4D, incorporating time or video) US, has provided a complementary tool to 2D US for assessing fetal morphology.[20] The management of fetal anomalies such as teratomas and lymphangiomas of the face and neck, incorporating volumetric determinations, has been enhanced by the use of prenatal 2D and 3D US.[21,22] In the adult head and neck region, 3D US has been evaluated in the measurement of cervical lymph node volume and found to be highly repeatable but with variable reproducibility of measurements depending on the level or location of the lymph nodes.[23] The clinical significance and application of this technique to lymph node assessment remains to be determined.

3D US may prove to be most useful in adults for needle placement for US-guided biopsies.[14]

Ultrasonographic (US) elastography is an emerging technique that combines the diagnostic advantages of high-frequency US examination with the assessment of a tissue's or lesion's stiffness to distinguish benign from malignant masses. US-elastography has been found to be useful in the differential diagnosis of breast and prostate cancers. Tissue strain imaging is a method of elastography whereby measurements of local displacements induced by a compressive force applied to the tissue surface are used to construct an elastogram, in which hard areas appear dark and soft areas appear bright. Correlation techniques track echo delays in segmented waveforms that are recorded before and after a quasistatic compression. Real-time elastograms and B-mode US images are superimposed to assess individual lesions within the field of view and compression. US-elastography may thus prove useful in the differential diagnosis of malignant thyroid lesions.[24]

Summary

Office-based ultrasonography has become an invaluable tool in the clinical management of patients with head and neck disorders. It provides a unique opportunity for the clinician to supplement the history and physical examination with detailed real-time anatomic imaging, and to perform guided procedures. It is quick, noninvasive, and relatively inexpensive. The equipment is becoming increasingly portable and affordable. Understanding the options and the functions available on US equipment enables optimal information acquisition. In time, office-based US will be considered an essential skill of the surgeon of the head and neck region.

Videos for This Chapter

Videos 3A and 3B: See DVD. Sonopalpation of a large neck mass can help identify the presence or absence of adherence to or invasion of surrounding structures (in this example, a large papillary thyroid carcinoma that does not invade the prevertebral fascia [video clip A] or the carotid artery [video clip B]).

Video 3C: See DVD. The patient can be asked to move their tongue during the examination to help delineate its boundaries and its symmetry.

Video 3D: See DVD. Laryngeal function and symmetry can be assessed by examining the larynx during respiration and phonation, where vocal fold abduction and adduction are observed.

References

1. Hegedus L. Thyroid ultrasonography as a screening tool for thyroid disease. *Thyroid.* 2004;14(11): 879–880.
2. Baskin HJ. Thyroid ultrasound: just do it. *Thyroid.* 2004;14(2):91–92.
3. Milas M, Stephen A, Berber E, Wagner K, Miskulin J, Siperstein A. Ultrasonography for the endocrine surgeon: a valuable clinical tool that enhances diagnostic and therapeutic outcomes. *Surgery.* 2005;138(6):1193–1200.
4. Milas M, Mensah A, Alghoul M, et al. The impact of office neck ultrasonography on reducing unnecessary thyroid surgery in patients undergoing parathyroidectomy. *Thyroid.* 2005;15(9):1055–1059.
5. Hegedus L. Thyroid ultrasound. *Endocrinol Metab Clin North Am.* 2001;30(2):339–360.
6. Senchenkov A, Staren ED. Ultrasound in head and neck surgery: thyroid, parathyroid, and cervical lymph nodes. *Surg Clin N Am.* 2004;84:973–1000.
7. Harness JK, Czako PF. Ultrasound of the thyroid and parathyroid glands. In: Harness JK, Wisher DB, eds. *Ultrasound in Surgical Practice: Basic Principles and Clinical Applications.* New York, NY: Wiley-Liss; 2001:237–263.
8. Kremkau FW. *Diagnostic Ultrasound: Principles and Instruments.* 7th ed. St. Louis, Mo: Elsevier; 2006.
9. Solbiati L, Osti V, Cova L, Tonolini M. Ultrasound of thyroid, parathyroid glands and neck lymph nodes. *Eur Radiol.* 2001;11(12):2411–2424.
10. Papini E, Guglielmi R, Bianchini A, et al. Risk of malignancy in nonpalpable thyroid nodules: predictive value of ultrasound and color-Doppler features. *J Clin Endocrinol Metab.* 2002;87(5):1941–1946.
11. Danese D, Sciacchitano S, Farsetti A, Andreoli M, Pontecorvi A. Diagnostic accuracy of conventional versus sonography-guided fine-needle aspiration biopsy of thyroid nodules. *Thyroid.* 1998;8(1): 15–21.
12. van den Brekel MW, Castelijns JA, Stel HV, Golding RP, Meyer CJ, Snow GB. Modern imaging techniques and ultrasound-guided aspiration cytology for the assessment of neck node metastases: a prospective comparative study. *Eur Arch Otorhinolaryngol.* 1993;250:11–17.
13. Stephen AE, Milas M, Garner CN, Wagner KE, Siperstein AE. Use of surgeon-performed office ultrasound and parathyroid fine needle aspiration for complex parathyroid localization. *Surgery.* 2005; 138(6):1143–1150.
14. Levine RA. Something old and something new: a brief history of thyroid ultrasound technology. *Endocr Pract.* 2004;10(3):227–233.
15. Marret H, Sauget S, Giraudeau B, Body G, Tranquart F. Power Doppler vascularity index for predicting malignancy of adnexal masses. *Ultrasound Obstet Gynecol.* 2005;25(5):508–513.
16. Grant EG. Sonographic contrast agents in vascular imaging. *Semin Ultrasound CT MR.* 2001;22:25–41.
17. Dayton PA, Ferrara KW. Targeted imaging using ultrasound. *J Magn Reson Imaging.* 2002;16: 362–377.
18. Zenk J, Bozzato A, Steinhart H, Greess H, Iro H. Metastatic and inflammatory cervical lymph nodes as analyzed by contrast-enhanced color-coded Doppler ultrasonography: quantitative dynamic perfusion patterns and histopathologic correlation. *Ann Otol Rhinol Laryngol.* 2005;114(1 pt 1):43–47.
19. Timor-Tritsch IE, Platt LD. Three-dimensional ultrasound experience in obstetrics. *Curr Opin Obstet Gynecol.* 2002;14:569–575.
20. Avni FE, Cos T, Cassart M, et al. Evolution of fetal ultrasonography. *Eur Radiol.* 2007;17(2):419–431.
21. Paladini D, Vassallo M, Sglavo G, Lapadula C, Longo M, Nappi C. Cavernous lymphangioma of the face and neck: prenatal diagnosis by three-dimensional ultrasound. *Ultrasound Obstet Gynecol.* 2005; 26(3):300–302.
22. Rahbar R, Vogel A, Myers LB, et al. Fetal surgery in otolaryngology: a new era in the diagnosis and management of fetal airway obstruction because of advances in prenatal imaging. *Arch Otolaryngol Head Neck Surg.* 2005;131:393–398.

23. Ying M, Pang SF, Sin MH. Reliability of 3-D ultrasound measurements of cervical lymph node volume. *Ultrasound Med Biol*. 2006;32(7):995–1001.

24. Lyshchik A, Higashi T, Asato R, et al. Thyroid gland tumor diagnosis at US elastography. *Radiology*. 2005;237:202–211.

Chapter 4

NORMAL HEAD AND NECK ULTRASOUND ANATOMY

Christine G. Gourin
Lisa A. Orloff

Introduction

Ultrasound imaging has been used medically for several decades. In recent years, the development of high-resolution transducers and color Doppler ultrasonography has improved the accuracy of ultrasound in the evaluation of head and neck pathology, and ultrasound has found an increasingly important role in the clinician's armamentarium. Ultrasound is the least expensive of all preoperative localization studies, does not involve ionizing radiation, is noninvasive, is reproducible and readily repeatable, and may offer some advantages over other localization tests in the setting of concomitant head and neck pathology. Fine-needle aspiration biopsy of suspected lesions is facilitated with the use of ultrasound, which allows accurate needle placement and confirmation. Ultrasound is easy to use and is cost-effective when performed as part of routine office practice.[1] Familiarity with the normal ultrasound appearance of head and neck structures is necessary for the clinician who wishes to incorporate ultrasound imaging into his or her practice.

Ultrasonography (US) is typically performed in the transverse and sagittal or longitudinal planes with the neck in mild extension. The examiner is positioned lateral to the patient's head or neck. Imaging in the transverse plane provides an axial image of head and neck structures whereas longitudinal imaging provides a sagittal view. Ultrasound evaluation should always progress in a systematic fashion with identification of normal landmarks such as the trachea (transverse) and superficial muscles and great vessels (longitudinal) to aid in identification of other head and neck structures, progressing from superficial (skin) to deep (viscera). High-frequency transducers in the range of 7 to 13 MHz offer optimal visualization of head and neck anatomy. Patients with short, thick, obese necks or those with large thyroid glands may require a lower frequency 5-MHz transducer with a larger footprint for penetration; however, use of lower frequency probes is associated with a decrease in resolution.[2] There is considerable variability in tissue characteristics, sound penetration, and anatomic definition from one patient to the next, even in nonobese individuals. Therefore, the examiner should freely adjust the settings on the ultrasound system as the examination proceeds.

This chapter aims to familiarize the reader with normal sonographic anatomy of the head and neck. Further highlights on examination of specific structures and characteristics of pathologic entities are described in greater detail in later chapters. It cannot be emphasized strongly enough that there is a loss of information when capturing and reviewing still images compared to performing and viewing dynamic US. Nevertheless, it is hoped that the descriptions, static images, plus video clips contained in this chapter and throughout this book will give the reader a hint of what can be gleaned from performing US examinations in "real time." As with the performance of US examinations, the reader is encouraged to view the video clips contained herein in a darkened room for maximum clarity.

Thyroid and Parathyroid Glands

Thyroid Gland

The thyroid gland has a superficial location in the central neck, with an isthmus that overlies the trachea at the level of the second or third tracheal rings. A pyramidal lobe arising from the superior aspect of the thyroid isthmus and projecting superiorly may be present in up to a third of patients. The thyroid lobes are situated anterior and lateral to the trachea and esophagus and medial to the carotid sheath. The sternohyoid and sternothyroid muscles lie anterior to the thyroid gland, whereas the sternocleidomastoid muscles are anterior and lateral to the gland. The thyroid gland is invested by the visceral layer of the pretracheal fascia, which is continuous with the superficial layer of the deep cervical fascia laterally which encloses the strap muscles. The pretracheal fascia attaches the thyroid gland to the trachea and larynx, which results in thyroid gland movement with laryngeal elevation during swallowing.

The thyroid gland arises from the medial thyroid anlage, a diverticulum of the endoderm of the primitive pharynx, which descends caudally to a final position anterior to the second to fifth tracheal rings in the 7th week of gestation. The gland remains connected to the foramen cecum of the tongue base during descent by the thyroglossal duct, which becomes solid and is reabsorbed by the 7th gesta-

tional week. Failure of reabsorption results in thyroglossal duct cysts, which usually present in the midline of the neck near the level of the hyoid bone. Failure of descent can result in a lingual thyroid gland, associated with the foramen cecum and located superior to the hyoid bone. Rarely, ectopic thyroid tissue may be present in the mediastinum as a result of displacement of thyroid tissue during descent of the heart and great vessels.

Ultrasound evaluation of the thyroid gland is best performed using a high-frequency linear transducer in the range of 7 to 12 MHz with the neck extended.[3] Patients with thick, obese necks or those with large thyroid glands may require a lower frequency 5-MHz transducer with a larger footprint for penetration, which results in a compensatory decrease in resolution.[2] Imaging in the transverse plane provides an axial view of the thyroid gland and the relationship of the thyroid compartment to the carotid sheath, strap muscles, trachea, and esophagus, often in a single wide-field image (Fig 4–1). Longitudinal

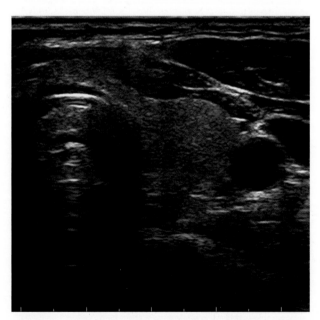

Fig 4–1. Midline transverse view of the normal thyroid. The relationship of the thyroid to the carotid arteries, strap muscles, trachea, and esophagus can be appreciated in this view, which is a common starting point for the US examination of the neck.

images allow visualization of the thyroid gland in a craniocaudal direction and differentiation of the thyroid from vascular structures and the esophagus (Fig 4–2 and Video 4A). Both transverse and longitudinal scanning is required for accurate imaging.

Scan interpretation is initially performed as a widefield survey, progressing from superficial to deep structures. Subcutaneous fat appears hypoechoic on US and is highly variable in quantity depending on body habitus. The overlying skin is often separated from the subcutaneous fat by a thin hyperechoic line. The strap muscles and sternocleidomastoid muscle are deep to the subcutaneous fat and appear hypoechoic on images, and may be separated from adjacent structures and the skin by thin, hyperechoic lines representing the cervical fascia (Fig 4–3 and Video 4B). The normal thyroid gland is homogeneous and hyperechoic relative to muscle. Nevertheless, pathology noted within the thyroid gland is described as hyperechoic, isoechoic, or hypoechoic with respect to the surrounding thyroid parenchyma. The trachea, located medial and deep to the thyroid lobes, is a useful reference point by virtue of its size and midline position: it is crescent shaped on imaging, representing the tracheal cartilage rings anteriorly, with an anechoic or black interior (due to air within its lumen not reflecting sound) and posterior shadowing (Fig 4–4). In contrast, the esophageal mucosa is highly echogenic, and is located posterior and normally to the left of the trachea (Fig 4–5 and Video 4C). The high echogenicity of the concentric esophageal mucosa results in a classic "bulls eye" target sign on transverse images. The carotid sheath is located lateral to the thyroid lobes and contains the anechoic carotid artery and internal jugular vein. These are distinguishable by the roundness and posterior enhancement associated with the carotid artery; the jugular vein, situated lateral to the carotid artery, lacks such enhancement, is more ovoid, and is easily compressible (Fig 4–6 and Video 4D).

Thyroid nodules are common and small nodules (<1 cm) not suspected clinically are present in as many as 70% of patients examined by US.[3] Nodules are usually multiple and often have cystic areas, with a capsule frequently demonstrated around the nodule.[4] A simple cyst appears anechoic, whereas a complex cyst appears hypoechoic and solid nodules are hypoechoic to hyperechoic. It has been reported that the incidence of malignancy is approximately 4% when a nodule is hyperechoic, whereas hypoechoic nodules have a 26% incidence of harboring malignancy.[3] However, hypoechogenicity alone is inaccurate in predicting malignancy, with poor specificity and a low positive predictive value.[3] Nodules with a large cystic component usually represent a benign cyst that has undergone hemorrhage or cystic degeneration. A peripheral halo with decreased echogenicity is seen surrounding hypoechoic or isoechoic nodules representing the capsule of the nodule or compressed thyroid tissue. The absence of such a halo is associated with an increased incidence of malignancy.[3] The comet tail sign within a thyroid nodule is associated with the presence of colloid in a benign nodule. Calcifications appear as echogenic foci: punctate calcifications do not exhibit shadowing and are associated with papillary carcinoma. Larger areas of calcification exhibit dense posterior shadowing secondary to acoustical impedance mismatch and are more commonly benign. For more details on thyroid US, the reader is referred to Chapter 5.

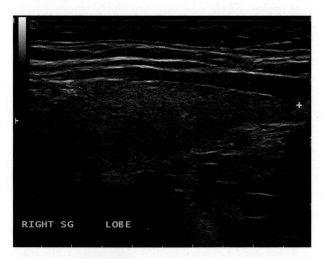

RIGHT SG   LOBE

Fig 4–2 and Video 4A. Sagittal view of the right thyroid lobe. The overlying strap muscles, platysma, and subcutaneous tissue are visible. The underlying spine can be better recognized in real time when the patient can be asked to swallow and the thyroid can be seen to slide over the vertebrae (**Video 4A**).

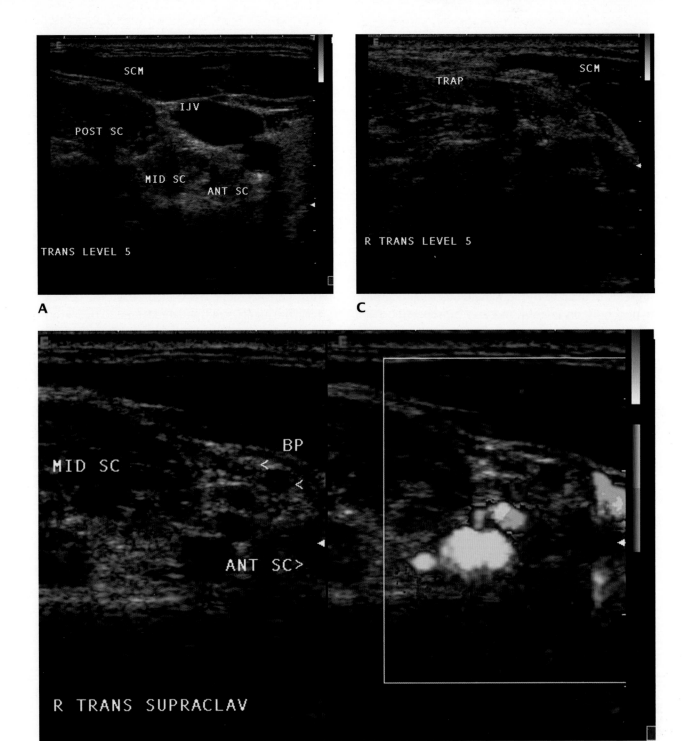

Fig 4–3 and Video 4B. A. Deep to the sternocleidomastoid (*SCM*) muscle and the carotid sheath are the scalene (*SC*) muscles (anterior, middle, and posterior) in the floor of the anterior neck. Vessels in this area can be distinguished from cords of the brachial plexus (*BP*) using color Doppler (**B**). More posteriorly (**C**), the trapezius (*TRAP*) can be seen extending behind the sternocleidomastoid (*SCM*) muscle. In real time, the anterior neck muscles can be followed along their course from origin to insertion, and it becomes easier to distinguish additional neck muscles such as the omohyoid muscle and the deep scalene muscles (**Video 4B**). The muscles are also distinguished from each other by thin, hyperechoic lines that represent the cervical fascia.

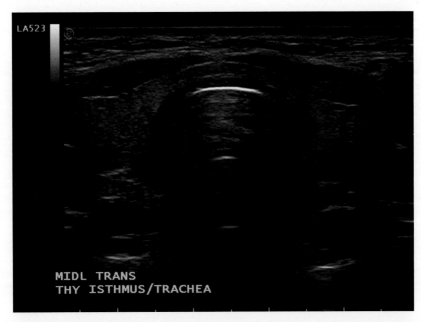

Fig 4–4. The anterior tracheal wall is easily recognized by its crescent shape and its midline position, but the lumen and posterior trachea are poorly visualized by US.

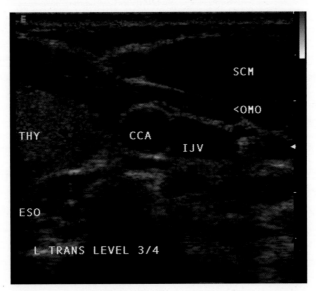

Fig 4–5 and Video 4C. The esophagus (*ESO*) is usually more visible on the left side in the transverse plane, posterolateral to the trachea and the thyroid, although it can change position with head movement and swallowing. Note the omohyoid (*OMO*) muscle in this figure crossing superficial to the internal jugular vein (*IJV*). The concentric rings of the esophagus seen at rest are accentuated when the patient is asked to swallow and the hyperechoic saliva passes (**Video 4C**). CCA = common carotid artery; THY = thyroid; SCM = sternocleidomastoid muscle.

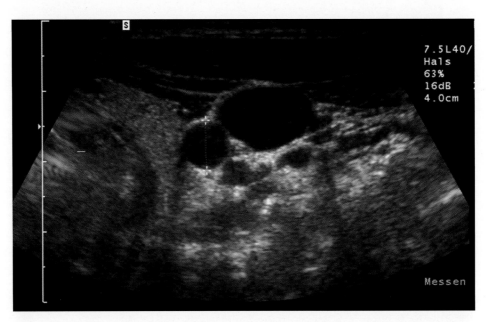

Fig 4–6 and Video 4D. The carotid artery (shown here with caliper marks) is one of the most reliable landmarks on either side of the neck, due to its round shape on transverse view, tubular shape on sagittal view, noncompressibility, pulsations, hyperechoic wall which causes the refractionlike "edge effect," anechoic lumen, and blood flow on color Doppler mode. The internal jugular vein on the other hand is compressible and changes diameter with maneuvers such as Valsalva (**Video 4D**). Note rounded structures from medial to lateral in this clip (left to right across the screen, from patient's right to left side): the esophagus, the left carotid artery, and the left internal jugular vein.

Color-flow Doppler imaging is a useful adjunct in imaging the thyroid gland and allows evaluation of thyroid vascularity. Patients with acute thyroiditis and Graves' disease show marked, diffusely increased glandular vascularity. Chronic and end-stage thryoiditis with atrophy are usually hypovascular by Doppler US. Benign hyperplastic nodules are associated with an absence of flow within the nodule or exclusively perinodular flow signals; marked intranodular flow is associated with an increased likelihood of malignancy.[3] Inability to visualize the thyroid gland by ultrasound in the absence of a history of prior thyroidectomy should alert the examiner to the possibility of an ectopic gland, either mediastinal, which is beyond the reach of ultrasonographic imaging, or to a lingual thyroid or thyroid agenesis. Color Doppler ultrasonography has been shown to be superior to gray-scale ultrasonography in detection of the lingual thyroid gland.[5]

Parathyroid Glands

A thorough knowledge of parathyroid embryology and location is key to successful parathyroid identification by US. Even so, normal parathyroid glands are rarely visible. Parathyroid US is usually performed in patients with hyperparathyroidism, for preoperative localization of the gland(s). Incidentally enlarged parathyroid glands are occasionally noted on neck US done for other purposes. The superior parathyroid glands are derived from the fourth branchial arch and are relatively constant in their location, on the posterior aspect of the superior pole of the thyroid gland near the cricothyroid junction and closely associated with the middle thyroid vein and recurrent laryngeal nerve.[6] The inferior parathyroids are derived from the third branchial arch and descend with the thymus, normally to the level of the inferior pole of the thyroid gland, and are usually located more anteriorly than the superior glands. However, their location is much more variable and they may be found anywhere along the path of descent of the thymus. Known ectopic locations of the inferior parathyroid glands in order of frequency are paraesophageal, intrathymic, anterior mediastinum, intrathyroidal, the carotid sheath, posterior mediastinum, aortopulmonary window, or high cervical location (undescended).[7] Although there are usually four glands, supernumerary glands may be present in 2 to 8%.[6] The blood supply to both the superior and inferior parathyroid glands arises from the inferior thyroid artery in the majority of cases.[8] Occasionally, the superior parathyroid glands receive their blood supply from the superior thyroid artery, or from anastomotic connections between the superior and inferior thyroid vessels.

Parathyroid US is performed with the patient's neck extended, which is facilitated by the use of a shoulder roll. A high-frequency linear transducer in the range of 7 to 12 MHz is used to scan, with 10-MHz probes most commonly used: the higher the frequency, the greater the resolution of small, superficially located glands.[9] Patients with thick, obese necks or those with large thyroid glands or deeply situated parathyroid glands may require a lower frequency 5-MHz transducer for penetration, with a compensatory decrease in resolution under these conditions.[2,9]

Imaging of parathyroid glands should begin in the transverse plane to provide a wide-field axial image that includes the carotid sheath, thyroid compartment and trachea, and esophagus. Sagittal or longitudinal images are most useful in imaging the entire length of the parathyroid gland and distinguishing it from vascular structures and the esophagus. Enlarged parathyroid glands are well circumscribed and oval, hypoechoic, and usually solid and homogeneous (Fig 4–7 and see Chapter 6). When smaller than 5 mm, they may be undetectable by ultrasound.[2] Color Doppler imaging can be used to demonstrate the parathyroid gland suspended by a vascular pedicle surrounded by fat, which may be useful in confirmation of parathyroid pathology and in distinguishing thyroid from parathyroid tissue.[9]

The accuracy of ultrasound imaging is limited by operator skill and experience, patient size, gland

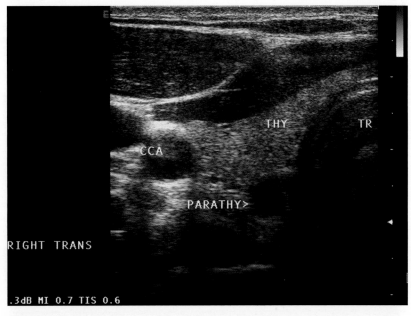

Fig 4–7. Although normal parathyroid glands are not usually visible, occasionally an incidental parathyroid adenoma can be detected on thorough routine neck US. The regions just posterior, posterolateral, and inferior to the thyroid gland are the sites of eutopic parathyroid glands.

size and ectopic location, concurrent thyroid pathology, and previous neck surgery. The experience of the ultrasonographer is the single most important determinant of parathyroid gland detection. An understanding of the limitations of US and the likely ectopic locations of parathyroid glands with evaluation of these sites is necessary for a successful ultrasound examination. The short, obese neck is more difficult to evaluate by US because of the need to use lower frequency, lower resolution transducers in this setting. Parathyroid glands less than 100 mg in weight or 1 cm in size are less likely to be accurately detected by US.

Ectopic locations are associated with reduced accuracy of detection by ultrasound, and require that a careful bilateral ultrasound neck examination that encompasses the entire cervical region from angle of mandible to thoracic inlet as well as lateral examination of the carotid sheath be performed to identify all parathyroid tissue. US has limited penetration of bone and air. The limitations of US in evaluating glands located behind bone or air columns results in a lower percentage of retrotracheal, retroesophageal, and mediastinal glands identified by ultrasound.[2] False-positive images can occur in the setting of concomitant thyroid pathology, in particular, multinodular goiter or a thyroid adenoma, because thyroid nodules can be difficult to distinguish from intrathyroidal parathyroid adenomas on US. However, US can detect a parathyroid gland obscured by an overlying nodular thyroid gland. Lymph nodes, blood vessels, and a collapsed esophagus can be mistaken for parathyroid glands.[9] Previous neck surgery is associated with poorer parathyroid gland detection rates.[2,10-12] US has been reported as less sensitive in this setting due to anatomic distortion and changes in the vasculature resulting from surgery. However, when US is performed by an experienced ultrasonographer with attention paid to potential ectopic cervical sites of parathyroid tissue, the accuracy of US is similar to its use in the unoperated neck.[10]

Trachea and Esophagus

The trachea is located in the midline of the neck and as such serves as a useful reference point for transverse ultrasound images. The trachea is deep to the thyroid gland and is crescent shaped on imaging due to incomplete tracheal cartilage rings posteriorly. The cricoid cartilage, which forms a complete ring, marks the superior limit of the trachea and is thicker vertically than the tracheal rings below. The first six tracheal rings can be imaged when the neck is in mild extension (Fig 4–8 and see Fig 4–4).

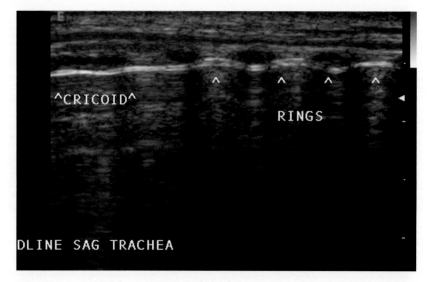

Fig 4–8. A midline superficial sagittal plane will reveal the upper tracheal cartilaginous rings and the cricoid cartilage more superiorly.

Between the trachea and the skin lie subcutaneous fat, the strap muscles (consisting of the sternohyoid, sternothyroid, and omohyoid muscles), and the isthmus of the thyroid gland. The strap muscles cover the trachea and the isthmus of the thyroid gland, which is located over the second or third tracheal rings in the midline. The strap muscles appear hypoechoic, and are encased by the thin, hyperechoic lines of the investing cervical fascia. The isthmus of the thyroid is more hyperechoic than muscle on US, in contrast to the trachea which has an anechoic or black interior and posterior shadowing (Fig 4–9). A high-riding innominate artery may be identified above the sternal notch as a transverse anechoic structure crossing the trachea, with a vascular origin confirmed with color Doppler, as well as by continuity with the right common carotid artery (Fig 4–10 and Video 4E).

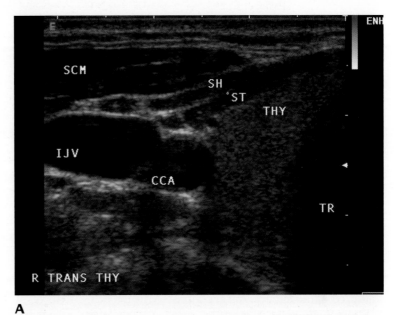

Fig 4–9. The sternohyoid (*SH*) and sternothyroid (*ST*) (strap) muscles and the sternocleidomastoid (*SCM*) muscle are easily recognized adjacent to the thyroid gland (*THY*) in the anterior and anterolateral neck. TR = trachea, CCA = common carotid artery, IJV = internal jugular vein, SUBQ = subcutaneous tissue. **A.** Transverse plane; **B.** Sagittal plane.

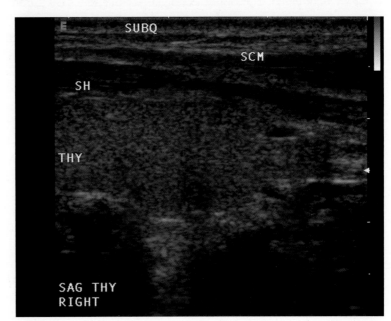

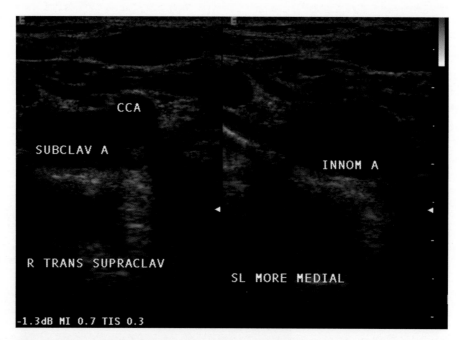

Fig 4–10 and Video 4E. The right subclavian artery can be traced to its junction with the right carotid artery at the innominate artery, a transverse anechoic structure crossing the trachea above the sternal notch. Its vascular origin is confirmed with color Doppler. The transverse cervical artery also runs across the surface of the scalene muscles in the supraclavicular region (**Video 4E**).

The cervical esophagus is located posteriorly and to the left of the trachea, and in contrast to the trachea, is highly echogenic. The bright echogenicity of the concentric esophageal mucosa results in a classic "bulls eye" target sign on transverse images that aids in identification. The esophagus can be seen to compress and expand with swallowing, which is a useful adjunct to accurate identification but can also confound the inexperienced examiner. With the patient's head turned to the left, the esophagus may also be seen posterior and to the right of the trachea (Fig 4–11 and Video 4F; also see Fig 4–5).

Salivary Glands

Submandibular Gland

The submandibular gland is located in the submandibular triangle, or level I of the neck, bounded by the anterior and posterior bellies of the digastric muscle anteriorly and posteriorly, by the hyoid inferiorly, by the body of the mandible superiorly, and by the mylohyoid and hyoglossus muscles medially. The submandibular gland is sometimes artificially divided into superficial and deep lobes, separated by the mylohyoid muscle with the deep lobe representing a projection of submandibular tissue superomedial to the muscle.[13] The sublingual space, containing the sublingual salivary gland, is deep to the mylohyoid, whereas the submental space, which contains lymph nodes and fat, is superficial to the mylohyoid and is bounded posteriorly by the anterior belly of the digastric muscle.

The submandibular space contains submandibular and submental lymph nodes which may be associated with the submandibular gland, but unlike the parotid gland, the submandibular glands do not contain lymph nodes within the gland parenchyma. Adipose tissue is present to a variable degree within the submandibular space. The inferior loop of the hypoglossal nerve is located inferior and deep to the submandibular gland, whereas the facial artery

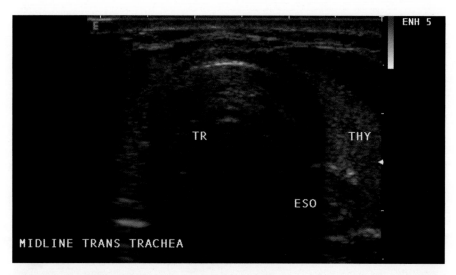

Fig 4–11 and Video 4F. Cervical esophagus in transverse view at rest and during swallowing (**Video 4F**).

courses deep to the anterior and superior portion of the gland before crossing the body of the mandible.[14] The anterior and posterior (or retromandibular) facial veins are superficial to the gland; the posterior facial vein distinguishes submandibular gland tissue (anterior to the vein) from parotid tissue which lies posterior to the vein.

US is the initial method of choice for imaging the submandibular glands, but evaluation of the deep lobe of the submandibular gland and the distal submandibular duct (Wharton's duct) is limited by the proximity of the mandible because of the inability of ultrasound to penetrate bone.[15,16] The patient is imaged with the neck extended and the head turned away from the side being examined. High-frequency linear transducers in the range of 7 to 12 MHz provide optimal visualization. Color-flow Doppler imaging assists in differentiating vascular structures from ductal structures. The hypoglossal nerve is difficult to image sonographically. Scanning should be performed in both the transverse and longitudinal planes progressing from superficial to deep structures using known landmarks for guidance. The overlying skin is often separated from the subcutaneous fat by a thin hyperechoic line. Subcutaneous fat appears hypoechoic. The thin platysma muscle lies immediately beneath the subcutaneous fat and, typical of muscle, is hypoechoic. Thin, hyperechoic lines representing the cervical fascia invest the cervical muscles and aid in distinguishing these from other structures.

The submandibular gland is homogeneous and hyperechoic relative to the adjacent muscles,[17] while being similar in echogenicity to the thyroid gland parenchyma (Figs 4-12A and 4-12B and Video 4G). The normal gland is notably homogeneous, even when enlarged due to benign hypertrophy; any deviation such as mixed echogenicity with solid (hyperechoic) or cystic (anechoic or hypoechoic) areas suggests pathology.[18] Wharton's duct arises from the deep aspect of the gland and may be easily visualized when dilated and appears as a hypoechoic structure. A normal duct is more difficult to visualize and is best seen on transverse images as a small linear, hypoechoic structure located between the mylohyoid and hyoglossus muscles[17] (Fig 4-13). Vascular structures are anechoic. The lingual vein courses parallel to the submandibular duct and can be differentiated by color-flow Doppler. Calculi, when present, appear as bright hyperechoic echogenic foci with posterior shadowing.[13] Distal stones in the floor of mouth are not imaged well by US. Normal sublingual gland visualization is similarly somewhat limited, but sublingual gland pathology can often be identified as asymmetry, presence of a mass, or abnormal hypoechogenicity (Fig 4-14). For additional examples of salivary gland pathology, the reader is referred to Chapter 7.

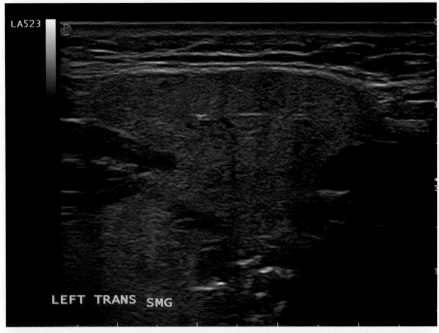

A

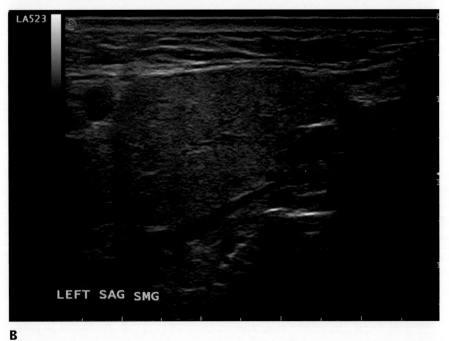

B

Fig 4–12 and Video 4G. The submandibular gland (*SMG*) is normally homogeneous and similar in echogenicity to the thyroid. Transverse (**A**) and sagittal (**B**) views, and ascending video (**Video 4G**) reveal the characteristic triangular or teardrop shape of the SMG.

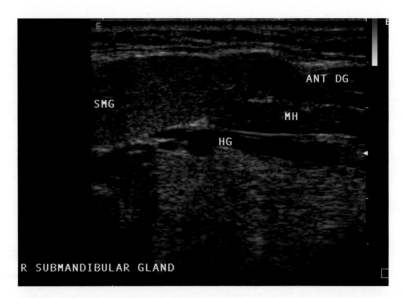

Fig 4–13. The submandibular (Wharton's) duct is not normally visible but it courses between the mylohyoid (*MH*) and hyoglossus (*HG*) muscles. DG = digastric muscle, anterior belly shown here; SMG = submandibular gland.

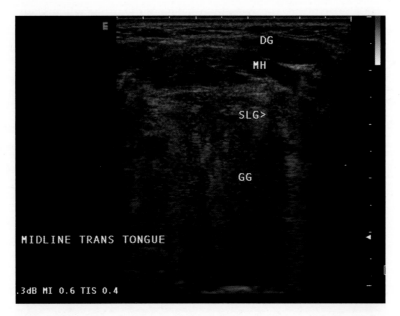

Fig 4–14. The sublingual gland (*SLG*) can sometimes be seen through the floor of the mouth, between the mylohyoid (*MH*) muscle and the tongue body. GG = genioglossus, DG = digastric. The SLG can also be seen as an extension of the SMG within the floor of the mouth on the oral side of the mylohyoid (Fig 4–12A).

Parotid

The parotid gland lies within the parotid space, a construct used mainly in radiology, which also contains the facial nerve, the retromandibular vein, the external carotid artery, and lymph nodes. The boundaries of the parotid space are the external auditory canal superiorly, the posterior belly of the digastric muscle inferiorly, and the mandible and medial pterygoid muscle medially. The buccinator and masseter muscles mark the anterior border of the parotid space. The posterior belly of the digastric muscle separates the parotid space from the carotid space inferiorly.[19] Similar to the submandibular gland, the parotid is artificially separated into deep and superficial lobes divided by the course of the facial nerve. Unlike the submandibular gland, the parotid gland contains lymph nodes within its parenchyma as well as having lymph nodes associated with the gland externally. The superficial location of the parotid makes all but the deepest portions of the gland easily accessible to ultrasound imaging.

As with the submandibular gland, the parotid gland is best imaged by having the patient turn their head away from the side being examined. Progressing from superficial to deep, the parotid gland lies beneath the skin, subcutaneous fat, and superficial musculoaponeurotic layer; fascial layers appear as hyperechoic lines and fat is hypoechoic (Fig 4–15A and 4–15B and Videos 4H and 4I). The masseter muscle lies anterior to the parotid gland and is hypoechoic. This muscle is also easily recognized by asking the patient to chew while observing contraction by US. Masseter asymmetry may be present between sides secondary to unilateral hypertrophy and is a normal variant.[20] The gland is homogeneous and relatively hyperechoic on US, similar to the submandibular gland. Fatty infiltration may result in diffuse increased echogenicity. Areas of decreased echogenicity within the gland are indicative of abnormal pathology.[21] The facial nerve is not visualized by sonography; however, the retromandibular vein lies parallel to and at the same depth as the facial nerve and can be used as a landmark to distinguish between superficial and deep lobe parotid tissue. The use of color Doppler and changing the angle of the probe when scanning in the longitudinal plane facilitates identification of the vein (Fig 4–16).

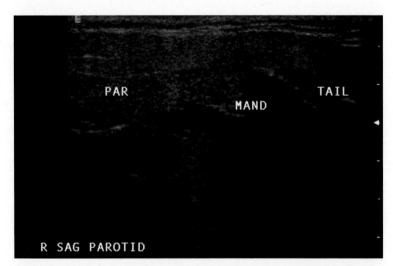

Fig 4–15 and Videos 4H and 4I. Right sagittal parotid (PAR), with its tail wrapping around the mandibular angle (MANO) inferiorly. **Video 4H** shows the parotid in sagittal plane moving from posterior to anterior, followed by masseter contraction due to chewing. A small intraparotid lymph node is noted. **Video 4I** shows the left masseter muscle (*to the left side of the screen*) and the parotid (*to the right*) in transverse plane.

Stenson's duct may be visualized within the superficial lobe of the gland, approximately 1 fingerbreadth below the zygomatic arch as thin echogenic lines, but is difficult to visualize beyond the gland parenchyma (Fig 4-17).[19] Normal lymph nodes are more abundant in the superficial lobe but are also present

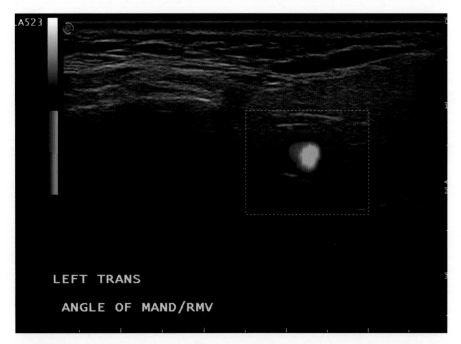

Fig 4–16. The retromandibular vein (*RMV*) is a well-recognized landmark for the plane of the facial nerve, which itself is not seen on US.

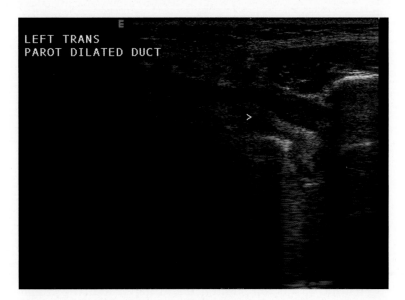

Fig 4–17. The normal parotid (Stenson's) duct is not usually seen but in this case of chronic sialadenitis, the duct was dilated and visible.

in the deep lobe and appear as small (<5 mm) oval structures with an outer hypoechoic cortex and an echogenic hilum representing the lymphatic sinuses (Figs 4-18A and 4-18B). The deep lobe of the parotid gland is difficult to image as deep lobe tissue extends through the stylomandibular ligament to lie medial to the mandible, which interferes with sonographic imaging.

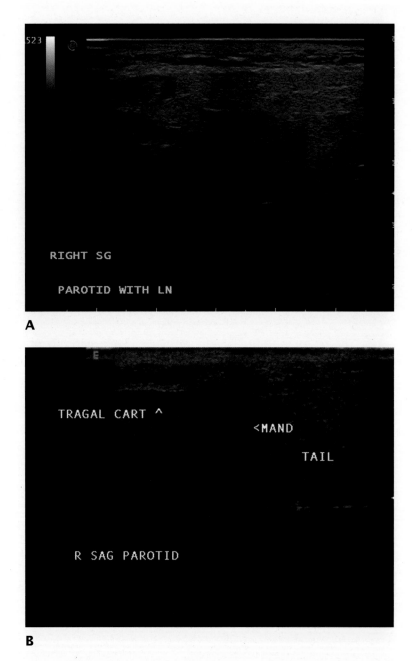

Fig 4-18. Benign lymph nodes (**A**) are frequently seen within the parotid gland (on sagittal plane here), and the tragal cartilage (**B**) appears as a hyperechoic line at the most posterior aspect of the gland.

Parapharyngeal Space

The parapharyngeal space (PPS) is a potential space lateral to the upper pharynx, shaped like an inverted pyramid extending from the skull base superiorly to the greater cornu of the hyoid bone inferiorly. The superior border of the PPS comprises a small area of the temporal and sphenoid bones, including the carotid canal, the jugular foramen, and the hypoglossal foramen. Anteriorly, the PPS is limited by the pterygomandibular raphe and pterygoid fascia, and posteriorly by the cervical vertebrae and prevertebral muscles. The medial border of the PPS is the pharynx and the lateral border is composed of the ramus of the mandible, the medial pterygoid muscle, and the deep lobe of the parotid gland. Below the level of the mandible, the lateral boundary consists of the fascia overlying the posterior belly of the digastric muscle.

The fascia from the styloid process to the tensor veli palatini divides the PPS into an anterolateral compartment, termed prestyloid, and a posterolateral, or poststyloid, compartment. The prestyloid compartment contains the retromandibular portion of the deep lobe of the parotid gland, adipose tissue, and lymph nodes associated with the parotid gland. The poststyloid compartment contains the internal carotid artery, the internal jugular vein, cranial nerves IX through XII, the sympathetic chain, and lymph nodes. These compartments are helpful in formulating differential diagnoses of masses, based on potential structures of origin within their spaces.

Transcervical or transcutaneous ultrasound imaging of the PPS is limited by its bony borders, which cannot be penetrated adequately with current ultrasonic technology. A recent development is the advent of small 10-MHz high-frequency linear transducers which allow transoral ultrasound imaging of the PPS, as well as the deep lobe of the parotid gland and the retropharyngeal space.[22] The probe is placed over the lateral pharyngeal wall, and thus the PPS is imaged through the pharynx. The pharyngeal mucosa is highly echogenic; just posterior to the mucosa lie the great vessels, cranial nerves, and lymph nodes, whereas slightly anterior and laterally the deep lobe of the parotid, fat, and lymph nodes may be visualized. Imaging is limited by the small space in which to work, as well as by patient tolerance of the procedure including the gag reflex, which limit the extent to which the probe can be angled.

Cervical Lymph Nodes

It has been estimated that there are 300 lymph nodes in the cervical region.[23] The cervical lymphatics extend from the level of the skull base to the clavicle and are divided into six nodal levels by clinicians[23,24] (Fig 4–19). Describing lymph nodes imaged by nodal level not only provides anatomic information but also has clinical and prognostic significance, as different pathology affects different nodal levels based on known patterns of lymphatic drainage.[25]

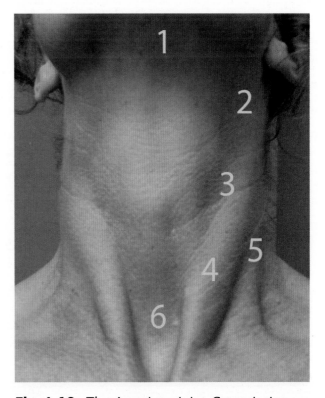

Fig 4–19. The American Joint Commission on Cancer (AJCC) classification system for cervical lymph node levels is depicted here.

Level I includes the submandibular and submental nodes, and is further subdivided into IA and IB to differentiate between these. The submental nodes (IA) occupy the space between the anterior midline and the anterior bellies of the right and left digastric muscles, bounded by the mandible superiorly and the hyoid bone inferiorly. The submandibular nodes (IB) are bounded by the anterior and posterior bellies of the digastric muscle anteriorly and posteriorly, respectively, with the hyoid bone defining the inferior limit and the body of the mandible defining the superior limit. The hyoglossus and mylohyoid muscles define the deep or medial limit of level I. Facial nodes that are closely associated with the facial artery as it courses over the body of the mandible drain into the submandibular nodes and are commonly included in level I.

The sternocleidomastoid muscle separates levels II to IV from level V. Levels II to IV nodes are deep to the sternocleidomastoid muscle and occupy the anterior triangle of the neck, posterior to the posterior belly of the digastric muscle. The anatomic landmark that separates levels II from III is the hyoid bone, whereas the omohyoid muscle and cricoid cartilage are both used as landmarks to delineate between level III superiorly and level IV inferiorly, which extends to the level of the clavicle. Level II is further

subdivided into IIA and IIB based on the relationship of the nodes to the internal jugular vein and spinal accessory nerve: level IIB is posterior to the internal jugular vein and superior to the XI nerve, although this subdivision is rarely made on US examinations as the XI nerve is not sonographically visible. Level V, also termed the posterior triangle, encompasses all nodal tissue between the posterior border of the sternocleidomastoid anteriorly and the trapezius muscle posteriorly. The deep limit of levels II to IV are the scalene muscles, whereas the splenius capitus and levator scapulae mark the deep limit of level V. The deep layer of the deep cervical fascia enveloping these deep neck muscles serves as the floor of the cervical lymphatics. Level VI includes all midline nodes between the hyoid superiorly and the manubrium or the innominate artery inferiorly, and between the common carotid arteries laterally.

Normal lymph nodes are oval shaped and have a central fatty hilum, through which blood vessels and efferent lymphatic drainage passes, surrounded by germinal centers which drain into sinuses that converge to form the efferent lymphatic vessels at the hilum. On US, the echogenic hilum is visualized as a hyperechoic linear structure passing directly into the lymph node, whose outer cortex is hypoechoic[24] (Fig 4-20). In most lymph nodes, the longi-

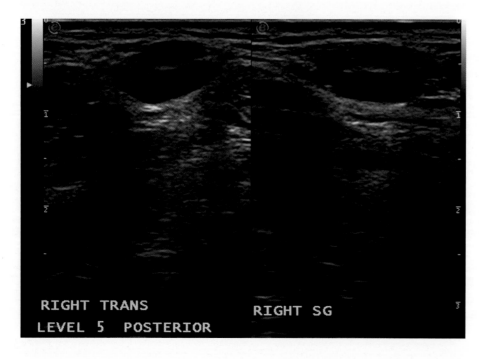

Fig 4-20. Benign lymph node with visible hilum.

tudinal axis is greater than the transverse axis with the exception of level I nodes, which usually have a larger axial diameter[24] (Fig 4–21 and Video 4J). The majority of benign lymph nodes are 5 mm or less in maximum diameter. Size criteria for normal versus pathologic lymph nodes vary in the literature, with

Fig 4–21 and Video 4J. Benign ovoid level 2 (**A**) and more rounded level 1 (**B**) lymph nodes. SMG = submandibular gland. **Video 4J** shows several benign lymph nodes in the left levels 4 through 2 as the transducer ascends. Note bean-shaped lymph node at the level of the carotid bifurcation.

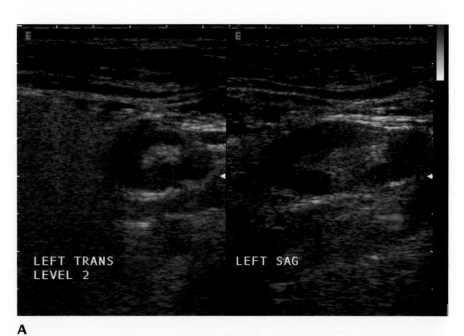

A

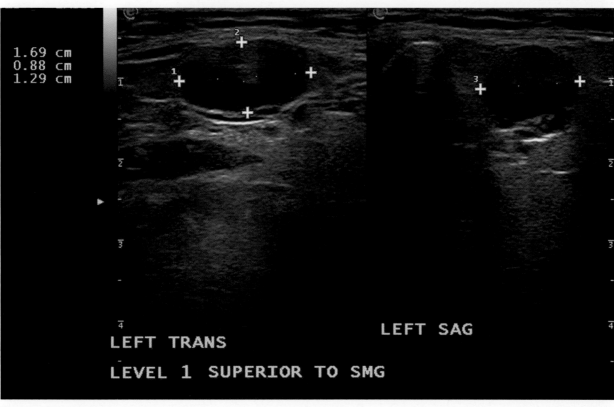

B

1 cm most commonly used as the starting point for suspicion of malignancy based on size: however, when a primary head and neck malignancy is known to be present, nodes >6 mm are considered suspicious.[23,25] Benign reactive lymph nodes undergo hyperplasia of the germinal center and pulp along with histiocytosis of the marginal sinus.[26] The normal architecture is not destroyed, and therefore an echogenic hilum and an outer hypoechoic cortex should still be visible (Fig 4–22). However, inflammatory nodes may have hyperemia and areas of echogenicity due to coagulation necrosis which can make them difficult to distinguish from metastatic lymph nodes harboring cancer.[27]

US of the cervical lymphatics is performed with a high-frequency linear transducer in the range of 7 to 12 MHz: as with the parathyroid glands, the higher the frequency, the greater the resolution of small lymph nodes. The neck should be scanned in a systematic fashion beginning in the transverse plane, followed by imaging in the longitudinal plane. The sequence is less important than the consistency and thoroughness of the examination. If the submental region is evaluated first, with the patient's head in the midline with chin and neck extended, then the patient's head is turned away from the side of the neck being imaged to allow assessment of the submandibular triangle (level I) and subsequently the anterior triangle of the neck (levels II–IV), proceeding in a sweeping motion from superior to inferior.[27] The sternocleidomastoid is easily visualized because of its large size, superficial location, and elongated shape; it has a solid hypoechoic ultrasound pattern characteristic of muscle and the medial boundary of the muscle separating this from the lymphatics is identifiable as a dense hyperechogenic line representing the investing deep cervical fascia[10] (Fig 4–23 and Videos 4K and 4L). The carotid artery and jugular vein, which is distinguished by compression, are important landmarks. In the postoperative neck, the jugular vein may be absent or thrombosed. The anterior cervical chain (levels II–IV) lymph nodes are medial to the carotid artery and superficial and adjacent to the juglar vein, but when

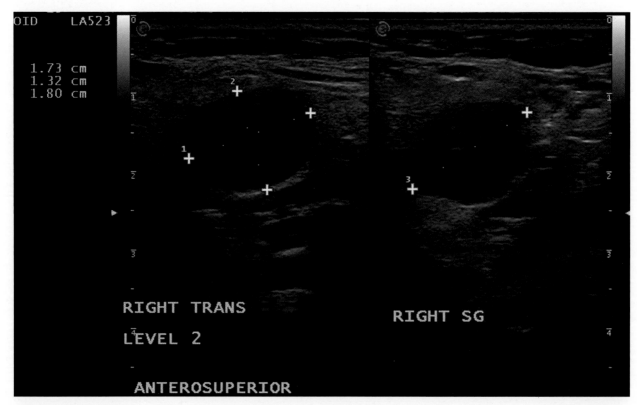

Fig 4–22. A benign reactive lymph node that shares features with malignant nodes including round shape, absent hilum, hypoechogenicity, and enlargement.

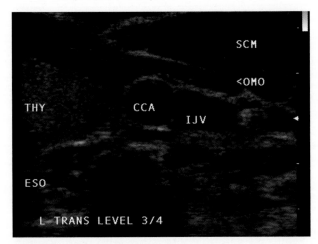

Fig 4–23 and Videos 4K and 4L. The carotid artery (*CCA*) and internal jugular vein (*IJV*) are seen deep to the sternocleido-mastoid (*SCM*) and omohyoid (*OMO*) muscles. ESO = esophagus, THY = thyroid. **Video 4K** demonstrates the carotid artery first in the transverse plane and then rotating the transducer 90 degrees to view the sagittal plane. Video 4L shows how compressible (with gentle transducer pressure) and distensible (with Valsalva maneuver) the internal jugular vein is.

involved with pathology often extend posterior to the vessels.

Changing the angle of the probe to obtain sagittal images is useful in imaging the longitudinal length of identified lymph nodes and distinguishing these from vascular structures and the overlying sternocleidomastoid and omohyoid muscles (Fig 4-24). The vagus nerve may sometimes be identified as a thin hypoechoic line coursing parallel to the carotid artery. Ultrasound identification of the spinal accessory nerve is poor. Level V is scanned by beginning at the mastoid tip and scanning along a line extending from the mastoid process to the acromion.[27] Finally, level VI is scanned beginning at the hyoid bone and proceeding inferiorly, starting in the midline and moving from side to side. Normal pretracheal and paratracheal lymph nodes may be obscured by air from the adjacent trachea,[27] as well as by the thyroid gland itself. Examinaton of level VI is facilated by having the patient extend their neck as much as tolerated and turning their head away from the side being examined.

Normal retropharyngeal nodes cannot be assessed by ultrasound, although enlarged lymph

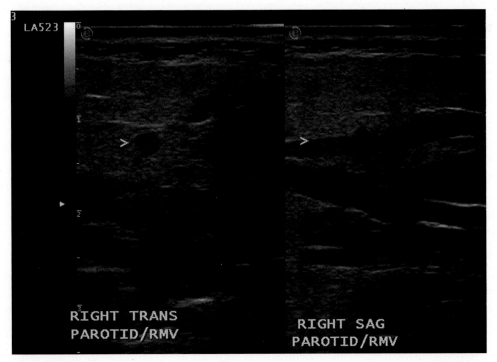

Fig 4–24. Examining structures in two perpendicular planes (such as this retromandibular vein, *RMV*) distinguishes nodular structures from tubular ones.

nodes larger than 1.5 cm have been imaged transcutaneously using 3.5-MHz probes placed behind the angle of the mandible, while the patient protrudes the mandible anteriorly.[28] Transoral US is a newer means of assessing pathologic retropharyngeal nodes[12]; further experience with this technique is needed.

The Carotid Sheath

The contents of the carotid sheath include the carotid artery, the internal jugular vein, lymph nodes, the vagus nerve, and the sympathetic chain which bifurcates at the carotid bulb to become the external carotid artery medially and the internal carotid artery laterally and posteriorly. The internal carotid does not have any extracranial branches, in contrast to the external carotid artery. The vagus nerve lies medial to the carotid, whereas the sympathetic chain is deep. As mentioned previously, the vagus nerve may sometimes be identified as a thin hypoechoic line coursing parallel to the carotid artery on longitudinal images or a punctate dot on transverse images between the carotid artery and jugular vein. The sympathetic chain is difficult to image sonographically.

The carotid sheath is best examined with the patient's neck in mild extension and the head turned away from the side being examined. On transverse US, the carotid artery is round and anechoic with posterior enhancement secondary to wall thickness, and pulsations may be seen (Fig 4–25 and Video 4M). The internal jugular vein is anechoic and compressible, located lateral and anterior to the carotid artery. The relative position of the internal jugular vein to the carotid artery varies with head position. The greater the extent of head rotation away from the side of the neck being examined, the greater the degree of overlap of the carotid artery by the internal jugular vein (Video 4N). With the head in the midline position, there is 1 cm of distance between the vessels, whereas this distance decreases to 1 mm with the head rotated away from the neck by 90 degrees.[29]

Color-flow Doppler imaging is the sonographic equivalent of intravenous contrast in computed to-

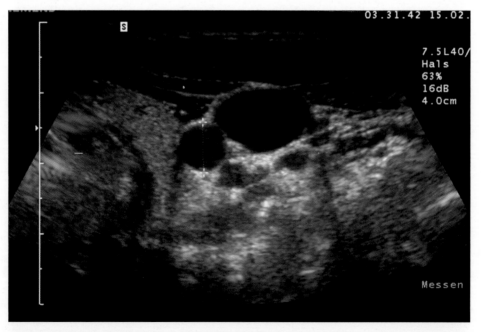

Fig 4–25 and Video 4M. The carotid artery in transverse view is characteristically round, with a bright wall and an anechoic lumen along with posterior enhancement.

mography or magnetic resonance imaging. It allows delineation of vessels and tissue characterization not possible with the use of gray-scale sonography alone and is invaluable in evaluating the contents of the carotid sheath. Normal carotid flow on color Doppler imaging is characteristically brisk, accelerates during systole, and reverses during diastole. At the level of the carotid bulb, flow becomes turbulent with disruption of normal laminar flow because of the abrupt vessel widening at this point.[30] In contrast, color Doppler applied to the jugular vein shows a low-flow venous pattern which is not biphasic (Video 40 and see Chapter 13).

Severe carotid stenosis is associated with a reduction in the color Doppler flow signal. Carotid occlusion can be diagnosed by the absence of pulsations and color Doppler flow and the presence of echogenic material filling the lumen.[31] Carotid plaques may be identified by US and may be hypo- or hyperechoic. Solid plaques are fibrous and contain abundant collagen, and are hyperechoic on imaging. These are believed to be less thrombogenic than soft hypoechoic or echolucent plaques which are rich in lipids, contain little collagen, and are less stable, prone to intraplaque hemorrhage and embolism[32] (see Chapter 13). Previous irradiation to the head and neck produces a significant and accelerated increase in the intima-media thickness of the carotid artery wall with concomitant luminal narrowing.[32,33] However, measurement of the intima-media thickness by US does not distinguish between intimal atherosclerosis and medial hypertrophy.[32] No difference has been found in the incidence of atherosclerotic plaques between irradiated and unirradiated patients, suggesting that carotid injury from radiation causes intimal-medial thickening with a reduction in the carotid artery lumen but not intimal atherosclerosis.[32] Identification of plaque ulcerations is poor with B-mode US.[30]

Lack of compressibility of the internal jugular vein suggests thrombosis. The thrombus appears echogenic on US with absence of flow on color Doppler images and may be mistaken for a lymph node[30] (Fig 4–26). Slow venous flow may sometimes cause internal echoes and be mistaken for a thrombus. The use of color Doppler or a Valsalva maneuver can differentiate between this normal condition and thrombosis.[30]

Larynx and Hypopharynx

The larynx is a midline structure located between the hyoid bone superiorly and the trachea inferiorly. The thyrohyoid ligament suspends the larynx from the hyoid bone. The laryngeal skeleton, consisting of the thyroid and cricoid cartilages, undergoes ossification with advancing age. Covering the laryngeal framework anteriorly are the sternohyoid and omohyoid muscles; deep to these are the extrinsic laryngeal muscles that attach directly to the laryngeal cartilage (the sternothyroid and posterolaterally the inferior pharyngeal constrictor, plus the cricothyroid muscles).

The interior of the larynx contains the epiglottis, aryepiglottic folds, the true and false vocal folds (or cords), and the arytenoid cartilages. The laryngeal vestibule is the recess formed between the epiglottis, aryepiglottic folds, and false vocal folds, whereas the ventricle is a recess between the true and false vocal folds that projects laterally into the laryngeal saccule. The arytenoid cartilages support the true vocal folds posteriorly and articulate with the posterior aspect of the cricoid cartilage. The vocal ligaments of the true vocal folds attach to the inner thyroid lamina anteriorly in the midline; this attachment is termed Broyle's ligament. The epiglottis is contiguous with the false vocal folds in the midline superiorly at the petiole and projects superiorly, above the laryngeal cartilage. It is attached to the thyroid cartilage by the thyroepiglottic ligament and to the hyoid bone superiorly by the hyoepiglottic ligament. The pre-epiglottic space is anterior to the epiglottis and is contained by the thyroid cartilage and hyoid bone anteriorly, the thyroepiglottic ligament inferiorly, and the hyoepiglottic ligament superiorly. This space is largely composed of fat and is contiguous laterally and inferiorly with the paraglottic space, lateral to the vocal folds. The paraglottic space is bounded laterally by the thyroid cartilage and inferiorly by the vocalis and cricoarytenoid muscles and similarly contains abundant loose areolar tissue as well as the projection of the laryngeal saccule.

Ossification of the laryngeal skeleton results in differing acoustic impedances which can confound imaging.[34] The echogenic laryngeal mucosa contrasts with the anechoic intraluminal air column forming

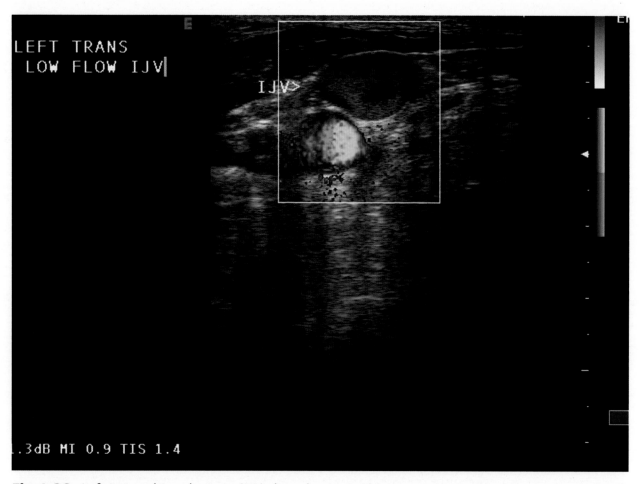

Fig 4–26. Left internal jugular vein (*IJV*) thrombosis, in this case associated with metastatic papillary thyroid carcinoma.

a mucosa-air column interface which facilitates identification of the internal laryngeal structures and allows differentiation between the mucosal surfaces and the hypoechoic internal laryngeal musculature. Ossification of the thyroid cartilage results in a bright echogenic signal that limits visualization of internal laryngeal structures. However, this limitation can be circumvented by scanning the vocal folds through the cricothyroid membrane.[35] The arytenoid cartilages are identified, and by angling the probe superiorly, the entire endolarynx can be visualized, including the vocal folds and anterior commissure (Fig 4–27). Similar to the laryngeal framework cartilages, the arytenoid cartilages are echogenic, whereas the vocalis muscles have a homogeneous, hypoechoic appearance. The false vocal folds overlie the echogenic fat of the paraglottic space, in contrast to the true vocal folds which overlie the thin hypoechoic vocalis muscle. The patient's head may be turned to either side to improve visualization of the ipsilateral vocal fold. The epiglottis and pre-epiglottic space can be visualized through the thyrohyoid membrane: the pre-epiglottic fat is echogenic, whereas the epiglottic cartilage is sonolucent (Fig 4–28). Chapter 9 addresses laryngeal ultrasonography and pathology in greater detail.

The hypopharynx extends from the level of the hyoid to the inferior margin of the cricoid cartilage and includes the postcricoid region and the posterior and lateral pharyngeal walls which merge with the piriform sinus on either side. Sonographic evaluation of the hypopharynx is limited because of the overlying laryngeal structures and the fact that this area is usually effaced when the patient is supine.

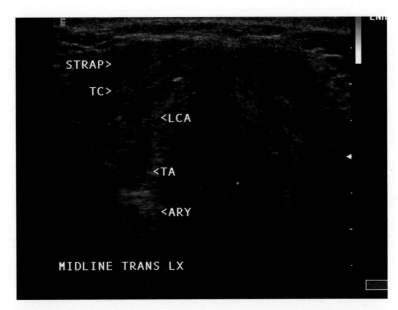

Fig 4–27. In quiet respiration, the hypoechoic lateral crico-arytenoid (*LCA*) and thyroarytenoid (*TA*) muscles can be seen inside the thyroid cartilage (*TC*) of the larynx (*LX*) and extending anteriorly from the arytenoid cartilages (*ARY*).

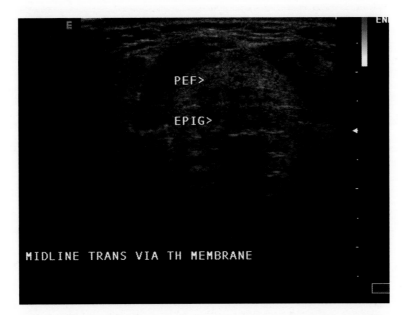

Fig 4–28. The hyperechoic pre-epiglottic fat (*PEF*) and the hypoechoic epiglottis (*EPIG*) are seen with the transducer applied and angled at the thyrohyoid membrane (*THM*).

US can be useful in imaging pharyngeal musculature movement during swallowing by indirectly measuring the extent of displacement of echogenic overly- ing pharyngeal mucosa and laryngeal elevation (see Chapter 14), but yields limited anatomic informa-tion (Video 4P).[36,37]

Tongue, Floor of Mouth, and Oropharynx

The tongue is composed of both extrinsic and intrinsic musculature. The extrinsic muscles of the tongue are the genioglossus, hyoglossus, and styloglossus. The intrinsic muscles of the tongue (the inferior lingual, vertical, and transverse muscles) consist of bundles of interlacing fibers with dense connective tissue septa which are avascular in the midline. The lingual mucosa covering the mobile tongue is continuous with the mucosa of the floor of mouth. Underlying this is the muscular support of the floor of mouth which is formed by the genioglossus in the midline where this muscle attaches to the genial tubercle of the mandible, and the geniohyoid and mylohyoid muscles laterally.

Ultrasound imaging of the tongue and floor of mouth is performed through the submental space with the patient's head positioned in the midline and the chin extended, sweeping from the mandible superiorly to hyoid bone inferiorly with the probe angled superiorly toward the vertex of the scalp. Useful landmarks are the lingual septum for transverse imaging and the geniohyoid muscle medially and mylohyoid laterally on sagittal images[38] (Figs 4-29A, 4-29B, and 4-29C). The tongue musculature is dense and hypoechoic with a hyperechoic midline septum. The floor of mouth musculature can be demonstrated as hypoechogenic structures surrounded by thin hyperechoic bands of investing fascia, and the anatomy is best demonstrated on transverse images. The overlying mucosa is highly echogenic. The sublingual salivary glands are sometimes visible at the lateral and superficial aspect of the ventral tongue as seen from the submental perspective (see Figs 4-12 and 4-14). Evaluation of the floor of mouth mucosa and the surface of the tongue may be limited by sonographic artifacts caused by impedance

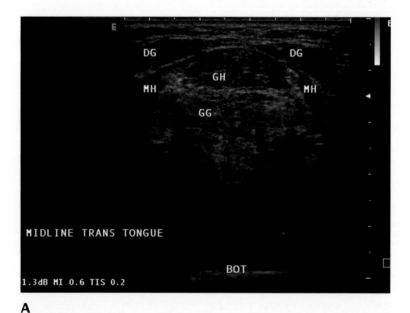

A

Fig 4–29. A. The structures of the tongue and floor of mouth are clearly identified via a submental approach. GH = geniohyoid, GG = genioglossus, MH = mylohyoid, DG = digastric (anterior belly here), BOT = base of tongue. The same approach using a larger and lower frequency curvilinear transducer can achieve greater sound penetration and greater resolution of the deep aspects of the tongue in both transverse (**B**) and sagittal (**C**) views. MAND = mandible, HY = hyoid. *continues*

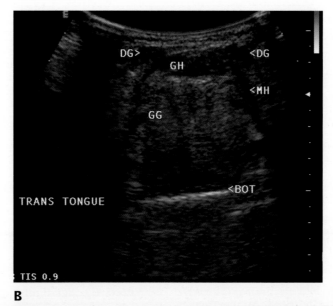

B

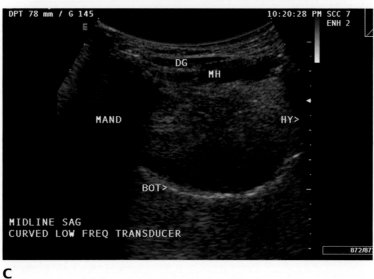

C

Fig 4–29. *continued*

differences between saliva and mucosa, and air bubbles may result in recurrent acoustical signals or ring artifact.[39]

The oropharynx consists of the soft palate and lateral palatine arches, the palatine tonsils, lingual tonsils, tongue base, and oropharynx wall. The tongue base musculature can be visualized by angling a probe positioned above the hyoid toward the occiput, and asking the patient to protrude the tongue (Figure 4–30 and Video 4Q). Real-time US examination obviously enhances dynamic assessment and image interpretation. The lingual tonsils

consist of nonencapsulated lymphoid tissue, with hypoechoic regions corresponding to germinal centers and prominent hyperechoic areas corresponding to areas of fat and sinuses that demonstrate marked variation in size. Sonographic evaluation of the tongue base and lingual tonsils may be limited in obese patients because of the need to use a lower frequency probe with a corresponding decrease in resolution.

Transcutaneous ultrasound imaging of the tonsils and lateral pharyngeal walls is subject to the same limitations as imaging of the PPS and is limited

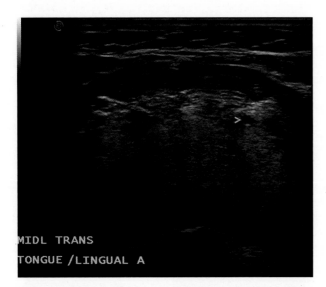

Fig 4–30 and Video 4Q. Midline transverse view of the tongue clearly reveals the lingual arteries (*carat*) along with the soft tissues. **Video 4Q** shows transverse rotating to sagittal views of tongue movement with good symmetry.

by the bone of the mandible, which cannot be penetrated adequately. Transoral small 10-MHz high-frequency linear transducers may facilitate imaging of the lateral pharyngeal walls and tonsils in the future.[12]

Summary

US is a useful diagnostic tool in the evaluation of head and neck anatomy. Technologic advances in ultrasound imaging capabilities have led to dramatically increased interest in and utilization of this technology so that ultrasound has an increasingly important role in the clinician's armamentarium. Acquiring familiarity and skill with this technology is necessary for the clinician wishing to stay abreast of modern imaging techniques and incorporate ultrasound imaging into his or her practice. Familiarity with the normal sonographic anatomy of the head and neck is the foundation on which performing diagnostic head and neck ultrasonography can be built.

Videos in This Chapter

Videos 4A–4M. See figure legends.

Video 4N. The left internal jugular vein position changes in relation to the left carotid artery as the patient's head is turned from left to right in this example.

Video 4O. Color Doppler at the level of the carotid bulb shows biphasic pulsation with turbulence.

Video 4P. During swallowing the esophagus can be seen to move in continuity with the bulging piriform sinus.

Video 4Q. See figure legends.

References

1. Akbar NA, Bodenner DL, Kim LT, Suen JY, Kokoska MS. Considerations in incorporating office-based ultrasound of the head and neck. *Otolaryngol Head Neck Surg.* 2006;135:884–888.
2. Khati N, Adamson T, Johnson KS, Hill MC. Ultrasound of the thyroid and parathyroid glands. *Ultrasound Q.* 2003;19:162–176.
3. Wong KT, Ahuja AT. Ultrasound of thyroid cancer. *Cancer Imaging.* 2005;5:167–176.
4. McCaffrey TV. Evaluation of the thyroid nodule. *Cancer Control.* 2000;7:223–228.
5. Onishi H, Sato H, Noda H, Inomata H, Sasaki N. Color Doppler ultrasonography: diagnosis of ectopic thyroid gland in patients with congenital hypothyroidism caused by thyroid dysgenesis. *J Clin Endocrinol Metab.* 2003;88:5145–5149.
6. Rice DH. Surgery of the parathyroid glands. *Otolaryngol Clin North Am.* 1996;29:693–699.
7. Shen W, Duren M, Morita E, et al. Reoperation for persistent or recurrent primary hyperparathyroidism. *Arch Surgery.* 1996,131:861–869.
8. Shaha AR, Jaffe BM. Parathyroid preservation during thyroid surgery. *Am J Otolaryngol.* 1998;19:113–117.
9. Meilstrup JW. Ultrasound examination of the parathyroid glands. *Otolaryngol Clin North Am.* 2004;37:763–778.

10. Ghaheri BA, Koslin B, Wood AH, Cohen JI. Preoperative ultrasound is worthwhile for reoperative parathyroid surgery. *Laryngoscope*. 2004;114: 2168–2171.

11. Feingold DL, Alexander HR, Chen CC, et al. Ultrasound and sestamibi scan as the only preoperative imaging tests in reoperation for parathyroid adenomas. *Surgery*. 2000;128:1103–1110.

12. Rotstein L, Irish J, Gullane P, Keller MA, Sniderman K. Reoperative parathyroidectomy in the era of localization technology. *Head Neck*. 1998;20: 535–539.

13. Howlett DC, Alyas F, Wong KT, et al. Sonographic assessment of the submandibular space. *Clin Radiol*. 2004; 59:1070–1078.

14. Evans RM. Anatomy and technique. In: Ahuja A, Evans R, eds. *Practical Head and Neck Ultrasound*. London, England: Greenwich Medical Media Ltd; 2003:1–16.

15. Facius M, Malich A, Schnieder G, et al. Electrical impedance scanning used in addition to ultrasound for the verification of submandibular and parotid lesions. *Invest Radiol*. 2002;37:421–427.

16. Yasumoto M, Shibuya H, Suzuki S, et al. Computed tomography and ultrasonography in submandibular tumors. *Clin Radiol*. 1992;46:114–120.

17. Alyas F, Lewis K, Williams M, et al. Diseases of the submandibular gland as demonstrated using high resolution ultrasound. *Br J Radiol*. 2005;78:362–369.

18. Bialek E, Jakubowski W, Karpinska G. Role of ultrasonography in diagnosis and differentiation of pleomorphic adenomas. *Arch Otolaryngol Head Neck Surg*. 2003;129:929–933.

19. Bradley MJ. Salivary glands. In: Ahuja A, Evans R eds. *Practical Head and Neck Ultrasound*. London, England: Greenwich Medical Media Ltd; 2003:17–32.

20. Ernshoff R, Bertram S, Strobl H. Ultrasonographic cross-sectional characteristics of muscles of the head and neck. *Oral Surg Oral Med Oral Pathol Oral Radiol Endod*. 1999;87:93–106.

21. Zajkowski P, Jakubowski W, Bialek EJ, et al. Pleomorphic adenoma and adenolymphoma in ultrasonography. *Eur J Ultrasound*. 2000;12:23–29.

22. Wong KT, Tsang RKY, Tse GMK, Yuen EHY, Ahuja AT. Biopsy of deep-seated head and neck lesions under intraoral ultrasound guidance. *Am J Neuroradiol*. 2006;27:1654–1657.

23. Castelijns JA, van den Brekel MWM. Imaging of lymphadenopathy in the neck. *Eur Radiol*. 2002;12:727–738.

24. Krestan C, Herneth AM, Formanek M, Czerny C. Modern imaging lymph node staging of the head and neck region. *Eur J Radiol*. 2006;58:360–366.

25. Van den Brekel MWM, Castelijns JA. What the clinician wants to know: surgical perspective and ultrasound for lymph node imaging of the neck. *Cancer Imaging*. 2005;5:S41–S49.

26. Görges R, Eising EG, Fotescu D, et al. Diagnostic value of high-resolution B-mode and power-mode sonography in the follow-up of thyroid cancer. *Eur J Ultrasound*. 2003;16:191–206.

27. Ahuja A, Ying M. Grey-scale sonography in assessment of cervical lymphadenopathy: review of sonographic appearances and features that may help a beginner. *Br J Oral Maxillofacial Surg*. 2000;38:431–459.

28. Miyashita T, Takeno A, Ablimit I, et al. Ultrasonographic demonstration of retropharyngeal lymph nodes: preliminary report. *Ultrasound Med Biol*. 2003; 633–636.

29. Wang R, Snoey ER, Clements RC, Hern HG, Price D. Effect of head rotation on vascular anatomy of the neck: an ultrasound study. *J Emerg Med*. 2006; 31:283–286.

30. Ahuja AT. Lumps and bumps in the head and neck. In: Ahuja A, Evans R, eds. *Practical Head and Neck Ultrasound*. London, England: Greenwich Medical Media Ltd; 2003:87–104.

31. Sellar RJ. Imaging blood vessels of the head and neck. *J Neurol Neurosurg Psychiatry*. 1995;59:225–237.

32. Cheng SW, Ting AC, Wu LL. Ultrasonic analysis of plaque characteristics and intimal-medial thickness in radiation-induced atherosclerotic carotid arteries. *Eur J Endovasc Surg*. 2002;24:499–504.

33. Muzaffar K, Collins SL, Labropoulos N, Baker WH. A prospective study of the effects of irradiation on the carotid artery. *Laryngoscope*. 2000;110: 1811–1814.

34. Arens C, Eistert B, Glanz H, Waas W. Endolaryngeal high-frequency ultrasound. *Eur Arch Otorhinolaryngol*. 1998;255:250–255.

35. Rubin JS, Lee S, McGuinness J, et al. The potential role of ultrasound in differentiating solid and cystic swellings of the true vocal fold. *J Voice*. 2004; 18:231–235.

36. Kuhl V, Eicke BM, Dieterich M, Urban PP. Sonographic analysis of laryngeal elevation during swallowing. *J Neurol*. 2003;25:333–337.

37. Miller JL, Watkin KL. Lateral pharyngeal wall motion during swallowing using real time ultrasound. *Dysphagia*. 1997;12:125–132.

38. Bressman R, Thind P, Uy C, et al. Quantitative three-dimensional ultrasound analysis of tongue protrusion, grooving, and symmetry: data from 12 normal speakers and a partial glossectomee. *Clin Linguistics Phonetics*. 2005;19:573–588.

39. Arens C, Glanz H. Endoscopic high-frequency ultrasound of the larynx. *Eur Arch Otorhinolaryngol*. 1999;256:316–322.

Chapter 5

THYROID ULTRASONOGRAPHY

Theresa B. Kim
Lisa A. Orloff

Introduction

Ultrasonography of the thyroid gland is perhaps the most well-known and long-practiced application of US in the head and neck. The thyroid gland is relatively superficial and easily accessible, it has a distinctive echotexture, and the degree of detail obtainable by US is actually much greater than that with CT or MRI. Goals and indications for thyroid US include, but are not limited to, the following:

1. To clarify or better assess palpable thyroid nodules.
2. To assess the remainder of the thyroid gland in the patient with a palpable thyroid nodule.
3. To determine whether nodularity is present in the patient with an equivocal or difficult physical examination, and to characterize such nodularity if present.
4. To objectively monitor nodules, goiters, or lymph nodes in patients undergoing treatment or observation of thyroid disease.
5. To determine whether characteristics associated with malignancy are present.
6. To screen for thyroid lesions in patients who have been exposed to radiation.
7. To screen for thyroid lesions in patients with other diseases in the neck, such as hyperparathyroidism, who are undergoing treatment planning.

8. To facilitate fine-needle aspiration biopsy of a nodule.
9. To assess the thyroid and the extrathyroidal neck in the patient with thyroid cancer prior to treatment.
10. To monitor treated thyroid cancer patients for early evidence of recurrence in the thyroid bed and cervical lymph nodes.
11. To identify thyroid features associated with diseases including thyroiditis and Graves' disease.
12. To refine management of patients on therapy such as antithyroid medications.
13. To help teach regional anatomy and the art of thyroid palpation.
14. To detect undescended thyroid or thyroid agenesis.
15. To monitor fetal thyroid development in utero.
16. To assess the size and location of the neonatal thyroid.
17. To detect goiter as a sign of iodine deficiency.
18. To facilitate therapeutic procedures such as sclerotherapy or laser ablation of thyroid nodules.
19. To screen family members of patients with familial forms of thyroid cancer.

The value of the thyroid US examination depends on the skill, the experience, and the motivation of the examiner, as well as on the quality of the equipment used. As clinicians have become increasingly familiar with the advantages of thyroid and neck ultrasonography, the use of radionuclide thyroid scans in the initial workup of thyroid lesions has become less and less common. Still, US and radioiodine thyroid scans are complementary, and US better delineates anatomic detail in patients who have areas of relatively increased or decreased iodine or other isotope uptake on nuclear scanning (Figs 5–1A and 5–1B).

Anatomy

Gland, Blood Supply, Lymphatics

The thyroid gland is a richly vascular structure composed of two lobes with an adjoining midline isthmus. Approximately 40% of patients also have a pyramidal lobe originating from the right or left lobe or the isthmus and extending superiorly. Accessory collections of thyroid tissue may be present as remnants along the thyroglossal duct between the foramen cecum at the base of the tongue and the thyroid isthmus.

The arterial blood supply to the thyroid is provided by the superior thyroid artery arising from the external carotid artery and the inferior thyroid artery arising from the thyrocervical trunk. Occasionally, a thyroid ima artery may arise from the innominate artery, carotid artery, or aortic arch and supply the thyroid gland near the midline.[1] Venous drainage of the gland is more variable, with a network of veins in the thyroid capsule draining into the superior, middle, and inferior thyroid veins and eventually leading into the internal jugular or the innominate veins.

Lymphatic drainage of the thyroid gland consists of an extensive network of channels draining eventually into the jugular or mediastinal lymph nodes. The superior pole and lateral lobes drain toward the jugular lymph node chain, whereas the remainder of the gland drains into the prelaryngeal (Delphian), pretracheal and paratracheal lymph nodes (Fig 5–2).

Relations to Surrounding Structures

The thyroid gland has a tightly adherent true capsule and is surrounded by a looser layer of visceral

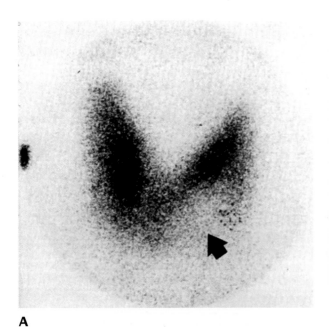

A

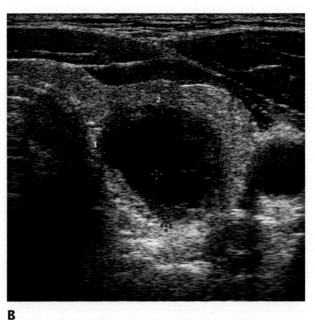

B

Fig 5–1. Iodine scan (**A**) and corresponding transverse ultrasound image (**B**) demonstrating cold nodule in left inferior thyroid pole (*left transverse view*).

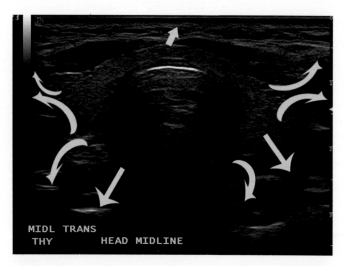

MIDL TRANS
THY   HEAD MIDLINE

Fig 5–2. Lymphatic drainage of the thyroid gland is to the prelaryngeal (Delphian), pretracheal, paratracheal, jugular, and mediastinal nodes (*midline transverse view*).

fascia which is a division of the middle layer of the deep cervical fascia. Berry's ligament is the posteriorly placed suspensory ligament which attaches the gland to the cricoid cartilage and first and second tracheal rings.

The strap muscles overlie the gland anteriorly and laterally with the sternohyoid and sternothyroid muscles joined in the midline by a thin layer of fascia at the median raphe. This fascia can be divided to allow the strap muscles to be retracted laterally during a thyroidectomy. The sternocleidomastoid muscle lies anterior and lateral to the strap muscles, and the superior belly of the omohyoid runs obliquely lateral to the gland. Posterior and lateral to the thyroid is the carotid sheath, which contains the common carotid artery, internal jugular vein, and vagus nerve. The parathyroid glands are usually found along the posterolateral portion of the gland and are discussed separately.

Technique and Measurements

US of the thyroid is a painless and relatively quick procedure that does not require any preparation such as hormone withdrawal or fasting. The exam is best performed with the patient in a supine position with the neck extended, although it can be performed on the seated patient. Images are obtained in the transverse and sagittal planes, noting first the overall dimensions of each thyroid lobe. By convention the left end of the probe is directed to the patient's right side for the transverse plane, and in a cranial direction for the sagittal plane (Fig 5-3). Attention is given to the echogenicity and vascularity of the tissue as well as the presence of any discrete nodules.

A normal thyroid lobe consists of a superior and inferior pole, and measures approximately 1.5 to 2 cm in the transverse dimension, 4 to 5 cm in the sagittal plane, and 2 cm in the anterior-posterior dimension. If the sagittal dimension or length is greater than the width of the ultrasound transducer and its borders extend beyond the image, the length can be approximated by using the dual-screen option when available and "splicing" together the superior and inferior portions of the lobe (Fig 5-4). The thyroid isthmus has an average length of 1.2 to 1.5 cm in the sagittal plane, and the pyramidal lobe is seldom visible. Rarely, the isthmus is absent and the gland consists of two individual lobes. The size and weight of the thyroid gland varies in women with the menstrual

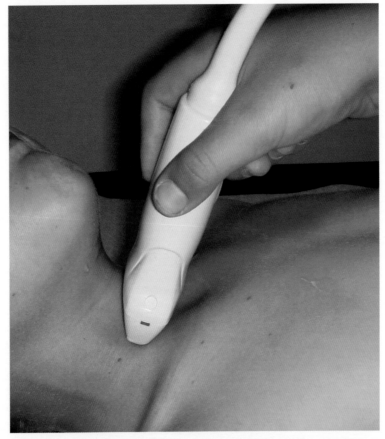

A

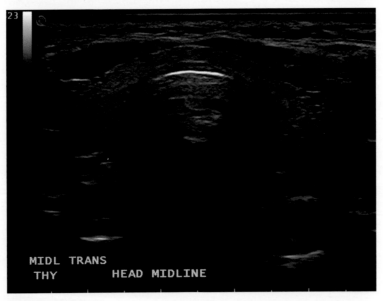

MIDL TRANS
THY   HEAD MIDLINE

B

Fig 5–3. Conventional orientation for performing and displaying US images of the neck. Transverse application of the transducer (**A**) yields a transverse (axial) image of the site of application (in this case the thyroid), with the patient's right side toward the left side of the screen (**B**). *continues*

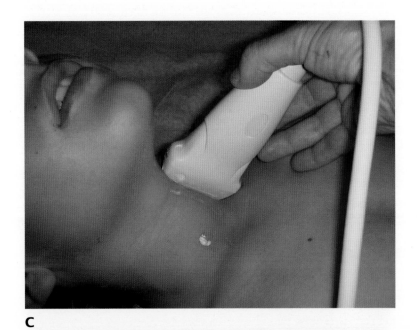

C

D

Fig 5–3. *continued* Sagittal (longitudinal) application of the transducer (**C**) yields a sagittal image of the thyroid lobe with the cranial aspect to the left of the screen and the caudal aspect to the right (**D**).

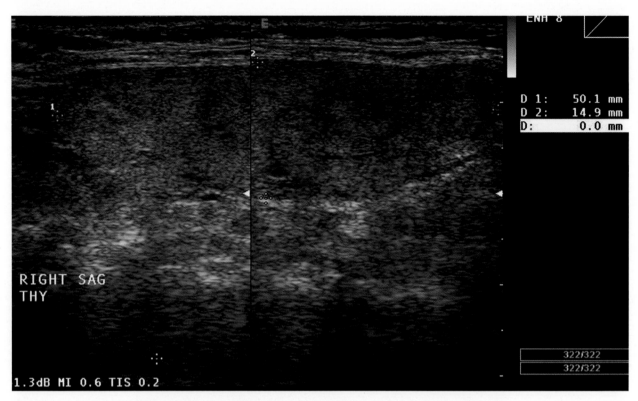

Fig 5–4. Sagittal view of thyroid lobe with superior and inferior portions spliced together using the split-screen feature.

cycle and pregnancy, but the average gland weighs approximately 25 to 30 g. Normal thyroid parenchyma echoes are fine, uniform, and slightly hyperechoic when compared to the surrounding muscles due to the gland's iodine content (Figs 5-5A, 5-5B and 5-6).[2,3]

Methods for estimating thyroid volume by applying a mathematical formula to measurements obtained from ultrasound have been described.[4,5] The World Health Organization advocates a formula for calculating the volume of each lobe based on an elliptical model: Volume = 0.479 [L × D × W] where L = length or sagittal diameter, D = depth or anteroposterior diameter, and W = width or transverse diameter.[5] However, prospective studies have shown high interobserver variability in estimating thyroid nodule volume[6] and poor correlation between predicted and actual thyroid volumes.[7] Nevertheless, thyroid volume is used by some to facilitate [131]I

dosimetry in patients with thyrotoxicosis.[8] Thus, one should use caution in making clinical decisions about management of thyroid nodules based on volumetric calculations.

A complete ultrasound examination of the thyroid gland should also include examination of the regional lymphatics, noting any abnormally enlarged lymph nodes. Lymphatic metastases of thyroid carcinoma most often occur in the pretracheal and paratracheal lymph nodes or along the jugulodigastric chain.[3] Absence of a cervical thyroid gland in an untreated patient or presence of a thyroglossal duct cyst should also prompt ultrasound inspection of the midline neck from the base of the tongue to the sternum, to assess for possible lingual or undescended thyroid (Figs 5-7A, 5-7B, and 5-7C). Ultrasound-guided biopsy and other procedures for thyroid disorders are discussed in Chapter 12.

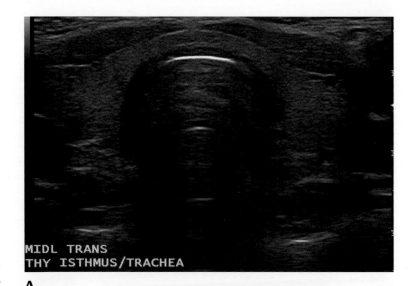

Fig 5–5. Normal thyroid gland. **A.** Normal gland without nodules (*midline transverse view*). **B.** Small nodule within right lobe in an otherwise homogeneous thyroid gland (*midline transverse view*).

A

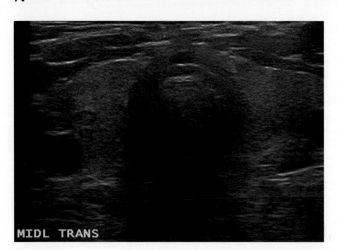

B

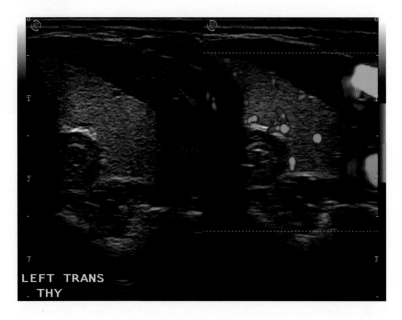

Fig 5–6. Normal thyroid vascularity in the left thyroid lobe, without and with Doppler overlay. Note esophagus immediately posterior to the left thyroid lobe (*left transverse view*).

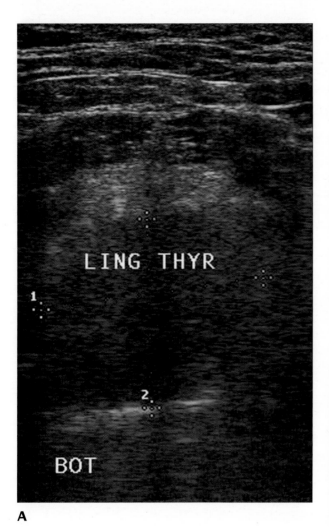

A

B

C

Fig 5–7. Lingual thyroid gland. **A.** Midline transverse US image demonstrating hypoechoic mass in the base of the tongue. **B.** Absent cervical thyroid by US (*left transverse view*). **C.** Flexible fiberoptic laryngoscopy showing mass in the tongue base (lingual thyroid) and the downturned epiglottis distal to the mass.

Ultrasound Features of Thyroid Nodules

Thyroid nodules are common in the general population, occurring in 50% or more of normal adults.[9] Most are discovered incidentally, although palpable nodules have a reported prevalence of 4 to 7%.[9,10] Risk factors for development of a thyroid nodule include iodine deficiency, female gender, advancing age, and radiation exposure. True thyroid nodules must be differentiated from other findings such as thyroid hemiagenesis, thyroglossal duct cyst, and processes involving the entire gland such as Hashimoto's thyroiditis.

Ultrasonography is a powerful tool in the diagnosis and management of thyroid nodules. Many studies have attempted to identify features which are associated with malignancy; however, there are as yet no universally accepted or pathognomonic criteria for distinguishing a malignant versus benign nodule on ultrasound. Despite this controversy, ultrasound is very helpful in identifying those lesions which warrant further investigation with fine-needle aspiration biopsy. The number and size of nodules, echogenicity, heterogeneity, the presence of solid or cystic components and calcifications, margins, and vascularity aid the clinician in determining appropriate management of a thyroid nodule.

Benign Thyroid Nodules

The most common types of nodules are benign hyperplastic (colloid) nodules or benign follicular adenomas (Figs 5–8A, 5–8B, and 5–8C, Video 5A). Colloid nodules consist of colloid and benign follicular cells

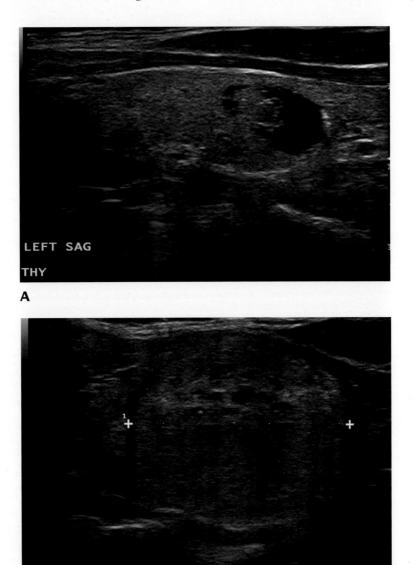

Fig 5–8 and Video 5A. Colloid nodules. **A.** Colloid nodule, left sagittal view. **B.** Colloid nodule, right sagittal view. *continues*

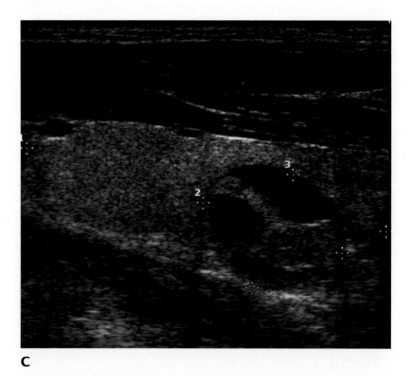

C

Fig 5–8 and Video 5A. *continued* **C.** Heterogeneous colloid nodule, right sagittal view. **Video 5A:** Same patient as in (A), with multiple colloid nodules seen on ascending transverse view of right thyroid lobe.

and are associated with small, hyperechoic, internal lucencies on ultrasound, known as the "comet tail" sign (Fig 5-9).[11] Follicular adenomas are the most common type of thyroid neoplasm and are, with few exceptions, not considered a forerunner of carcinoma (Fig 5-10).[12] They are typically round, well-encapsulated lesions with a clear margin or "halo" distinguishing them from the surrounding normal thyroid tissue (Fig 5-11). Spontaneous or traumatic hemorrhage may occur into the nodule (Fig 5-12).

Size

Although palpable thyroid nodules occur in up to 7% of the general adult population, the incidence of nonpalpable thyroid nodules visible by US is up to 10 times greater (ie, 70%).[13] The risk of malignancy for palpable thyroid nodules is approximately 10%, but several studies suggest that a similar incidence

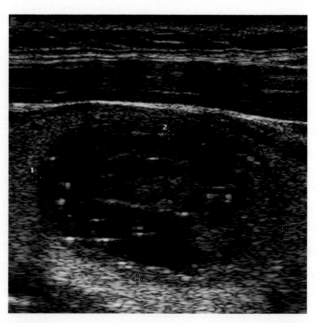

Fig 5–9. Comet tail echoes within a colloid nodule (*left sagittal view*).

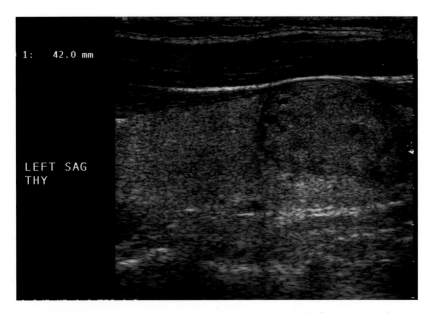

Fig 5–10. Follicular adenoma of the thyroid (*left sagittal view*).

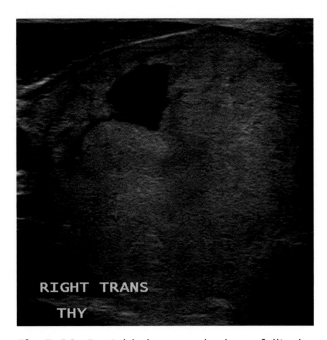

Fig 5–11. Partial halo around a large follicular adenoma (*right transverse view*).

of malignancy may be found among nodules smaller than 1 cm in diameter or "incidentalomas."[14-16] The ability to detect thyroid nodules as small as 2 mm in diameter carries with it the dilemma of how best to manage, and not overmanage, such lesions. As it is rare for a micronodule to become a clinically significant malignancy, a conservative but conscientious approach is to perform periodic ultrasound surveillance and further evaluation, such as by ultrasound-guided FNA, if growth is observed over time.[2]

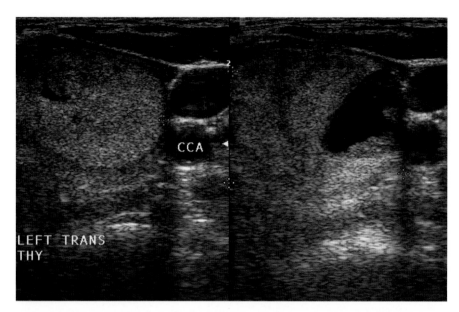

Fig 5–12. Hemorrhage into a follicular adenoma, (*left transverse view at two levels within the nodule*). Note halo surrounding the nodule.

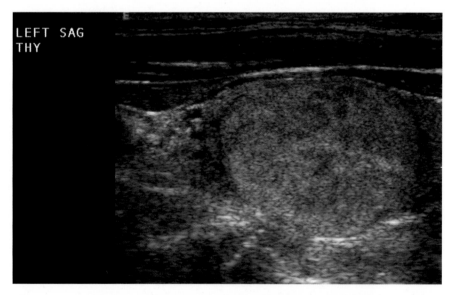

Fig 5–13. Single, well-circumscribed thyroid nodule (*left sagittal view*). This nodule proved to be follicular variant of papillary of carcinoma.

Single/Multiple

Thyroid nodules may be single (Fig 5-13) or multiple (Figs 5-14A and 5-14B, and Video 5B). Up to 50% of patients who present with a single palpable thyroid nodule are found on US to, in fact, have multiple nodules; moreover, many patients with suspected diffuse goiter are discovered to have discrete

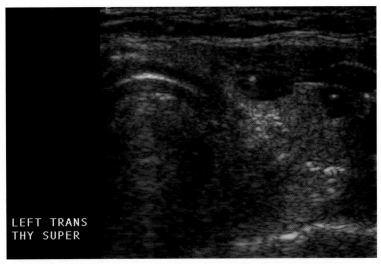

LEFT TRANS
THY SUPER

A

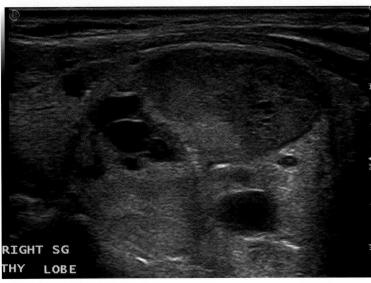

RIGHT SG
THY LOBE

B

Fig 5–14 and Video 5B. Multiple nodules. **A.** Multiple small nodules with single comet tail echoes, suggestive of colloid. **B.** Multiple colloid nodules of varying sizes. **Video 5B:** Transverse ascending view of multiple nodules within a right thyroid lobe.

nodules requiring biopsy.[13] Although the number of nodules present has not been demonstrated to correlate with the risk of malignancy,[17] each nodule must be evaluated independently and any nodule larger than 1 cm in size, or even smaller nodules with sus-picious features, may warrant cytologic evaluation by fine needle aspiration (Fig 5-15).

The term "multinodular goiter" is used to describe a gland containing multiple nodules, but it does not distinguish between an enlarged thyroid

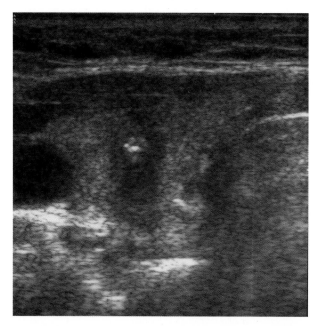

Fig 5–15. Subcentimeter but suspicious nodule with microcalcifications, warranting FNA biopsy. This nodule proved to be a papillary thyroid carcinoma.

and a normal-sized thyroid with multiple nodules. Each individual nodule may be solid or cystic, with or without calcifications. If a single, large nodule is present it is termed the dominant nodule.

Echogenicity

The echogenicity of a nodule should be compared to that of the surrounding thyroid tissue. Most benign adenomas or adenomatous nodules are slightly hypoechoic when compared to normal thyroid tissue (Figs 5–16A and 5–16B). Marked hypoechogenicity may be a risk factor for malignancy.[18] Heterogeneity should be noted.

Solid/Cystic

True epithelial-lined thyroid cysts are rare, but many thyroid nodules are cystic or have cystic components, such as cystic degeneration of a follicular adenoma or in the setting of multinodular goiter (Fig 5–17).[12]

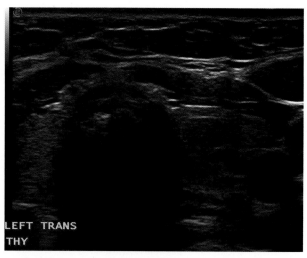

LEFT TRANS
THY

A

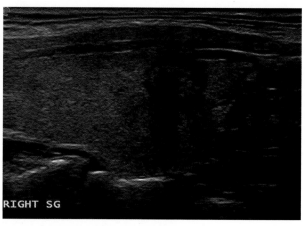

RIGHT SG

B

Fig 5–16. Hypoechoic nodules. **A.** Homogeneous mildly hypoechoic nodule (*left transverse view*). **B.** Heterogeneous hypoechoic nodule (*right sagittal view*).

Occasionally, a parathyroid gland or thyroglossal duct cyst may be mistaken for a thyroid cyst.[1] Solid nodules may sometimes be difficult to distinguish from the gland itself (Figs 5–18A and 5–18B).

Calcifications

Debate exists regarding the significance of calcification within a thyroid nodule. Peripheral calcification, also known as "eggshell calcification," is typically

Fig 5–17. Cystic degeneration of a thyroid nodule (*left transverse view*).

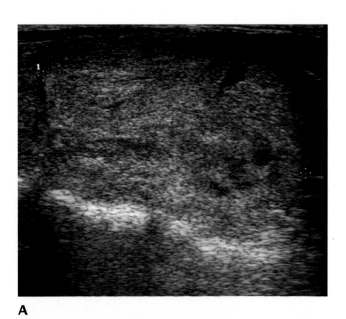

Fig 5–18. Solid nodules can be difficult to distinguish from the background thyroid parenchyma. **A.** Isoechoic thyroid nodule (*right sagittal view*). **B.** Subtle solid isoechoic nodule (*right transverse view*).

A

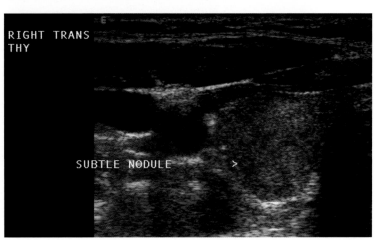

B

considered a benign feature and reflects previous hemorrhage and degenerative change (Fig 5–19). Microcalcification, on the other hand, may be a predictor of malignancy. Some studies have reported that 45 to 60% of malignant nodules and only 7 to 14% of benign nodules are associated with microcalcifications (Figs 5–20A and 5–20B, and Video 5C).[18,19] Another study reported that 62% of patients with microcalcification had cancer but that as many as 38% of patients with microcalcification had benign pathology.[20] The overall specificity of microcalcifications for thyroid carcinoma (most often attributed to psammoma bodies in papillary carcinoma) has been reported as 95.2% but with a low sensitivity of 59.3% and a diagnostic accuracy rate of 83.8%.[21] Macrocalcifications are often seen in medullary thyroid carcinoma.[22]

Definition/Margins

Benign lesions are often associated with a hypoechoic circumferential "halo" thought to represent a capsule and compressed thyroid tissue.[23] However, because thyroid neoplasms may have a partial halo this should not be considered a pathognomonic feature of a benign nodule (Fig 5–21). Mobility of the nodule with respect to surrounding thyroid tissue or adjacent structures such as the carotid sheath vessels or the prevertebral fascia should be assessed, as fixation suggests malignant invasion of the surrounding tissue (Fig 5–22A and Videos 5D and 5E).

Shape

Alexander et al performed a retrospective analysis of the relationship of nodule shape with malignancy. They reported that nodules with a more spherical shape had a higher incidence of cancer.[24] In contrast, Kim et al found that nodules which are more tall than wide were more likely to harbor malignancy.[18] Thus, the shape of a thyroid nodule may have prognostic but as yet unclear significance.

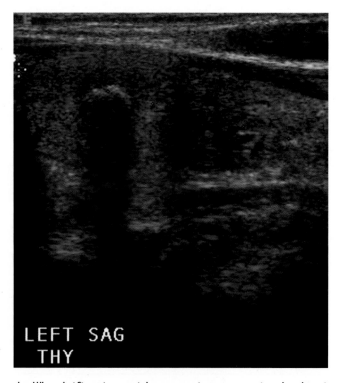

Fig 5–19. Coarse "eggshell" calcification with posterior acoustic shadowing (*left sagittal view*).

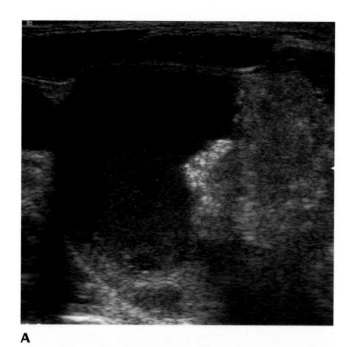

A

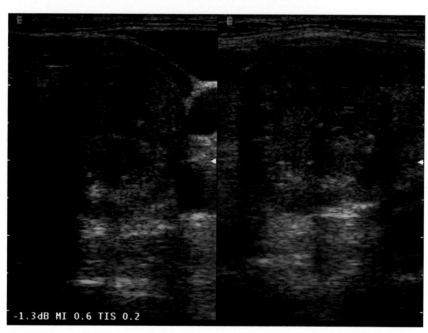

-1.3dB MI 0.6 TIS 0.2

B

Fig 5–20 and Video 5C. Microcalcifications. **A.** Cystic and solid papillary thyroid carcinoma with microcalcifications (*right transverse view*). **B.** Papillary thyroid carcinoma with microcalcifications (*left transverse and sagittal views*). **Video 5C:** papillary thyroid carcinoma with microcalcifications (*left sagittal view*).

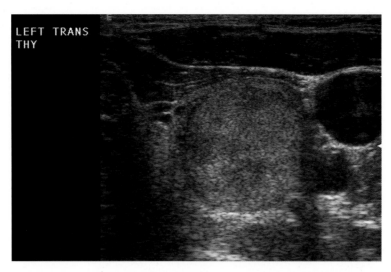

Fig 5–21. A well-defined halo is not always indicative of a benign thyroid nodule, as shown in this papillary thyroid carcinoma (*left transverse view*).

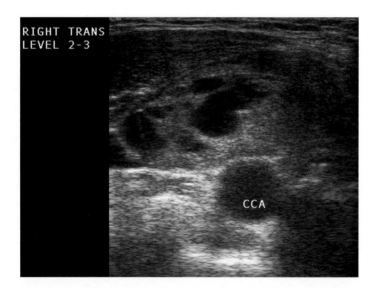

Fig 5–22 and Videos 5D and 5E. Sonopalpation. **A.** Lymph node metastasis from a follicular variant of papillary carcinoma to a right level 2 lymph node that abuts the common carotid artery (*right transverse view*). **Video 5D:** same patient as in Figure 5–22A, with mobility of the metastatic lymph node relative to the common carotid artery demonstrated by sonopalpation (*right transverse view*). **Video 5E:** large right superior thyroid mass that contains poorly differentiated thyroid cancer with extrathyroidal extension. This mass abuts the common carotid artery but is mobile by sonopalpation.

Vascularity

The presence and pattern of blood vessels around or within a nodule may correlate with malignant potential. Chammas et al classified thyroid nodules according to the pattern of vascularity seen with power Doppler into 5 types: absent blood flow, perinodular flow only, perinodular flow as great or greater than central blood flow, mainly central nodular flow, and central flow only.[17] Nodules with central blood flow greater than perinodular flow or exclusively central blood flow had a higher incidence of malignancy ($p = .001$) (Fig 5-23). Follicular carcinomas also tend to show a moderate increase in central vascularity by Power Doppler compared to follicular adenomas that favor peripheral flow.[25] In general, increased vascularity in a thyroid nodule is suggestive of malignancy but should not be considered a pathognomonic feature (Figs 5-24A, B,

and C). Of note, the amount of blood flow may have implications for fine-needle aspiration cytology, as more vascular lesions tend to yield a higher proportion of red blood cells with respect to thyroid epithelial cells, thereby increasing the difficulty of cytopathologic diagnosis.

Associated Findings

Other findings that should be considered in the interpretation of a thyroid nodule include the presence of abnormally enlarged or otherwise abnormal lymph nodes in the lateral neck (Fig 5-25). Thrombus within the nodule itself or in the internal jugular vein (Fig 5-26), or extrathyroidal spread of a thyroid nodule to the strap muscles, esophagus, or trachea are also features that are highly suggestive of malignancy (Figs 5-27A and 5-27B, and Video 5F).

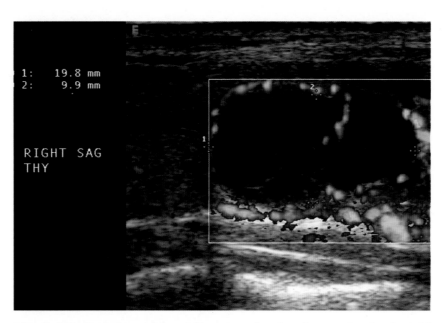

Fig 5–23. Peripheral blood flow in a benign hemorrhagic thyroid cyst (*right sagittal view*).

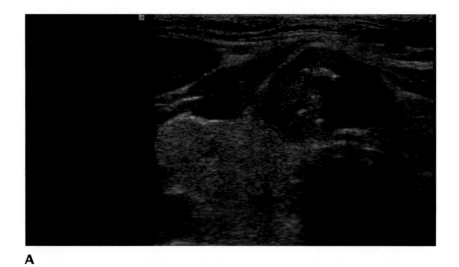

A

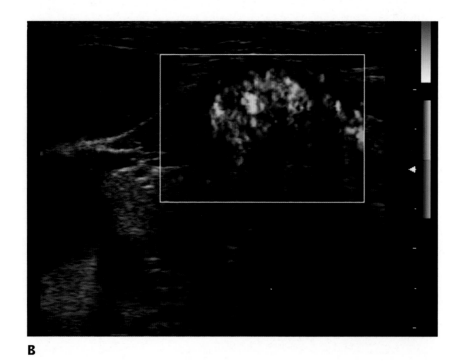

B

Fig 5–24. Increased vascularity in a lesion. **A.** Thyroid nodule with microcalcifications (*right transverse view*). **B.** Same nodule as in A, with color Doppler showing increased vascularity (*right transverse view*). *continues*

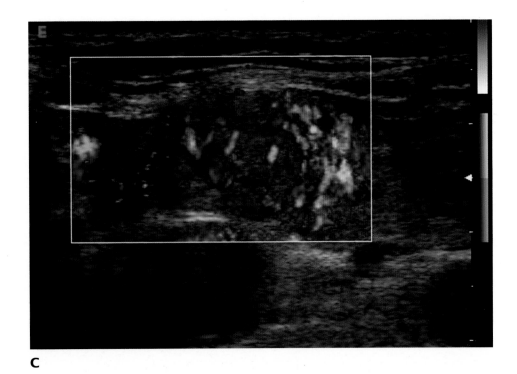

C

Fig 5–24. *continued* **C.** Hürthle cell adenoma with diffuse central and polar vascularity (*left transverse view*).

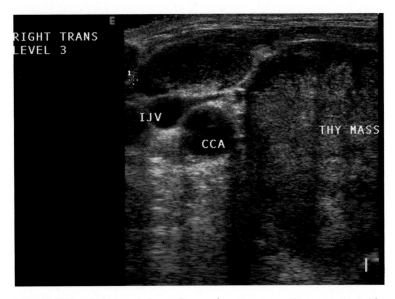

Fig 5–25. Enlarged lymph node representing metastatic disease in the setting of papillary thyroid carcinoma (*right transverse view of thyroid tumor and level 3 nodal metastasis*).

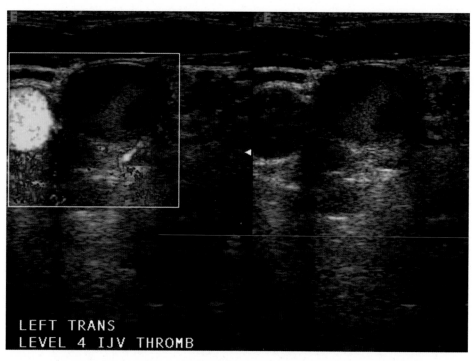

Fig 5–26. Thrombosed internal jugular vein with flow in the common carotid artery in the same patient as Figure 5–25 with papillary thyroid carcinoma (*left transverse view*).

Although paratracheal lymph nodes are a common site of early metastasis of thyroid carcinoma, these nodes are typically difficult to visualize by US in the presence of the thyroid gland itself. On the other hand, US is tremendously useful and sensitive in the evaluation of lateral cervical lymph nodes. The same characteristics that are suggestive of malignancy within a thyroid nodule may be found on US of cer-vical lymph node metastases from thyroid carcinoma, including microcalcifications, cystic degeneration, hypervascularity, enlargement, a rounded shape, and irregular borders with extracapsular extension (Figs 5–28A, B, and C, and Video 5G; Figs 5–29A, B, and C, and Videos 5H and 5I; Figs 5–30A and 5–30B). A more comprehensive discussion of cervical lymph node evaluation can be found in Chapter 15.

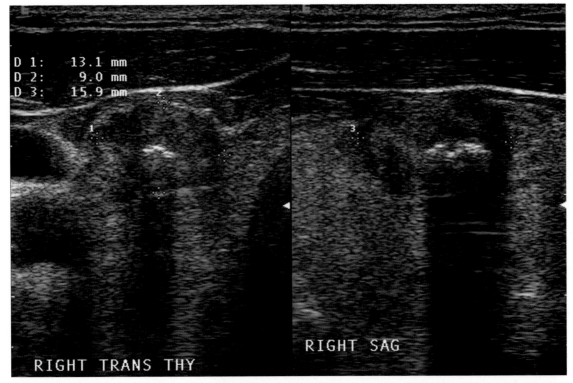

A

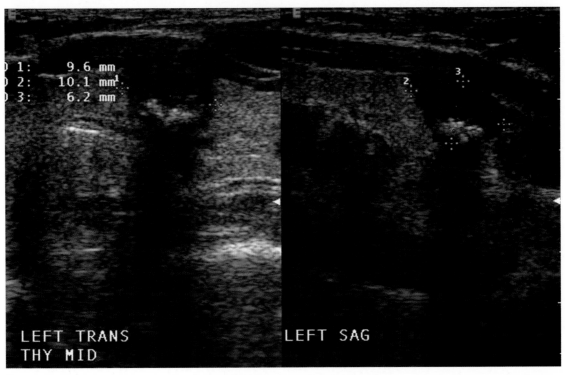

B

Fig 5–27 and Video 5F. Extrathyroidal spread. **A.** Papillary thyroid carcinoma with spread to the overlying strap muscles (*right transverse and sagittal views*). **B.** Papillary thyroid carcinoma with extrathyroidal spread to the strap muscles (*left transverse and sagittal views*). **Video 5F:** same patient as in Figure 5–27B, with extrathryroidal spread of papillary carcinoma (*transverse view*).

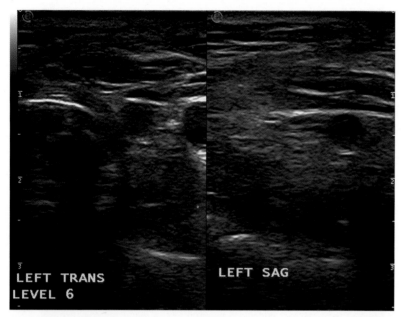

A

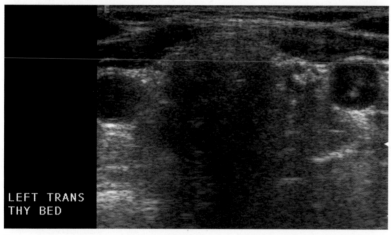

B

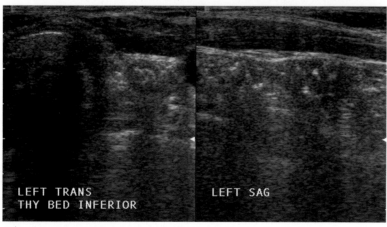

C

Fig 5–28 and Video 5G.
Recurrent papillary thyroid carcinoma. **A.** Small round hypoechoic nodule within the thyroid bed medial to the common carotid artery representing recurrent papillary carcinoma (*left transverse and sagittal views*). **B.** Poorly defined nodule of papillary carcinoma with microcalcifications within the left thryoid bed (*left transverse view*). Note blurring of tissue planes from prior surgery and ^{131}iodine therapy; **C.** Same patient as in (B), with additional inferior thyroid bed nodularity withmicrocalcifications (*left transverse and sagittal views*). **Video 5G:** Lefttransverse descending view of the left thyroid bed in the same patient as in Figures 5–28B and 5–28C, showing multiple nodules of recurrent papillary carcinoma.

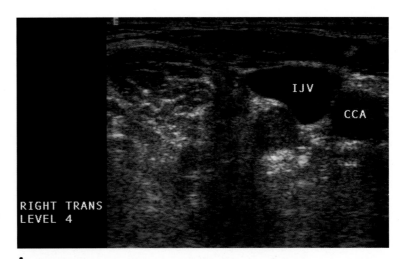

A

Fig 5-29 and Videos 5H and 5I. Lymph node metastases. **A.** Recurrent papillary carcinoma in a right level 4 lymph node (*right transverse view*). **B.** Hypervascular lymph node metastasis from papillary thyroid carcinoma, lateral to the internal jugular vein in the left level 3 region (*transverse view*). **C.** Anaplastic thyroid carcinoma metastatic to a level 2 lymph node (*left transverse and sagittal views*). Note hypoechoic, rounded appearance of node. **Video 5H:** left transverse ascending view through a left thyroid papillary carcinoma and associated lymph node metastases in levels 4, 3, and 2. **Video 5I:** primary papillary carcinoma in the left thyroid lobe with lymph node metastases shown here in levels 4 and 3 (*left transverse view*).

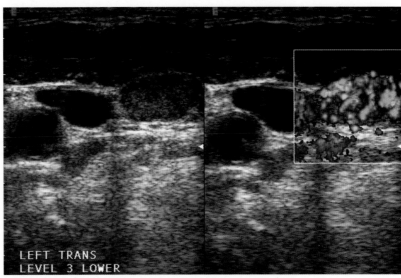

B

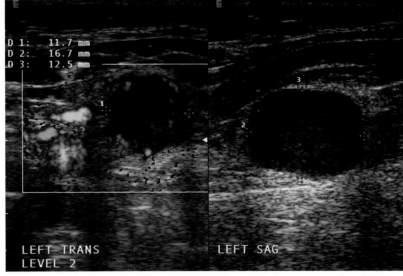

C

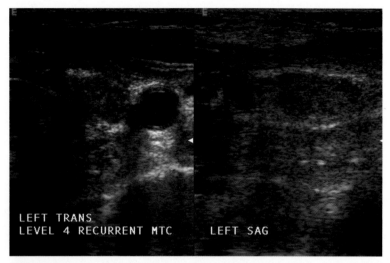

LEFT TRANS
LEVEL 4 RECURRENT MTC   LEFT SAG

A

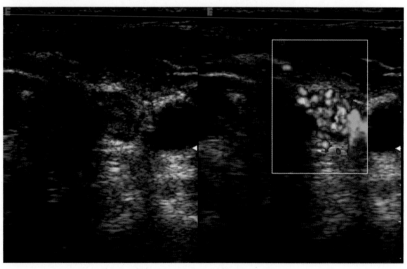

B

Fig 5–30. Recurrent medullary thyroid carcinoma. **A.** Level 4 lymph node recurrence of medullary thyroid carcinoma medial to the common carotid artery (*left transverse and left sagittal views*). **B.** Same patient as in (A) with color Doppler showing hypervascularity of the lymph node metastasis.

Thyroid Gland Diseases

Goiter

"Goiter" is a general term used to describe an enlarged thyroid gland. It may occur in the setting of multinodular goiter (Figs 5–31A and 5–31B), thyroiditis, thyrotoxicosis, or iodine deficiency. When evaluating a patient with goiter, it is important to note whether the gland is diffusely enlarged or if one lobe predominates, whether nodularity is present, and whether vascularity is increased, decreased, or average.

Thyroiditis

The most common types of thyroiditis are autoimmune or chronic lymphocytic thyroiditis (Hashimoto's disease), de Quervain's subacute thyroiditis, and acute suppurative thyroiditis. Hashimoto's thyroiditis has the highest incidence in women aged 40 to 60 years. It is also the most common cause of goitrous hypothyroidism when dietary iodine is sufficient,[26] with up to 50% of patients developing hypothyroidism.[3] The appearance on US is that of ill-defined hypoechoic areas separated by echogenic septa, with increased (early) or decreased (late) vascularity (Figs 5–32A through 5–32E). The thyroid has no native lymphoid tissue, but intrathyroid lymphoid tissue accumulates as a result of the autoimmune process in association with thyroid peroxidase antibodies (anti-TPO),[27] and patients with Hashimoto's thyroiditis have up to a 60-fold increase in the risk of developing lymphoma.[28,29]

The natural history of de Quervain's subacute thyroiditis consists of an acute period of neck pain, fever, and lethargy after an upper respiratory illness, followed by a subacute period of hypothyroidism which spontaneously resolves over 3 to 6 months. During the acute phase, patients present with a tender, palpable nodule which can be distinguished from an adenomatous nodule on ultrasound by the lack of calcification or halo, and surrounding heterogeneous thyroid tissue. In the subacute period, the affected lobe or sometimes the entire gland, is hypoechoic and enlarged. On resolution of the disease, the thyroid returns to normal although some patients may have a persistent nodule or atrophy of the gland.[3] Acute suppurative thyroiditis is a rare condition affecting children. Because the thyroid gland has a thick, fibrous capsule it is relatively resistant to infection.[3] The presence of an abscess can be confirmed on ultrasound as a hypoechoic fluid-filled collection that may contain pockets of gas.

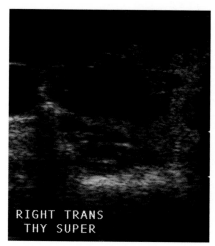
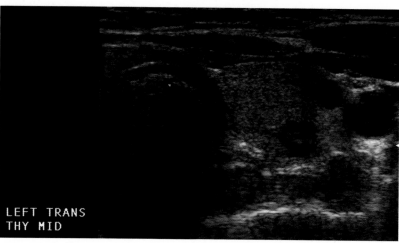

A **B**

Fig 5–31. Multinodular goiter. **A.** Multiple hypoechoic nodules (*right transverse view of superior thyroid pole*). **B.** Multiple small nodules within the mid-portion of the left thyroid lobe (*left transverse view*). Note the well-visualized esophagus.

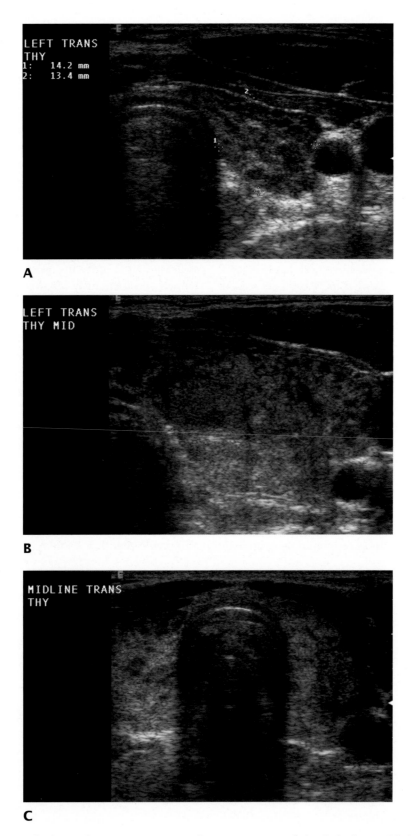

Fig 5–32. Hashimoto's thyroiditis. **A.** Honeycomb appearance of the left thyroid lobe in Hashimoto's thyroiditis (*left transverse view*). **B.** Solid nodule within a gland with Hashimoto's thyroiditis (*left transverse view*). **C.** Hashimoto's thyroiditis in a patient who proved also to have papillary thyroid carcinoma (*midline transverse view*). *continues*

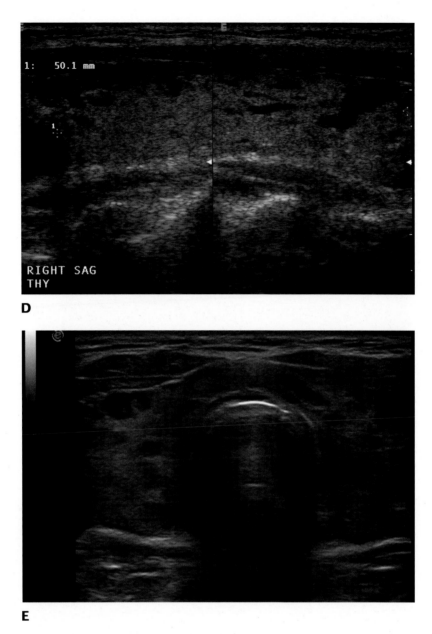

D

E

Fig 5–32. *continues* **D.** Spliced sagittal split-screen view of the right thyroid lobe in the same patient as (C). **E.** Midline transverse view of the thyroid of a patient with "Swiss cheese" appearance of chronic thyroiditis.

Thyrotoxicosis

Graves' disease is an autoimmune disorder occurring most commonly in women aged 30 to 60, but can also affect children or adults of any age. It is the single most common cause of thyrotoxicosis. Symptoms include hyperthyroidism, diffuse thyroid enlargement, infiltrative ophthalmopathy with exophthalmos, and skin changes from myxedema.[1]

Ultrasound features are well described and include heterogeneous tissue with diffuse hypoechogenicity and hypervascularity (Figs 5–33A through 5–33D, and Video 5J). In addition, studies suggest that the velocity of flow in the inferior thyroid

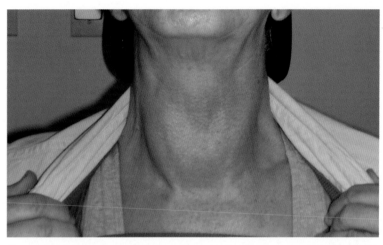

A

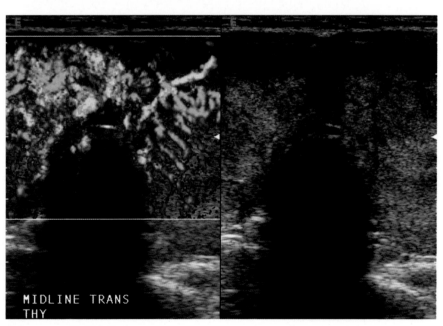

B

 Fig 5–33 and Video 5J. Graves' disease. **A.** Clinical photograph of a patient with Graves' thyrotoxicosis. **B.** Same patient as (A), showing midline transverse US view of her hypervascular thyroid gland with and without color Doppler. *continues*

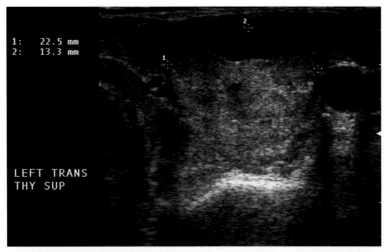

C

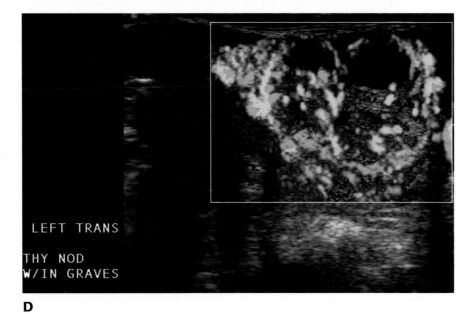

D

Fig 5–33 and Video 5J. *continued* **C** and **D**. Left transverse view of a Graves' thyroid without (C) and with (D) color Doppler, showing hypervascularity and nodularity; **Video 5J:** Right transverse view ascending through the right thyroid lobe in the same patient as in Figures 5–33A and 5–33B.

artery is markedly increased in Graves' disease.[30,31] Because thyroid cancer may coexist with Graves' disease, any palpable or atypical nodules must be carefully documented and further investigation is warranted if they exhibit any suspicious ultrasound characteristics (Fig 5–34). Color flow mapping may be useful in the selection of an optimal dose of anti-thyroid medication (eg, Methimazole) to achieve a euthyroid state,[32] and may also be predictive of the likelihood of relapse after the withdrawal of anti-thyroid medications.[33,34] More recently, transvaginal ultrasonography has been used as a noninvasive tool to monitor fetal thyroid size in the setting of maternal Graves' disease.[35]

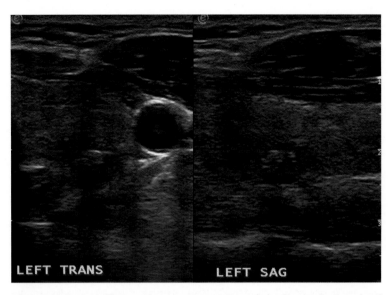

Fig 5–34. Papillary carcinoma within the thyroid gland of a patient previously treated with ^{131}I for Graves' disease (*left transverse and sagittal views*).

In amiodarone-induced thyrotoxicosis (AIT), US has been reported to have both diagnostic and therapeutic implications.[2] Doppler sonography patterns help distinguish between the two types of AIT and thus direct treatment.[36,37] Type I AIT occurs in patients with latent thyroid disease and Doppler sonography shows increased or normal blood flow. These patients respond to thionamide therapy. Type II AIT arises in previously normal thyroid glands and exhibits no demonstrable vascular flow; these patients are treated with glucocorticoid therapy.

Radiation Changes

Radiation exposure, whether in the form of external beam radiation or radioactive iodine (^{131}I), leads to atrophy and shrinkage of the gland as well as fibrosis in the thyroid parenchyma (Fig 5–35). Furthermore, external beam radiation causes similar fibrosis and blurring of tissue planes in the extrathyroidal neck including the salivary glands (Figs 5–36A and 5–36B).

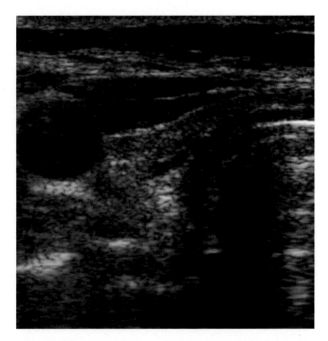

Fig 5–35. Atrophy and shrinkage of the right thyroid lobe after [131]Iodine radiation (*right transverse view*).

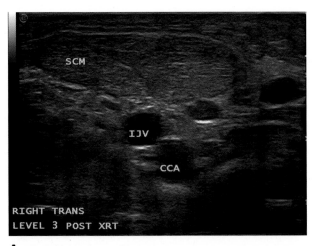

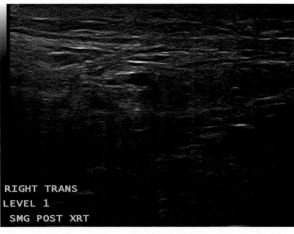

A   **B**

Fig 5–36. Blurring of tissue planes in the extrathyroidal neck. **A.** Blurred soft tissue planes in the right level 3 region in a patient treated with external beam radiation for squamous cell carcinoma of the tonsil (*right transverse view*). **B.** Fibrosis of the submandibular gland and level 1 region in the same patient as (**A**) (*right transverse view*).

Thyroid Cancer

The majority of thyroid nodules are benign, with malignancy rates near 10%.[38] Most thyroid cancers are of follicular cell origin (papillary, follicular, and Hürthle cell carcinoma), collectively called well-differentiated thyroid cancer (WDTC), whereas other malignancies such as medullary thyroid carcinoma, anaplastic carcinoma, lymphoma, and metastatic disease are much less common. Risk factors for cancer include female gender, advanced age, exposure to ionizing radiation, and family history of thyroid cancer.

Because most thyroid cancers present as a palpable nodule, distinguishing between benign and malignant thyroid masses is critical. As discussed earlier, there is controversy over how strongly certain ultrasound features correlate with malignancy. Although some characteristics, including the pattern of calcification, echogenicity, size and shape of the nodule(s), vascularity, and invasion of adjacent structures have been found to be associated with malignancy,[19,24,39,40] others have found that ultrasound does not reliably distinguish between benign and malignant lesions.[20,41] Ultrasound remains, how-

ever, an invaluable tool in identifying thyroid lesions and aids in determining which lesions should undergo further evaluation through biopsy or other imaging. In addition, US may be used to evaluate for regional lymphatic metastases or for local recurrence following thyroidectomy.

Papillary Carcinoma

Papillary thyroid carcinoma (PTC) is the most common thyroid malignancy and represents 70 to 80% of all thyroid cancers. The female/male ratio is 2:1, and the peak age at diagnosis is 20 to 30 years. Multifocal lesions are common as are regional nodal metastases. Distant metastases such as to bone or the lungs are less but not uncommon. Local invasion of the larynx, trachea, esophagus, spine, or soft tissues of the neck is seen only with the most aggressive of PTCs. Prognosis is excellent with up to 90% cure rate; poorer prognosis is associated with large size, advanced patient age, nodal involvement, extrathyroidal spread, male gender, and vascular invasion. Rarely, papillary carcinomas may degenerate into anaplastic carcinoma.

Ultrasound features typically seen in PTC include a solid, hypoechoic lesion with microcalcifications (Figs 5–37A and 5–37B, and Videos 5K and 5L). Cystic components may be present within a solid lesion, and although an incomplete halo may be seen, ill-defined margins are more common (Fig 5–38). Doppler examination may also reveal disorganized hypervascularity (Figs 5–39A and 5–39B). Of these

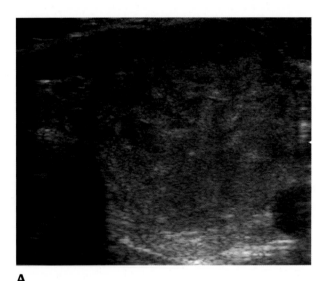

A

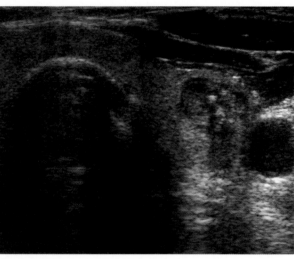

B

Fig 5–37 and Videos 5K and 5L. Papillary thyroid carcinoma. **A.** Large primary tumor within the left thyroid lobe (*left transverse view*). **B.** Small, nonpalpable primary papillary thyroid carcinoma (*left transverse view*). **Video 5K:** left transverse view ascending through the large primary tumor in the left thyroid lobe in the same patient as in Figure 5–37A. **Video 5L:** left transverse descending view through the primary tumor in the same patient as in Figure 5–37B.

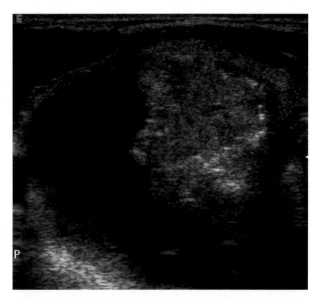

Fig 5–38. Cystic papillary thyroid carcinoma (*right transverse view*).

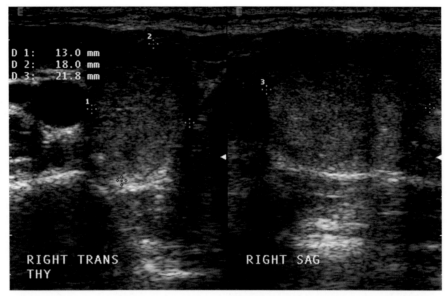

A

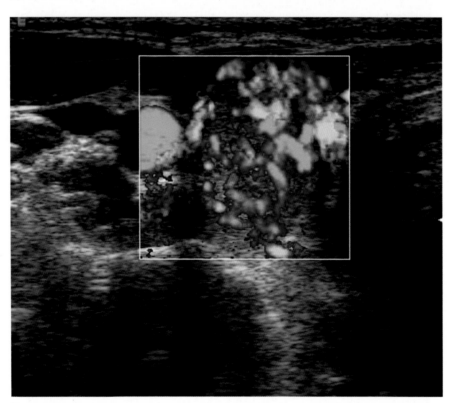

B

Fig 5–39. Papillary thyroid carcinoma with hypervascularity. **A.** Tumor without color Doppler (*right transverse and sagittal views*). **B.** Tumor with color Doppler overlay (*right transverse view*).

features, microcalcifications may be the most specific for PTC due to the fact that psammoma bodies are a histopathologic feature considered pathognomonic for PTC;[18] they are composed of tiny laminated, spherical collections of calcium which reflect sound waves and appear as tiny bright foci (Fig 5–40). Not all nodules that exhibit features typically associated with malignancy, such as microcalcifications, are actually malignant (Fig 5–41).

Follicular Carcinoma

Follicular carcinoma accounts for approximately 10% of thyroid malignancies. It is more common in older women, with a female/male ratio of 3:1 and mean age at diagnosis of 50 years.[1] Unlike PTC, follicular carcinoma is more likely to spread via hematogenous routes, accounting for a higher incidence of distant metastasis and poorer prognosis.

Follicular neoplasms, both benign and malignant, are typically solid, hypoechoic, and homogeneous lesions. As opposed to papillary carcinoma, cystic components and calcifications are rare and a halo is often seen (Figs 5–42A through 5–42E). Hypervascularity is common and FNA samples are often bloody. The most important prognostic feature is whether extracapsular and/or local invasion is present. Because follicular adenoma cannot be distinguished from follicular carcinoma on fine needle aspiration, the predominance of follicular cells on FNA, especially in sheets or microfollicles, often necessitates an excisional biopsy of the affected lobe.

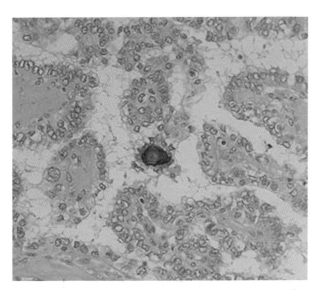

Fig 5–40. Histopathology of papillary thyroid carcinoma, with a psammoma body in the center of the photomicrograph.

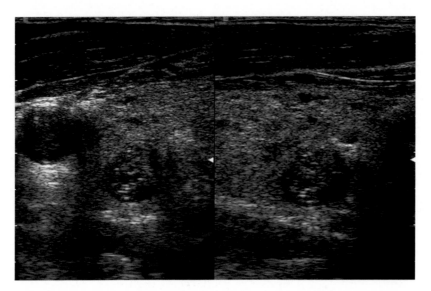

Fig 5–41. Echoes that appear to be microcalcifications in a nodule that proved to be benign (*right transverse and sagittal views*).

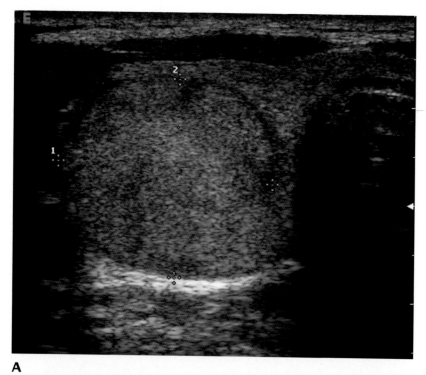

A

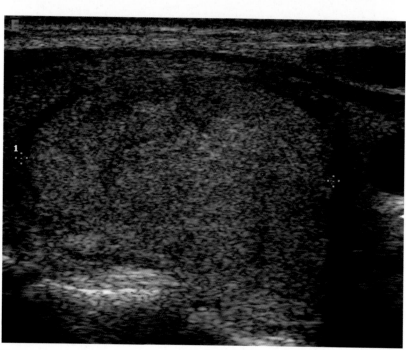

B

Fig 5–42. Follicular neoplasms. **A** and **B.** Right transverse (**A**) and sagittal (**B**) views of a minimally invasive follicular carcinoma. *continues*

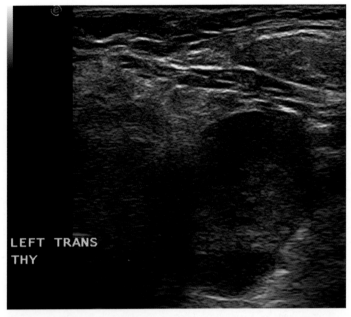

C

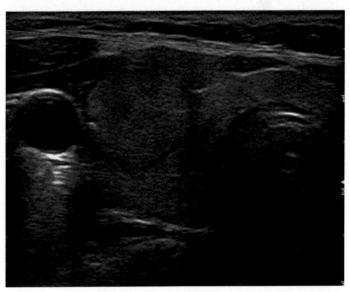

D

Fig 5–42. *continued* **C.** Follicular carcinoma in an inferior pole nodule (*left transverse view*). **D.** Follicular neoplasm that proved to be a benign follicular adenoma (*right transverse view*). *continues*

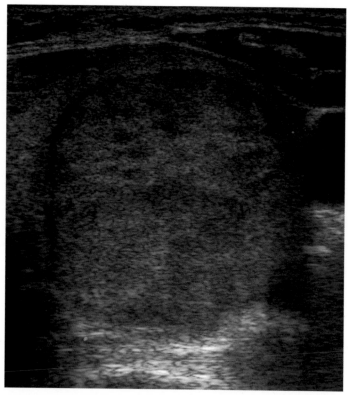

E

Fig 5–42. *continued* **E.** Minimally invasive follicular carcinoma (*left transverse view*). The thyroid lobe contained two foci of microscopic papillary carcinoma noted on left thyroid lobectomy.

Hürthle Cell Carcinoma

The World Health Organization classification of thyroid lesions considers Hürthle cell tumors to be a subtype of follicular cell neoplasm. Approximately 20% of Hürthle cell lesions are malignant, and Hürthle cell carcinoma accounts for only 3% of thyroid cancers. These tumors behave more aggressively than either PTC or follicular carcinoma, and often present with bilateral and multifocal lesions with a higher risk of regional lymph node and distant metastasis.

On ultrasound, Hürthle cell tumors are solid with both hypoechoic and hyperechoic components with an irregular border (Fig 5–43). Most do not have calcifications or a halo.

Medullary Carcinoma

Medullary thyroid carcinomas (MTC) account for 5% of thyroid cancers. They arise from parafollicular C cells which are primarily concentrated in the superior poles.[1] Women and men are affected equally, and although most cases are spontaneous, up to 30% are familial and may be associated with MEN syndromes type 2A and 2B. MTC occurring in the setting of an MEN syndrome is usually multifocal and bilateral. Spread to regional lymph nodes in the neck and/or mediastinum and hematogenous spread are common.

MTC appears solid and hypoechoic on ultrasound yet frequently has hyperechoic foci representing both

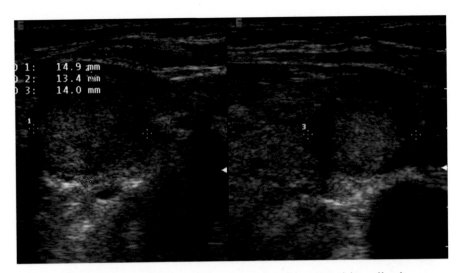

Fig 5–43. Hürthle cell lesion, that proved to be a Hürthle cell adenoma. (*left transverse and sagittal views*).

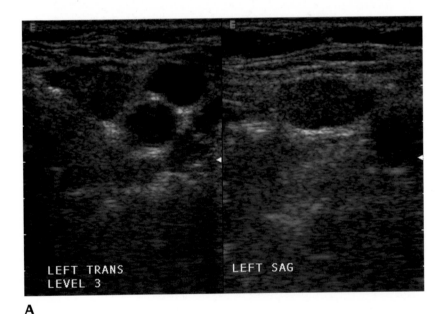

A

Fig 5–44. A. Medullary thyroid carcinoma. Recurrence within a level 3 lymph node (*left transverse and left sagittal views*). *continues*

amyloid deposition and calcification (Figs 5–44A through 5–44C). These foci may also appear within affected lymph nodes. As with papillary carcinoma, Doppler examination may reveal disorganized hypervascularity.[3]

Anaplastic Carcinoma

Anaplastic carcinoma is the most aggressive type of thyroid cancer, and although it accounts for less than 2% of all thyroid cancers it comprises up to

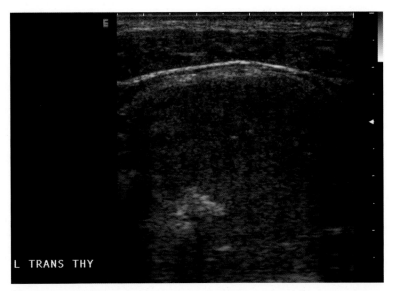

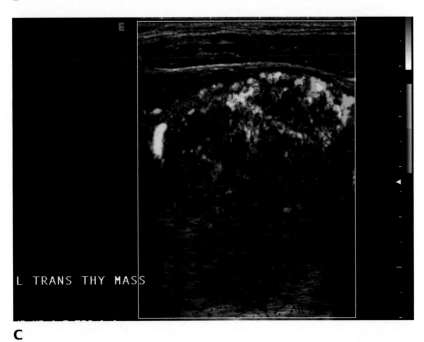

Fig 5–44. *continued* **B** and **C.** Medullary carcinoma with mass filling the left thyroid lobe, transverse view without (**B**) and with (**C**) color Doppler. Note area of calcification.

40% of deaths from thyroid cancer.[42] It is a disease of the elderly with very few cases occurring in patients younger than 50 years. Most anaplastic carcinomas develop in the setting of a pre- or coexisting thyroid cancer or goiter and may represent malignant transformation of a previously well-differentiated carcinoma. Patients typically present with a rapidly enlarging neck mass associated with pain, voice changes, dysphagia, or dyspnea. The majority of patients have lymph node involvement at the time of diagnosis.

Ultrasound demonstrates a diffusely hypoechoic lesion often infiltrating the entire lobe with areas of necrosis or ill-defined calcifications (Fig 5–45). Involved lymph nodes may also have necrotic changes. Invasion into surrounding vessels or soft tissue is often seen as well.

Lymphoma

Lymphoma involving the thyroid gland is rare, accounting for less than 5% of thyroid malignancies.[42] It may be primary or arise as part of a systemic lymphoma. Women are more often affected and age at diagnosis is usually greater than 50 years. Non-Hodgkin's lymphoma is the most common type and is usually associated with a history of Hashimoto's thyroiditis. In fact, the cytologic diagnosis can be easily mistaken for chronic lymphocytic thyroiditis. The clinical course of thyroid lymphoma may resemble anaplastic carcinoma with a rapidly enlarging neck mass, regional lymph node enlargement, and symptoms related to compression of the recurrent laryngeal nerve or trachea. Lymphoma, however, is usually not associated with pain. Local soft tissue invasion is common, as is vascular invasion.

Lymphoma may appear as a focal lesion within a lobe or as a diffuse abnormality involving the entire gland. The involved tissue is usually heterogeneous and hypoechoic and may be mistaken for anaplastic carcinoma (Fig 5–46). "Pseudocysts" with posterior enhancement are sometimes seen.[3]

Thyroid as a Site of Cancer Metastases

Metastases to the thyroid gland are uncommon, and usually arise from a primary melanoma, breast, lung, or renal cell carcinoma.[1,3] The origin of the tumor is usually identified by history, physical examination, FNA cytology, and adjunctive studies such as imaging (CT or PET) or laboratory testing. Thyroid metastases usually involve the inferior poles and are homogeneous, hypoechoic, and noncalcified (Fig 5–47).

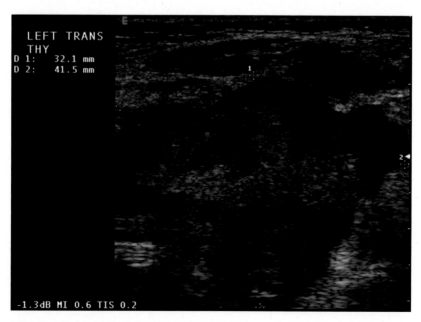

Fig 5–45. Anaplastic thyroid carcinoma. Note that the tumor is larger than the width of the US transducer (*left transverse view*).

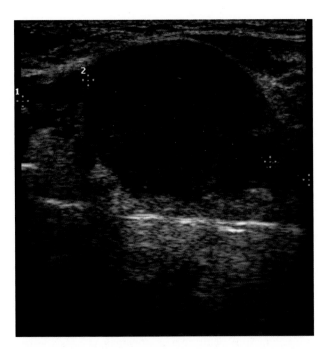

Fig 5–46. Lymphoma within a heterogeneous background of chronic thyroiditis (*right sagittal view*).

Extrathyroidal Neck

Metastasis to cervical and paratracheal lymph nodes is common in thyroid carcinomas, so it is vitally important to include the extrathyroidal neck when performing an ultrasound examination. Features that are characteristic of malignancy in the primary thyroid neoplasm are also seen in the involved lymph nodes. Microcalcifications, cystic degeneration, hypervascularity, enlargement, a rounded shape, irregular or indistinct margins, or extracapsular extension may be present. In addition, following surgical management of thyroid carcinoma, it is invaluable to perform US of the neck to monitor for recurrence in the thyroid bed as well as in the lateral cervical lymph nodes and soft tissues. US is increasingly replacing radioactive iodine scanning in the ongoing surveillance of the thyroid cancer patient, due to its superior anatomic resolution, ease of performance, and non-need for preparation and morbidity associated with thyroid hormone withdrawal or recombinant TSH injection and low-iodine diet limitations.

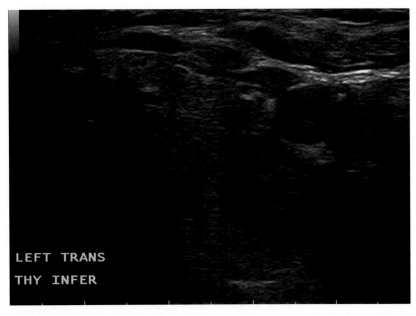

Fig 5–47. Metastasis to the thyroid gland (*left transverse view*). Patient with a history of primary malignant melanoma of the upper back, with prior axillary metastases, now with a PET/CT positive lesion in the left inferior thyroid lobe. This lesion actually proved not to be metastatic melanoma, but this conclusion could not be reached by US alone.

Summary

Improved US technology has led to the ability to detect even very small lesions in the thyroid gland as well as cervical lymph nodes, and metastases in the thyroid bed following thyroidectomy that previously went unrecognized. A recent study reported that preoperative US detected nonpalpable lymph nodes in 33% of patients, thereby defining the extent of lymphadenectomy performed.[43] Whether detection of these small lesions and "tailoring" of surgery based on US findings results in decreased rates of recurrence or increased survival rates remains a question to be answered. Nevertheless, improved detection of de novo disease and surveillance for recurrent disease by US, with its convenience, cost-effectiveness, safety, and interactive potential, greatly facilitates the thyroid patient's care.

Conclusion

Disorders affecting the thyroid gland range from benign to malignant and differ in their presentation, prognosis, and treatment. Ultrasound is an invaluable tool in both the diagnosis and management of this heterogeneous group of conditions.

Videos for This Chapter

Video 5A. See legend for Figure 5-8.

Video 5B. See legend for Figure 5-14.

Video 5C. See legend for Figure 5-20.

Video 5D. See legend for Figure 5-22.

Video 5E. See legend for Figure 5-22.

Video 5F. See legend for Figure 5-27.

Video 5G. See legend for Figure 5-28.

Video 5H. See legend for Figure 5-29.

Video 5I. See legend for Figure 5-29.

Video 5J. See legend for Figure 5-33.

Video 5K. See legend for Figure 5-37.

Video 5L. See legend for Figure 5-37.

References

1. Cummings CW, ed. *Cummings: Otolaryngology Head and Neck Surgery*. 4th ed. St. Louis, Mo: Mosby, Inc, 2005.
2. Blum, M. Ultrasonography of the Thyroid. [Thyroid Disease Manager, Ch. 6C]. Available at: http://www.thyroidmanager.org. Accessed August 2, 2006.
3. Ajuha A, Evans R, eds. *Practical Head and Neck Ultrasound*. London: Greenwich Medical Media Limited; 2000.
4. Shabana W, Peeters E, Verbeek P, Osteaux MM. Reducing inter-observer variation in thyroid volume calculation using a new formula and technique. *Eur J Ultrasound*. 2003;16(3):207–210.
5. *Assessment of Iodine Deficiency Disorders and Monitoring Their Elimination : A Guide for Programme Managers*. 2nd ed. World Health Organization. Dept. of Nutrition for Health and Development.
6. Brauer VF, Eder P, Miehle K, Wiesner TD, Hasenclever H, Paschke R. Interobserver variation for ultrasound determination of thyroid nodule volumes. *Thyroid*. 2005;15(10):1169–1175.
7. Miccoli P, Minuto MN, Orlandini C, Galleri D, Massi M, Berti P. Ultrasonography estimated thyroid volume: a prospective study about its reliability. *Thyroid*. 2006;16(1):37–39.
8. Lucas KJ. Use of thyroid ultrasound volume in calculating radioactive iodine dose in hyperthyroidism. *Thyroid*. 2000;10(2):151–155.
9. Mazzaferri EL. Management of a solitary thyroid nodule. *N Engl J Med*. 1993;25;328(8):553–559.
10. Tunbridge WM, Evered DC, Hall R, et al. The spectrum of thyroid disease in a community: the Whickham survey. *Clin Endocrinol* (Oxf). 1977; 7(6):481–493.
11. Ahuja A, Chick W, King W, Metreweli C. Clinical significance of the comet-tail artifact in thyroid ultrasound. *J Clin Ultrasound*. 1996;24(3):129–133.
12. Kumar V, Abbas AK, Fausto N. *Robbins and Cotran: Pathologic Basis of Disease*. 7th ed. St. Louis, Mo: Saunders; 2005.
13. Marqusee E, Benson CB, Frates MC, et al. Usefulness of ultrasonography in the management of

nodular thyroid disease. *Ann Intern Med.* 2000; 133(9):696–700.

14. Hagag P, Strauss S, Weiss M. Role of ultrasound-guided fine-needle aspiration biopsy in evaluation of nonpalpable thyroid nodules. *Thyroid.* 1998; 8(11):989–995.

15. Nam-Goong IS, Kim HY, Gong G, et al. Ultrasonography-guided fine-needle aspiration of thyroid incidentaloma: correlation with pathological findings. *Clin Endocrinol (Oxf).* 2004;60(1):21–28.

16. Papini E, Guglielmi R, Bianchini A, et al. Risk of malignancy in nonpalpable thyroid nodules: predictive value of ultrasound and color-Doppler features. *J Clin Endocrinol Metab.* 2002;87(5):1941–1946.

17. Chammas MC, Gerhard R, de Oliveira IR. Thyroid nodules: evaluation with power Doppler and duplex Doppler ultrasound. *Otolaryngol Head Neck Surg.* 2005;132(6):874–882.

18. Kim EK, Park CS, Chung WY, et al. New sonographic criteria for recommending fine-needle aspiration biopsy of nonpalpable solid nodules of the thyroid. *AJR Am J Roentgenol.* 2002;178(3): 687–691.

19. Kang HW, No JH, Chung JH, et al. Prevalence, clinical and ultrasonographic characteristics of thyroid incidentalomas. *Thyroid.* 2004;14(1): 29–33.

20. Seiberling KA, Dutra JC, Grant T, Bajramovic S. Role of intrathyroidal calcifications detected on ultrasound as a marker of malignancy. *Laryngoscope.* 2004;114(10):1753–1757.

21. Solbiati L, Volterrani L, Rizzatto G, et al. The thyroid gland with low uptake lesions: evaluation by ultrasound. *Radiology.* 1985;155(1):187–191.

22. Gorman B, Charboneau JW, James EM, et al. Medullary thyroid carcinoma: role of high-resolution US. *Radiology.* 1987;162(1 pt 1):147–150.

23. Baskin HJ, ed. *Thyroid Ultrasound and Ultrasound-Guided FNA Biopsy.* Norwell, Mass: Kluwer Academic Publishers; 2000.

24. Alexander EK, Marqusee E, Orcutt J, et al. Thyroid nodule shape and prediction of malignancy. *Thyroid.* 2004;14(11):953–958.

25. Miyakawa M, Onoda N, Etoh M, et al. Diagnosis of thyroid follicular carcinoma by the vascular pattern and velocimetric parameters using high resolution pulsed and power Doppler ultrasonography. *Endocr J.* 2005;52(2):207–212.

26. Larsen PR, Kronenberg HM, Melmed Shlomo, Polonsky KS, Wilson JD, Foster DW. *Williams Textbook of Endocrinology.* 10th ed. Philadelphia, Pa: Saunders; 2002.

27. Thieblemont C, Mayer A, Dumontet C, et al. Primary thyroid lymphoma is a heterogeneous disease. *J Clin Endocrinol Metab.* 2002;87(1):105–111.

28. Kato I, Tajima K, Suchi T, et al. Chronic thyroiditis as a risk factor of B-cell lymphoma in the thyroid gland. *Jpn J Cancer Res.* 1985;76(11):1085–1090.

29. Holm LE, Blomgren H, Lowhagen T. Cancer risks in patients with chronic lymphocytic thyroiditis. *N Engl J Med.* 1985;312(10):601–604.

30. Baldini M, Orsatti A, Bonfanti MT, Castagnone D, Cantalamessa L. Relationship between the sonographic appearance of the thyroid and the clinical course and autoimmune activity of Graves' disease. *J Clin Ultrasound.* 2005;33(8):381–385.

31. Caruso G, Attard M, Caronia A, Lagalla R. Color Doppler measurement of blood flow in the inferior thyroid artery in patients with autoimmune thyroid diseases. *Eur J Radiol.* 2000;36(1): 5–10.

32. Saleh A, Furst G, Feldkamp J, Godehardt E, Grust A, Modder U. Estimation of antithyroid drug dose in Graves' disease: value of quantification of thyroid blood flow with color duplex sonography. *Ultrasound Med Biol.* 2001;27(8):1137–1141.

33. Varsamidis K, Varsamidou E, Mavropoulos G. Doppler ultrasonography in predicting relapse of hyperthyroidism in Graves' disease. *Acta Radiol.* 2000;41(1):45–48.

34. Saleh A, Cohnen M, Furst G, Modder U, Feldkamp J. Prediction of relapse after antithyroid drug therapy of Graves' disease: value of color Doppler sonography. *Exp Clin Endocrinol Diabetes.* 2004;112(9):510–513.

35. Cohen O, Pinhas-Hamiel O, Sivan E, Dolitski M, Lipitz S, Achiron R. Serial in utero ultrasonographic measurements of the fetal thyroid: a new complementary tool in the management of maternal hyperthyroidism in pregnancy. *Prenat Diag.* 2003;23(9):740–742.

36. Bogazzi F, Bartalena L, Brogioni S, et al. Color flow Doppler sonography rapidly differentiates type I and type II amiodarone-induced thyrotoxicosis. *Thyroid.* 1997;7(4):541–545.

37. Eaton SE, Euinton HA, Newman CM, Weetman AP, Bennet WM. Clinical experience of amiodarone-induced thyrotoxicosis over a 3-year period: role of colour-flow Doppler sonography. *Clin Endocrinol (Oxf).* 2002;56(1):33–38.

38. Mandel SJ. A 64-year-old woman with a thyroid nodule. *JAMA.* 2004;292(21):2632–2642.

39. Roti E, Rossi R, Trasforini G, et al. Clinical and histological characteristics of papillary thyroid micro-

carcinoma: results of a retrospective study in 243 patients. *J Clin Endocrinol Metab*. 2006;91(6):2171-2178.

40. Shimura H, Haraguchi K, Hiejima Y, et al. Distinct diagnostic criteria for ultrasonographic examination of papillary thyroid carcinoma: a multicenter study. *Thyroid*. 2005;15(3):251-258.

41. Hegedus L. Thyroid ultrasound. *Endocrinol Metab Clin North Am*. 2001;30(2):339-360, viii-ix.

42. Green LD, Mack L, Pasieka JL. Anaplastic thyroid cancer and primary thyroid lymphoma: a review of these rare thyroid malignancies. *J Surg Oncol*. 2006;94(8):725-736.

43. Stulak JM, Grant CS, Farley DR, et al. Value of preoperative ultrasonography in the surgical management of initial and reoperative papillary thyroid cancer. *Arch Surg*. 2006;141(5):489-494; discussion 494-496.

Chapter 6

PARATHYROID ULTRASONOGRAPHY

David L. Steward
Mikhail Vaysberg

High-resolution ultrasound evaluation of the neck can be very sensitive in the detection of enlarged parathyroid glands in patients with known hyperparathyroidism, especially in the detection of solitary adenomas in primary hyperparathyroidism. Reported sensitivities range from 53 to 93% with experience of the sonographer as the most important factor.[1] Compared with sonographic evaluation of the thyroid gland, parathyroid detection and localization is relatively more challenging.[1,2]

Office-based ultrasonography (US) can reliably localize adenomas to correct side and location (right vs left and superior vs inferior) in 90% of cases, with greater sensitivity than sestamibi scanning. The greater anatomic detail of US provides significantly greater preoperative localization information for the surgeon than other radionuclide imaging, especially if performed personally.[3-5] Another advantage of US for parathyroid localization is identification of coexistent thyroid nodularity, permitting preoperative evaluation by US-guided fine needle biopsy that may lead to appropriate surgical or nonsurgical management of thyroid disease as indicated.[6-8] US-guided parathyroid fine needle biopsy (see Chapter 12) can occasionally be helpful but is not routinely necessary given the characteristic sonographic features in a patient with biochemical evidence of primary hyperparathyroidism.[9-11]

Normal-sized parathyroid glands (<40 mg) are not usually distinguishable with currently available equipment for high-resolution ultrasonography (7-15 MHz). Localization of enlarged parathyroid glands (>100 mg) begins with a careful and deliberately slow transverse (axial) scanning technique focusing first on one side of the neck and then the other. The entire anterior and lateral neck should be examined, but initial focus is in the central neck in the region of normal parathyroid gland distribution.[12,13]

Starting inferiorly on the right side, the linear transducer can be angled inferiorly to identify the innominate artery in the superior mediastinum and then follow the carotid artery takeoff superiorly focusing attention between the carotid on the left side of the screen and the midportion of the trachea on the right side of the screen (Fig 6-1). Transverse scanning should proceed slowly in the superior direction beyond the superior pole of the thyroid (Fig 6-2).[2]

Longitudinal (sagittal) scanning is sometimes a challenge for the novice sonographer but can occasionally detect adenomas missed with transverse/axial scanning; it is critical for accurate, three-dimensional localization, which facilitates easy surgical localization (Fig 6-3). Longitudinal scanning should start with visualization of the great vessels laterally followed by slow angling and/or moving of the transducer

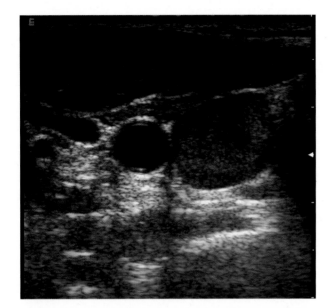

Fig 6–1. Transverse ultrasound image of a large right inferior parathyroid adenoma.

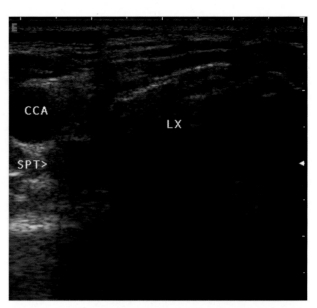

Fig 6–2. Transverse ultrasound image of a right superior parathyroid adenoma (*SPT*), just lateral to the larynx (*LX*) and deep to the common carotid artery (*CCA*).

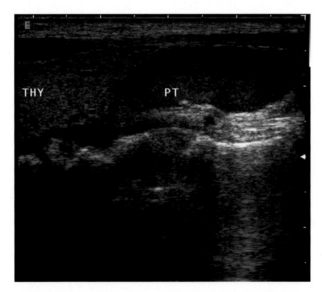

Fig 6–3. Longitudinal (*sagittal*) ultrasound image of the same right inferior parathyroid adenoma as in Figure 6–1.

medially until the trachea is visualized. Tilting the superior edge of the transducer into the patient will result in "toeing in" and permit better inferior imaging of the thoracic inlet. Allowing the inferior edge of the transducer to drop into the sternal notch will also help.

Transverse scanning on the left should begin by tilting the transducer inferiorly to visualize the subclavian vessels and then slowly proceeding superiorly with attention focused between the carotid laterally (right side of screen) and trachea and esophagus medially (left side of screen). Longitudinal scanning proceeds from lateral to medial as described above for the right side (Fig 6–4).

Parathyroid glands are most often hypoechoic relative to the thyroid gland (Figs 6–5A and 6–5B). They can rarely be nearly anechoic or cystic, and occasionally nearly isoechoic relative to the thyroid (Figs 6–6A and 6–6B, and Video 6A). Patients with thyroiditis will often have hypoechoic reactive lymph nodes adjacent to the thyroid gland which can be differentiated from parathyroid adenomas by their hyperechoic hilum and hilar rather than polar blood supply identified with color Doppler.[14-17] However, reactive paratracheal lymph nodes are often too small to display their hila (Fig 6–7A and 6–7B). Identification of irregular or enlarged, metastatic-appearing lymph nodes should raise suspicion for concomitant papillary or medullary thyroid carcinoma, or other malignancy. Such lesions should undergo fine needle biopsy and possibly serum calcitonin testing, along with even greater sonographic scrutiny of the thyroid gland. Parathyroid carcinoma is a much less likely possibility unless the thyroid has no evidence of nodularity and the enlarged parathyroid gland demonstrates irregular borders or evidence of invasion of adjacent structures.[18] Parathyroid carcinoma should likewise be suspected when clinical evidence includes an unusually high serum calcium level (ie, >14 mg/dL), a markedly elevated intact PTH level (3 or more times the upper limit of normal), significant elevation of serum alkaline phosphatase level, and even a palpable neck mass.[19,20]

When orthotopic in location, inferior parathyroid adenomas are most often visualized just inferior to the inferior lobe of the thyroid gland and sometimes just posterior to it. The superior parathyroid glands are almost always on the posterior aspect of the mid-portion of the thyroid gland, in a deeper plane than the inferior glands.[21] The distinction between superior and inferior parathyroid glands can at times be challenging, even during surgical exploration.[22] The inferior parathyroid glands lie anterior (ventral) to the plane of the recurrent laryngeal nerve whereas the superior parathyroid glands lie posterior (dorsal) to this plane. Using the inferior thyroid artery and/or the posterior surface of the common carotid artery as a surrogate marker for the plane of the recurrent laryngeal nerve, adenomas located entirely deep to the posterior surface of the artery are most often superior parathyroid glands even if located in a somewhat more inferior location than typical.[23,24]

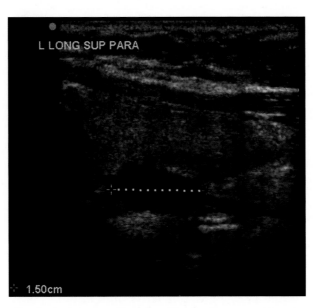

Fig 6–4. Longitudinal (*sagittal*) ultrasound image of a left superior parathyroid adenoma.

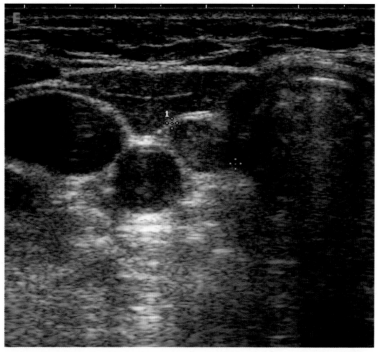

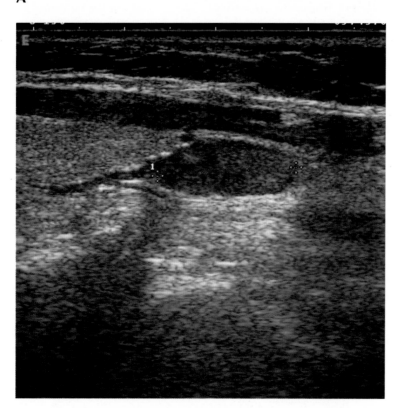

Fig 6–5. Parathyroid adenomas are usually homogeneous and hypoechoic relative to thyroid parenchyma. Transverse (**A**) and sagittal (**B**) views of a large right inferior parathyroid adenoma.

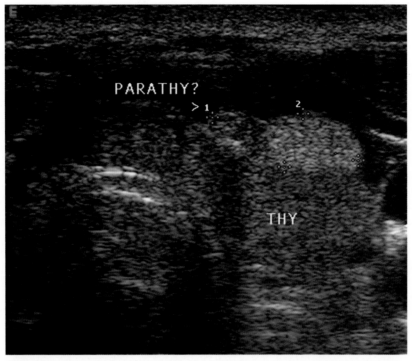

A

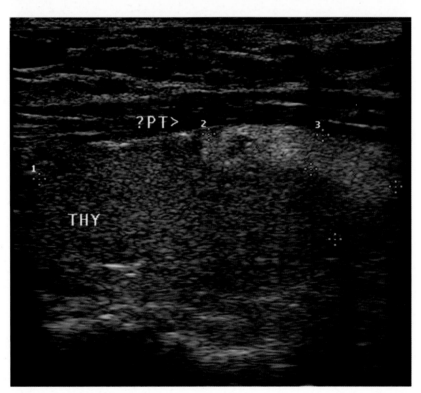

B

Fig 6–6 and Video 6A. A relatively hyperechoic parathyroid adenoma on the anterior surface of the left thyroid lobe, confirmed by surgery. Left transverse (**A**) and left sagittal (**B**) views, and ascending left transverse view (**Video 6A**).

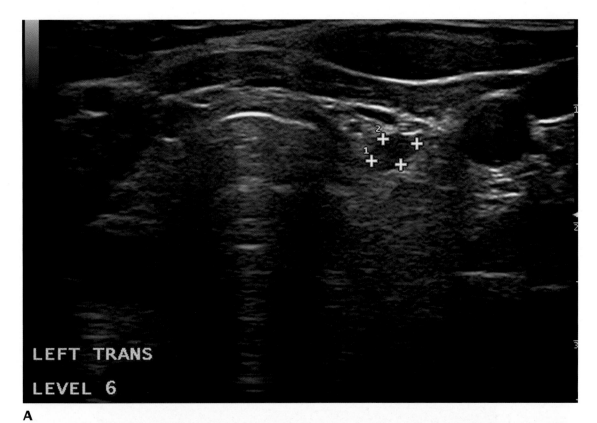

A

B

Figs 6–7A and B. Reactive lymph nodes in the level 6 region, such as those seen in this patient with Hashimoto's thyroiditis, can appear similar to enlarged parathyroid glands.

If an enlarged parathyroid gland is not identified on either side of the neck using transverse and longitudinal scanning, then the possibility of an ectopic location is raised. First, however, the far-field and/or overall gain of the US system should be increased and the frequency decreased to improve sound penetration and be sure that a deep superior adenoma has not been missed or obscured by the prevertebral musculature (Fig 6–8). An adenoma can be clearly distinguished from prevertebral muscles in "real time" by slowly scanning back and forth and seeing the hypoechoic ovoid mass come into and out of view (Video 6B). The prevertebral muscles run longitudinally and continue to be visualized throughout.[25]

Knowledge of common ectopic locations for both superior and inferior parathyroid glands is helpful when searching for an as yet nonlocalized adenoma.[23,26-28] Superior glands can be in a posterior plane from the hyoid to the posterior mediastinum, in positions that include: posterior to the carotid sheath; intrathyroidal, most often posterior,

when "caught" by the ultimobrachial body (Fig 6–9); and retropharyngeal, retroesophageal, and retrotracheal. Ectopic adenomas in the posterior mediastinum are not likely to be identified with cervical ultrasound and are more conducive to radionuclide imaging, but most other ectopic locations are readily identifiable. To overcome shadow artifact related to the carotid artery and trachea, scanning from a more lateral position will often reveal the hidden adenoma. Manipulating the patient's head position can also help expose parathyroid glands that are hidden behind these structures. Suspected intrathyroidal parathyroid adenomas can undergo ultrasound-guided fine needle biopsy with cytology to rule out thyroid malignancy; furthermore, needle rinsing with 0.5 to 1 cc of saline for chemical identification of intact parathyroid hormone is better able to discriminate parathyroid from thyroid (Fig 6–10 and Video 6C).[12,18]

Inferior ectopic parathyroid glands can be in an anterior plane from the hyoid to the anterior mediastinum, with the majority being within or in close

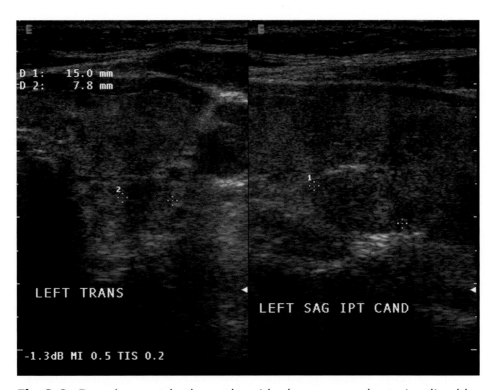

Fig 6–8. Deep/prevertebral parathyroid adenomas are best visualized by increasing the far-field gain and decreasing the US frequency.

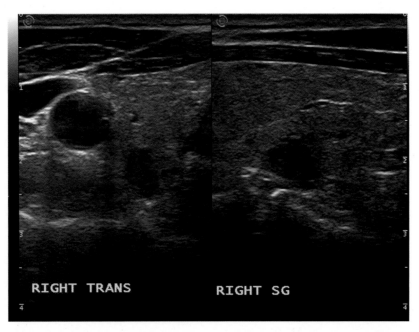

Fig 6–9. Intrathyroidal right superior parathyroid adenoma (transverse and sagittal views). Initial negative right-sided parathyroid exploration followed by right thyroid lobectomy led to an appropriate decline in intraoperative parathyroid hormone (IOPTH) level and subsequent sustained normocalcemia.

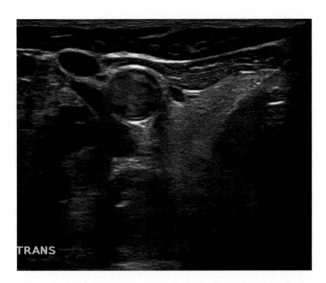

Fig 6–10. Ultrasound-guided FNA of a right inferior parathyroid adenoma. The sample is analyzed both by cytology and for parathyroid hormone. Note needle shaft passing through thyroid, and bright bevel of needle tip within parathyroid.

proximity to the thymus at the thoracic inlet or superior mediastinum Such glands are still often amenable to identification with US and resection through a cervical approach.[29-31]

Parathyroid hyperplasia can be seen in primary hyperthyroidism and is more common in patients with a positive family history and/or multiple endocrine neoplasia (MEN) syndromes I and IIa (Fig 6–11A–D).[32] Parathyroid hyperplasia is expected in secondary and tertiary hyperparathyroidism and is usually easily identified by US if the hyperparathyroidism is severe enough to warrant surgical intervention (Fig 6–12). Hyperplastic parathyroid glands have the same sonographic features and locations as parathyroid adenomas described above.[29,33] However, sporadic hyperplasia is sometimes difficult to identify with US, especially if one gland is predominately larger and suspected of being an adenoma. Sporadic primary parathyroid hyperplasia should be suspected in patients with both negative (nonlocalizing) cervical US exam and negative (nonlocalizing) sestamibi scans

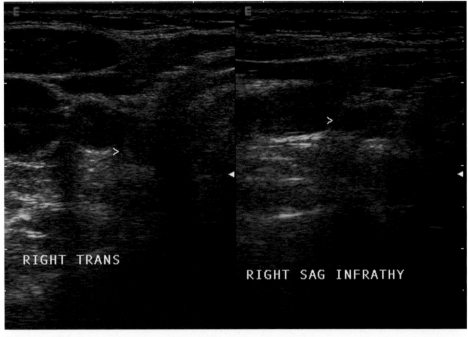

A

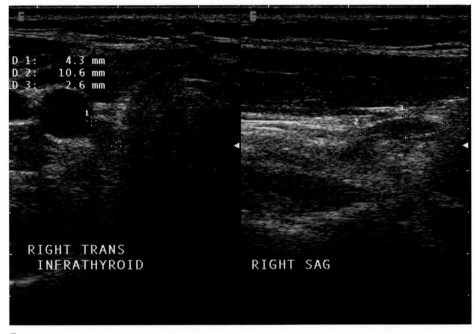

B

Fig 6–11. Parathyroid hyperplasia in a patient with MEN I syndrome. **A.** transverse and sagittal views of right inferior parathyroid gland. **B.** Transverse and sagittal views of relatively low-lying right superior parathyroid gland. *continues*

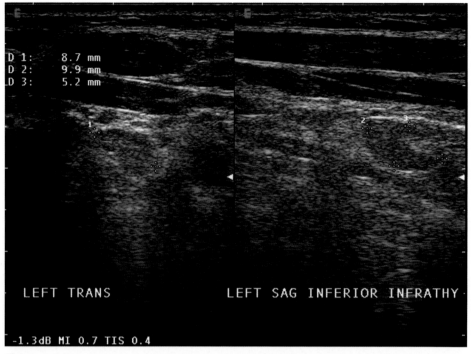

D 1:   8.7 mm
D 2:   9.9 mm
D 3:   5.2 mm

LEFT TRANS   LEFT SAG INFERIOR INFRATHY

-1.3dB MI 0.7 TIS 0.4

C

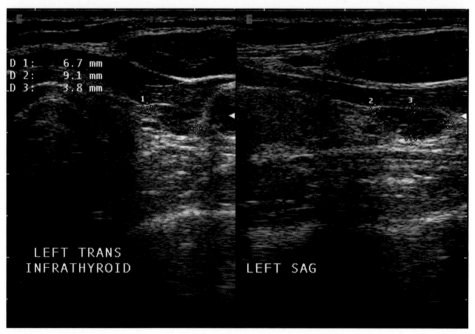

D 1:   6.7 mm
D 2:   9.1 mm
D 3:   3.8 mm

LEFT TRANS
INFRATHYROID   LEFT SAG

D

Fig 6–11. *continued* **C.** Transverse and sagittal views of left inferior parathyroid gland. **D.** Transverse and sagittal views of left superior parathyroid gland.

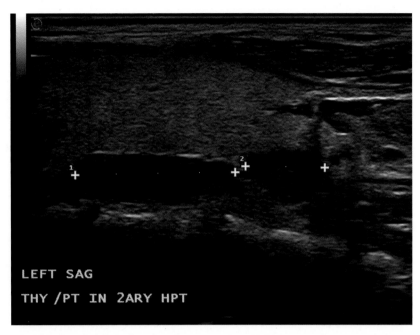

LEFT SAG

THY /PT IN 2ARY HPT

Fig 6–12. Left sagittal view of hyperplastic superior and inferior parathyroid glands in secondary hyperparathyroidism.

as these glands, in spite of their collective hyperfunction, can remain too small for accurate localization.[22,34] Even when asymmetric hyperplasia is present and fewer than four enlarged parathyroid glands are identified, the presence of two or more candidate glands by US may be sufficient to prepare the surgeon for a higher likelihood of bilateral exploration being necessary.

US can be used intraoperatively to reconfirm parathyroid location and guide incisions for minimally invasive parathyroidectomy. Real-time US allows the surgeon performing parathyroidectomy to visualize the parathyroid lesion(s) in the context of the surrounding anatomy that is beyond the ultrasound transducer's field of view by captured images. US can also be repeated following sestamibi scanning to corroborate findings or occasionally to identify a parathyroid lesion that was previously missed on initial US exam. US and sestamibi scanning are thus complementary localization techniques, and are ideally used in conjunction with one another.

Summary

Office-based US for parathyroid localization is a conceptually and logistically simple and rewarding technique that is enhanced by experience and motivation. Surgeons who perform parathyroid surgery are familiar with the pertinent anatomy and distribution of parathyroid glands, and should easily be able to translate such knowledge into sonographic skill as well. It stands to reason that the surgeon caring for the patient with hyperparathyroidism is ideally situated to perform US examinations and utilize the information obtained in the course of managing parathyroid and concomitant disease.

Videos for This Chapter

Video 6A. See legend for Figure 6–6.

Video 6B. Scanning over a parathyroid adenoma, the lesion will come in and out of view whereas the underlying prevertebral musculature appears continuous.

Video 6C. Ultrasound-guided FNA of a left inferior parathyroid adenoma, performed in an "inverted" position (examiner/operator standing at the patient's head facing toward the feet).

References

1. Petti G, Kirk G, Parathyroid imaging. *Otolaryngol Clin North Am*. 1996;29(4):681–691.

2. Reading C, Charboneau J, James E, et al. High resolution parathyroid sonography. *Am J Radiol*. 1982;139:539–546.

3. Steward D, Danielson G, Afman C, Welge J. Parathyroid adenoma localization: surgeon-performed ultrasound versus sestamibi. *Laryngoscope*. 2006;116:1380–1384.

4. Solorzano C, Carneiro D, Ramirez M, et al. Surgeon-performed ultrasound in the management of thyroid malignancy. *Am Surg*. 2004;70(7):576–580; discussion 580–582.

5. Yeh M, Barraclough B, Sidhu S, et al. Two hundred consecutive parathyroid ultrasound studies by a single clinician: the impact of experience. *End Pract*. 2006:12(3):257–263.

6. Tomimori E, Bisi H, Medeiros-Neto G, et al. Ultrasonographic evaluation of thyroid nodules: comparison with cytologic and histologic diagnosis. *Arq Bra Endocrinol Metabol*. 2004;48(1):105–113.

7. Gooding G, Clark O. Use of Doppler imaging in distinction between thyroid and parathyroid lesions. *Am J Surg*. 1992;164:51–56.

8. Milas M, Mensah A, Alghoul M, et al. The impact of office neck ultrasonography on reducing unnecessary thyroid surgery in patients undergoing parathyroidectomy. *Thyroid*. 2005;15(9):1055–1059.

9. Baskin H. New applications of thyroid and parathyroid ultrasound. *Minerva Endocrinolog*. 2004;29(4):195–206.

10. Stephen A, Milas M, Garner C, et al. Use of surgeon-performed office ultrasound and parathyroid fine needle aspiration for complex parathyroid localization. *Surgery*. 2005;138(6):1143–1150; discussion 1150–1151.

11. Tseng F, Hsiao Y-L, Chang T-C. Ultrasound-guided fine needle aspiration cytology of parathyroid lesions. A review of 72 cases. *Acta Cytolog*. 2002;46(6):1029–1036.

12. Kane R. Ultrasound of the thyroid and parathyroid glands: controversies in the diagnosis of thyroid cancer. *Ultrasound Q*. 2003;19(4):177–178.

13. Rewerk S, Post S, Willeke F. Sonographic localisation procedures in hyperparathyroidism—persistent hyperparathyroidism after removal of four parathyroid glands. *Ultraschall in der Medizin*. 2005;26(2):146–149.

14. Ahuja A, Evans R, eds. *Practical Head and Neck Ultrasound*. London: Greenwich Medical Media Limited; 2000:37–75.

15. Jun P, Chow L, Jeffrey R. The sonographic features of papillary thyroid carcinomas. *Ultrasound Q*. 2005;21(1):39–45.

16. Pierre-Yves M, Dassonville O, Demard F. High frequency ultrasound (HFU) helps differentiating cervical lymph nodes from parathyroid adenomas. *Med Sci Monitor*. 2003;9(9): 21–22.

17. Rickes S, Neye H, Ocran K, Wermke W. High-resolution ultrasound in combination with colour-Doppler sonography for preoperative localization of parathyroid adenomas in patients with primary hyperparathyroidism. *Ultraschall in der Medizin*. 2003;24(2):85–89.

18. Kebebew E, Arici C, Duh Q, Clark O. Localization and reoperation results for persistent and recurrent parathyroid carcinoma. *Arch Surg*. 2001; 136(8):878–885.

19. Fyfe ST, Zuckerbraun L, Hoover, LA, Goodman MD. Parathyroid carcinoma: Clinical presentation and treatment. *Am J Otolaryngol*. 1990;11:268–273.

20. Barczynski M. Parathyroid neoplasm—diagnostic challenge and therapeutic difficulty. *Przeglad Lekarski*. 2000;57(3):165–167.

21. Ahuja A, Wong K, Ching A, et al. Imaging for primary hyperparathyroidism—what beginners should know. *Clin Radiol*. 2004;59(11):967–976.

22. Thompson C. Localization studies in patients with hyperparathyroidism. *Br J Surg*. 1988; 75: 97–98.

23. Gilmour J. Gross anatomy of the parathyroid glands. *J Pathol Bacteriol*. 1937;44:431–462.

24. Fallo F, Camporese G, Capitelli E, et al. Ultrasound evaluation of carotid artery in primary hyperparathyroidism. *J Clin Endocrinol Metab*. 2003;88(5): 2096–2099.

25. Barraclough B, Barraclough B. Ultrasound of the thyroid and parathyroid glands. *World J Surg*. 2000;24(2):158–165.

26. Wang C. The anatomic basis of parathyroid surgery. *Ann Surg.* 1976;183:271–275.

27. Nazarenko G, Arablinskii A, Romanov R, Bogdanova E. Current complex noninvasive diagnosis of parathyroid tumors. *Vestnik Rentgenologii i Radiologii.* 1999;(6):4–10.

28. Rewerk S, Roessner E, Freudenberg S, Willeke F. Morphological features of enlarged parathyroid glands in B-mode-ultrasound. *Ultraschall in der Medizin.* 2006;27(3):256–261.

29. Khati N, Adamson T, Johnson K, Hill M. Ultrasound of the thyroid and parathyroid glands. *Ultrasound Q.* 2003;19(4):162–176.

30. Hoover L, Blacker J, Zuckerbraun L, et al. Surgical strategy in hyperparathyroidism. *Otolaryngol Head Neck Surg.* 1987;96:542–547.

31. Meilstrup J. Ultrasound examination of the parathyroid glands. *Otolaryngol Clin North Am.* 2004; 37(4):763–778.

32. Gollini P, Cataldi A, Fava C. MEN 1 and 2: the role of diagnostic imaging. *Radiologia Medica.* 2004; 107(1–2):78–87.

33. Shaha A. Localization studies for hyperparathyroidism: implications for surgery. *Acta Oto-Rhino-Laryngologica Belgica.* 2001;55(2):139–145.

34. Solbiati L, Cova L, Tonolini M. Ultrasound of thyroid, parathyroid glands and neck lymph nodes. *Eur Radiol.* 2001;11(12):2411–2424.

Chapter 7

SALIVARY GLAND ULTRASONOGRAPHY

Peter Jecker
Lisa A. Orloff

Introduction

Ultrasonography (US) is underutilized in most North American sites for imaging of the salivary glands, yet US is the first imaging method of choice in much of Europe and Asia.[1-5] With adequate training and experience, clinicians can perform and interpret salivary gland US and frequently obviate the need for MRI or CT imaging. Due to their superficial anatomic position and their fairly homogeneous soft tissue density, the major salivary glands lend themselves well to ultrasound examination. Sialography is rarely necessary in this era of high-resolution modern US, CT, and MRI. In the case of deep lobe parotid lesions, US may not afford complete visualization due to acoustic shadowing by the mandible as well as limited sound penetration. Likewise, in certain cases of malignant salivary gland lesions, cross-sectional imaging is complementary to US and is appropriate for the assessment of tumor margins and infiltration of bone, skull base structures, and the parapharyngeal space, as well as deep lymph node metastases. On the other hand, US can easily be performed by the clinician at the time of initial evaluation for salivary gland dysfunction or distortion, and more costly imaging studies can frequently be avoided or ordered more selectively. Also, ultra-sound-guided procedures including biopsy, sclerotherapy, and therapeutic injection are quite convenient and highly successful. The physician who has familiarity with the diagnosis and management of common salivary gland diseases is ideally situated to utilize US in his or her office practice.

Anatomy

Parotid Gland

The parotid gland is located anterior to the ear and the sternocleidomastoid muscle within the face and upper neck (Fig 7–1). Parts of the normal gland overlie the mandible and the masseter muscle, and the occasional accessory parotid gland can extend anterior to the masseter within the cheek. At the anterior border of the masseter muscle and about 1 cm inferior to the zygomatic arch, the main excretory parotid duct (Stenson's duct) drains the parotid by crossing the buccinator muscle and entering the mucosa of the cheek opposite the second maxillary molar. The normal nonobstructed Stenson's duct is usually not visible by US but measures between 3 and 5 cm in length.

Fig 7–1. Normal sagittal US image of the right parotid gland with medium homogeneous echogenicity. The parotid overlies and extends posteriorly and inferiorly around the mandible.

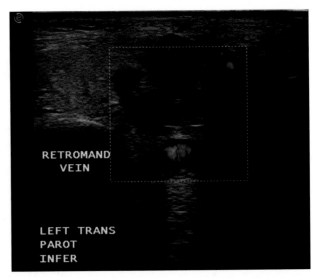

Fig 7–2. Retromandibular vein (*RMV*) immediately deep to an invasive malignant tumor of the left parotid gland (squamous cell carcinoma), seen on transverse view. The RMV can serve as a marker for the facial nerve.

The parotid gland itself is divided into superficial and deep lobes by the facial nerve and its branches, which cannot be seen by US. Visualization of the trunk of the facial nerve with high-frequency US (above 10 MHz) has been described[6] but is not expected. In comparison, MRI has attained limited views of the facial nerve trunk but it is often mistaken for salivary ducts.[7,8] As an alternative, the retromandibular vein, which lies directly in contact with the trunk of the facial nerve or its main branches,[9-11] is used as an US landmark for the facial nerve and the division between the superficial and deep parotid lobes (Fig 7–2). The retromandibular vein is similarly used as an anatomic landmark in CT and MRI imaging of the parotid gland.[11] The external carotid artery runs parallel and deep to the retromandibular vein but is usually not seen during parotid US. The deep parotid lobe is only partially visible by US due to the intervening position of the mandibular ramus. Also, the potentially high fat content of the parotid gland can render it relatively hyperechoic in comparison to adjacent muscles, and poorly penetrated by sound waves, making the retromandibular vein and other vessels and deep structures within the gland invisible on gray-scale US.

The parotid gland contains 20 to 30 lymph nodes,[12] mainly within the superficial lobe, which receive lymphatic drainage from the skin of the face, the auricle, and the external auditory canal. Normal intraparotid lymph nodes are rounded to oval and contain a relatively prominent and hyperechoic hilum (Fig 7–3). Their short axis in the benign state should not exceed 5 to 6 mm.[5,6]

Submandibular Gland

The submandibular gland lies within the posterior aspect of the submandibular triangle that is created by the anterior belly of the digastric muscle, the posterior belly of the digastric muscle, and the mandibular body. This region is also defined as level I in terms of the lymph node zones of the neck, and lymph nodes and connective tissue occupy the space anterior and superior to the submandibular gland. In transverse view, the submandibular gland is usually triangular to teardrop shaped, and may be seen to merge with the parotid or sublingual gland by parenchymal extensions (Fig 7–4). The deep part of the gland is separated from the palatine tonsil by

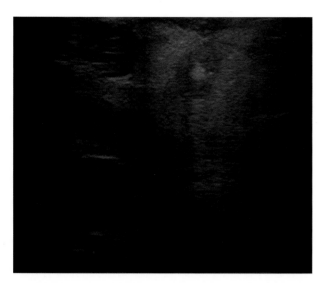

Fig 7–3. It is common to see benign intraparotid lymph nodes such as this one within normal glands.

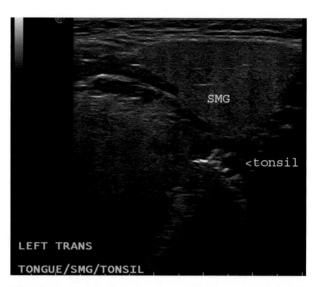

Fig 7–4. Normal transverse US image of the left submandibular gland (*SMG*), with medium echogenicity. The echogenicity may differ slightly from that of the parotid. Note the proximity to the tonsil and tongue.

the mylohyoid, hyoglossus and digastric muscles. The facial artery takes a tortuous course directly through or next to the submandibular gland, and the lingual artery may be seen medial to the gland. The facial vein runs along the anterosuperior part of the gland and may be seen to connect with the retromandibular vein posteriorly.

The submandibular duct (Wharton's duct) exits the submandibular gland near the gland's border with the mylohyoid muscle, around which it bends to course along the medial aspect of the sublingual gland to enter the floor of mouth near the anterior midline. A nondilated duct is generally not visible by US except in rare cases in thin individuals.

Sublingual Gland

The sublingual gland is less commonly affected by disease than the parotid or submandibular glands. It lies deep to the mylohyoid muscle from a submental approach, between the mandible laterally and the muscles of the floor of the mouth medially: the geniohyoid, intrinsic tongue, and hyoglossus muscles. On transverse US view it is relatively oval and on longitudinal view it is more lens-shaped (Fig 7-5). The submandibular (Wharton's) duct runs along its medial aspect. As is true during surgery, the sublin-

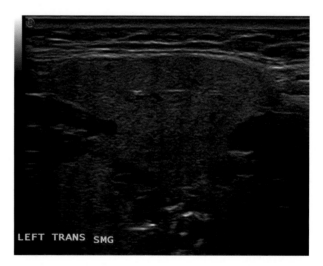

Fig 7–5. Normal sublingual gland, continuous with normal submandibular gland (*left transverse view*).

gual gland may be difficult to distinguish from the superior or deep portion of the submandibular gland, which extends superomedial to the mylohyoid muscle into the sublingual space.

The normal echogenicity of the major salivary glands is generally homogeneous and varies from very bright and hyperechoic to only slightly hyper-echoic in comparison to adjacent muscles. The echogenicity of the parenchyma depends on the amount of intraglandular fat. Salivary glands with a high fat content may be so hyperechoic that structures within their substance may be poorly penetrated and visualized on gray-scale US. Similarly, in patients who have undergone head and neck irradiation, sound penetration and anatomic definition may be poor.

The minor salivary glands are not typically distinguished by US from their harboring structures, such as the pharynx and tongue base, unless they are involved with pathologic enlargement or neoplastic growth. In such instances, minor salivary gland tumors may be visible by US depending on their size and location.

Technique

US examination of the salivary glands should be performed using a high-frequency linear array transducer, typically 7 to 12 MHz or greater. Lower frequencies may be useful in the assessment of large tumors and lesions located in the deep aspects of the glands. The salivary glands and all lesions within them should be evaluated in at least two perpendicular planes. Standard planes for major salivary gland US are the sagittal (longitudinal) plane and the transverse plane. During the US examination, the actual transducer orientation may need to be tilted slightly off true horizontal or vertical to navigate around the mandible. Also, the patient's head position can be turned and extended to improve visualization of the deep portion of the gland.

As these are paired glands, the contralateral gland should always be examined for comparison and differentiation of individual differences, unilateral diseases, and systemic processes. Furthermore, the echogenicity of the parotid glands and the submandibular glands can differ from each other physiologically within an individual patient without any disorder. The entire neck of the patient with a salivary gland disorder should be scanned to assess lymph nodes and search for concomitant or related disease.

Pathology

Because of the parotid gland's border with the masticator, parapharyngeal, and carotid spaces, it is important to consider pathologies arising from these spaces when examining the "parotid mass."

Inflammatory Conditions

Acute Inflammation

Acute sialadenitis causes painful swelling of the affected salivary gland(s). Viral sialadenitis, especially with mumps virus and cytomegalovirus, is usually bilateral and is the more common cause of acute inflammation in children.[13] Acute bacterial sialadenitis is more often unilateral and is usually caused by Staphylococcus aureus or oral flora.[14]

In acute sialadenitis, the salivary glands are enlarged and hypoechoic. They tend to be inhomogeneous, have increased blood flow, and may contain multiple small, oval, hypoechoic areas[15-19] (Figs 7–6A and 7–6B). Often there is associated cervical lymphadenopathy with enlarged nodes with increased central vascularity.

Abscess

Abscess formation may occur as a sequela of acute sialadenitis. Predisposing factors include dehydration, excretory duct obstruction by stones or fibrosis, and immunocompromise. Abscesses may be difficult to distinguish clinically from inflammation alone, as palpable fluctuance is masked by swelling in the majority of patients.[20] There may be accompanying tenderness and skin erythema.

US of salivary gland abscesses reveals hypoechoic or anechoic lesions with posterior acoustic enhancement and indistinct borders.[16,20] Central liquefaction may be recognized by avascularity or by floating debris.[15] Hyperechoic foci due to gas formation may be seen within the abscess.[12] Organized abscesses may show a surrounding hyperechoic "halo."[16] Therapeutic US-guided needle aspiration and drainage can be performed at the same time as diagnostic US.[20,21]

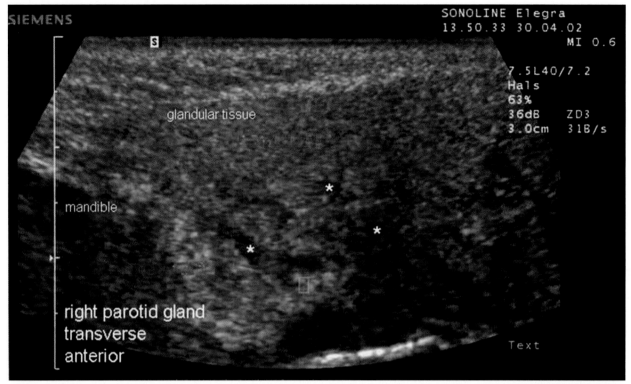

A

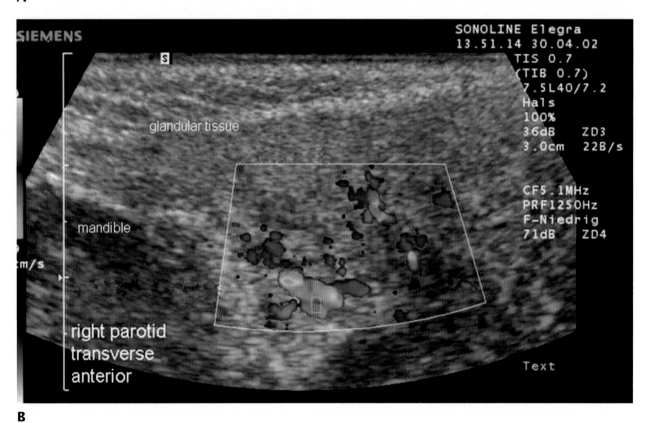

B

Fig 7–6. Acute sialadenitis of the right parotid gland. The areas of low echogenicity (**A**, *stars*) are not due to salivary stasis but to increased vascularization, as seen in the duplex mode (**B**).

Chronic Sialadenitis

The symptoms of chronic sialadenitis include intermittent, often painful, salivary gland swelling, that may or may not be associated with eating.[22] US reveals glands that are normal to small in size, hypoechoic, and heterogeneous[15,16,18] (Fig 7–7). Vascularity is usually decreased by Doppler US, but may be increased in the case of granulomatous diseases such as Heerfordt's syndrome, or parotid sarcoidosis.[23] Often seen are multiple small, round or oval, hypoechoic areas representing ectatic ducts scattered throughout the gland parenchyma (Figs 7–8A and 7–8B). Furthermore, with progression of the disease, the glandular tissue becomes increasingly hypoechoic. At the late end of the spectrum of chronic sialadenitis, the same sonographic pattern of hypoechoic glandular tissue and many lymph nodes can be seen as in patients with progressive Sjögren's syndrome. The differential diagnosis in such cases also includes granulomatous diseases such as sarcoidosis, and HIV infection.[24-27]

A unique form of chronic sialadenitis of the submandibular gland that may mimic a malignant mass is the Küttner's tumor, or chronic sclerosing sialadenitis.[28,29] Although diffuse involvement of the entire submandibular gland may occur, there may be only focal involvement with a hypoechoic, heterogeneous area within a normally shaped gland. The comparison of both submandibular glands is helpful, and whenever there is any doubt, US-guided fine needle aspiration biopsy is recommended.[30,31]

Mycobacterial disease of the major salivary glands may also present as a salivary gland mass and mimic malignancy.[32] In tuberculosis, caseous necrosis may produce focal hypoechoic to anechoic zones without color flow by Doppler.[33] Actinomycosis of the salivary glands can also manifest as a hypoechoic area with poorly defined margins.[34]

In chronic sialadenitis, intraparotid and cervical lymphadenopathy may be present, but the normal sonographic nodal architecture (homogeneous cortex, hyperechoic hilum) is preserved.[35]

Sjögren's Syndrome

Sjögren's syndrome is a chronic autoimmune disorder that is characterized by intense lymphocytic and

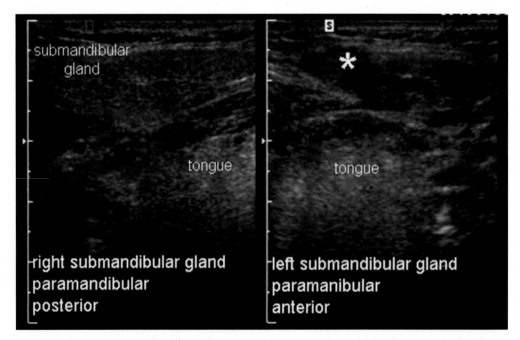

Fig 7–7. Chronic sialadenitis of the left submandibular gland. The comparison to the normal right submandibular gland reveals relative atrophy and poor echogenicity on the left.

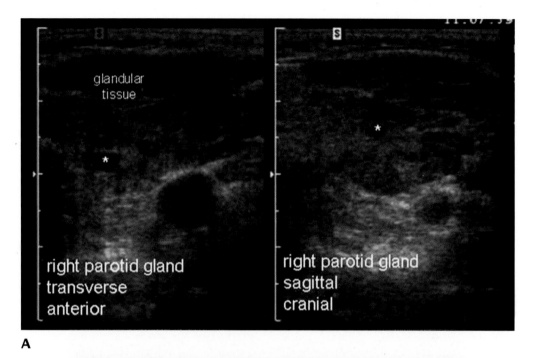

A

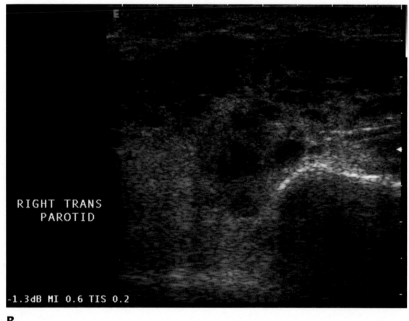

B

Fig 7–8. Chronic parotitis. **A.** Chronic right parotitis, shown in transverse and sagittal planes. The atrophied gland is hypoechoic with an enlarged ductal system (*stars*). **B.** Right transverse view of parotid with chronic parotitis in a patient with systemic lupus erythematosis.

plasma cell infiltration and destruction of the salivary and lacrimal glands.[36] It predominantly affects women over the age of 40 years, and causes clinical symptoms of dry mouth and dry eyes. US features of advanced Sjögren's syndrome include heterogeneity of the salivary glands with scattered multiple small, oval or round, hypoechoic or anechoic areas (Fig 7–9). There is also increased blood flow as noted by Doppler sonography.[15,24,37] Hypoechoic areas are believed to represent destroyed salivary parenchyma, infiltration by lymphoid cells, and dilated ducts.

Sjögren's syndrome is associated with reactive and neoplastic lymphoproliferative disease.[38] US monitoring of patients with Sjögren's syndrome is appropriate for the early detection of lymphoma,[39,40] and a low threshold should be maintained for US-guided biopsy of enlarging lesions.[15]

Calculous Disease

Sialolithiasis

Salivary stones or sialoliths occur far more often in the submandibular glands (up to 90% of cases[41–44]) than in the parotid glands (10–20% of cases[45]), due to the greater mucus content of the submandibular saliva. Calculi are usually single but can be multiple. Sialolithiasis causes partial or complete mechanical obstruction of the salivary duct, leading to recurrent swelling of the salivary gland during eating and pre-disposition to bacterial infection.[42] Submandibular sialoliths in the distal part of Wharton's duct may be palpable in the floor of the mouth. Stones within the proximal duct or the parenchyma itself require diagnostic imaging for detection.

Plain radiography, including occlusal view dental x-rays, can detect large radioopaque stones,[46] but do not provide useful information about the host salivary gland. CT reveals large stones and their surrounding gland but does not enable assessment of the ducts nor precise localization of stones within the ductal system.[47] MR sialography is a newer technique for assessing salivary ducts and stones.[1,48,49] Digital sialography remains the standard against which other methods of salivary duct imaging are compared. Sialendoscopy is yet another newer method of internally examining the salivary duct system, using miniaturized fiberoptic endoscopes, but even this procedure is invasive, albeit potentially therapeutic.[44] US is a noninvasive, well-established,

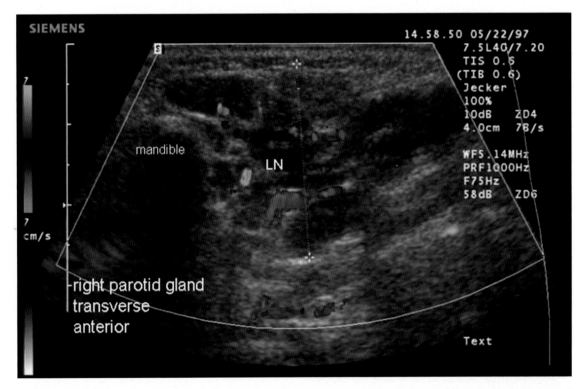

Fig 7–9. Sjögrens syndrome (advanced stage): Similar to Figure 7–8, the atrophied parotid gland is hypoechoic, and an enlarged intraglandular lymph node (*LN*) is detectable.

and painless method for detecting salivary stones, with high sensitivity (up to 94%), specificity (100%), and accuracy (96%).[50,48] Although stones smaller than 2 to 3 mm may be easily overlooked because of the absence of acoustic shadow,[51,52] if meticulous US technique is applied, intraglandular and even intraductal stones can usually be identified. Also, US can demonstrate inflammatory changes within the sali-vary gland parenchyma, which occur in about 50% of patients with sialolithiasis.[17] One must be careful not to misinterpret hyperechoic bubbles of air mixed with saliva within Wharton's duct as calculi.[12]

On US, sialoliths appear as hyperechoic lines or points with posterior acoustic shadowing[16] (Figs 7–10A, 7–10B, and 7–10C). When the duct is completely occluded, proximal ductal dilatation

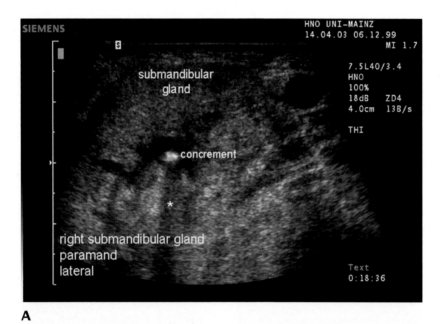

A

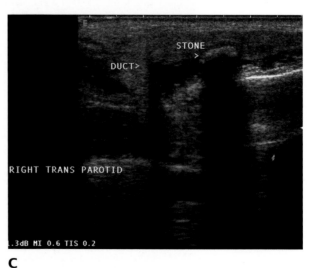

B   **C**

Fig 7–10. Sialolithiasis. **A.** The acoustic shadow (*star*) of the stone is a key to the diagnosis of submandibular sialolithiasis. This right submandibular gland itself is enlarged. **B.** Distal stone, with posterior shadow, within Stensen's duct overlying the masseter muscle. **C.** Intraparotid stone with posterior shadow and proximal ductal dilatation (*right transverse view*).

will be visible as a hypoechoic tubular structure that is distinguished from blood vessels by the absence of color flow by Doppler sonography. When chronic duct obstruction leads to chronic inflammation, the gland may lose its secretory function, in which case its ductal system may not be dilated and therefore will be difficult to visualize.[53]

Scarring of Wharton's or Stenson's duct can also result in ductal obstruction and the typical clinical symptoms, but in this situation, the duct is dilated proximal to the stenosis but appears to end abruptly at the area of stenosis without a visible calculus (Fig 7-11). If the patient's history is suspect for sialolithiasis but US is unrevealing, as part of the examination the patient can be given sialagogues such as lemon drops to stimulate saliva secretion and to enhance visualization of Wharton's duct as it retains saliva and dilates. Furthermore, bimanual palpation during US (digital palpation of the floor of the mouth with one hand while applying external application of the transducer with the other hand) can facilitate visualization of ductal stones.

Sialolithiasis of the parotid gland involving Stenson's duct can be detected over the masseter mus-cle, exiting the parotid gland (Fig 7-12). The small, more proximal ductal system within the gland is difficult to differentiate from enlarged blood vessels during acute sialadenitis. Here, the use of duplex sonography is very helpful (see Fig 7-6B).

Benign and Malignant Salivary Tumors

The majority of salivary gland tumors are benign (70-80%) and located in the parotid glands (80-90%). Conversely, although a minority of tumors are located in the submandibular glands, almost half of these are malignant.[54,55] Although it is not possible to definitively distinguish benign from malignant salivary gland tumors using US, tumor characteristics such as size, shape, location, borders, and vascularity can be assessed, and US-guided fine needle biopsy can often be easily performed.

Benign Neoplasms

The most common benign neoplasms of the major salivary glands are pleomorphic adenomas (benign mixed tumors). Clinically, these tumors present as

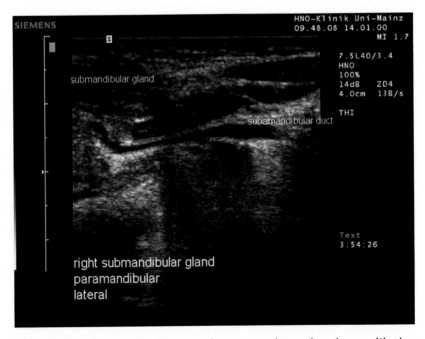

Fig 7-11. Stasis of saliva within an enlarged submandibular duct without a stone.

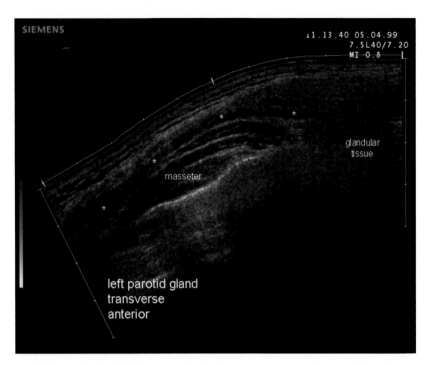

Fig 7–12. Enlarged Stenson's duct (*stars*) in a patient with salivary stasis of the parotid.

slowly growing, painless masses. Smaller tumors and deep lobe parotid tumors may be detected incidentally by US or by cross-sectional imaging performed for other purposes. Most pleomorphic adenomas arise in the parotid gland (60–90%), and are solitary and unilateral. They may occur at any age but their peak incidence is in the fourth and fifth decades of life, and they occur somewhat more often in women than in men.[54,55] Untreated pleomorphic adenomas may undergo malignant transformation (carcinoma ex pleomorphic adenoma) or behave in a clinically aggressive and metastasizing manner even when appearing histologically benign.[13,56] Surgically treated pleomorphic adenomas that experience intraoperative rupture or transection have a very high rate of multifocal local recurrence.[57]

On US, pleomorphic adenomas are hypoechoic, well-defined, lobulated tumors with posterior acoustic enhancement (Figs 7-13A, 7-13B, and 7-13C). Lobulation is one of their more distinctive features.[58] They may be homogeneous or inhomogeneous and may contain calcifications.[58-61] Vascularity is usually but not always poor or absent.[58-61]

Recurrent pleomorphic adenomas appear as multiple hypoechoic nodules within the salivary gland bed by US (Fig 7-14).

Warthin tumor (papillary cystadenoma lymphomatosum) is the second most common benign salivary neoplasm (5–10% of all salivary neoplasms).[55] These tumors occur most often in the parotid glands of male smokers in the fifth and sixth decades of life,[55,62] and not infrequently, they occur bilaterally, either simultaneously or metachronously.[54,63,64]

Sonographically, Warthin tumors appear as oval, hypoechoic, well-circumscribed tumors that may contain multiple anechoic areas.[19,61,64,65] They may or may not show hypervascularity, and they generally show posterior acoustic enhancement (Figs 7-15A and 7-15B and Video 7A). Warthin tumors may also appear as a simple cyst by US and require differentiation from other benign and malignant cystic lesions of the salivary glands.[58,66]

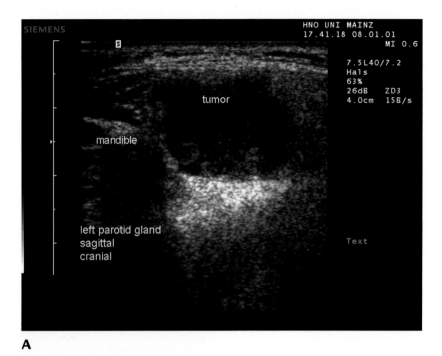

A

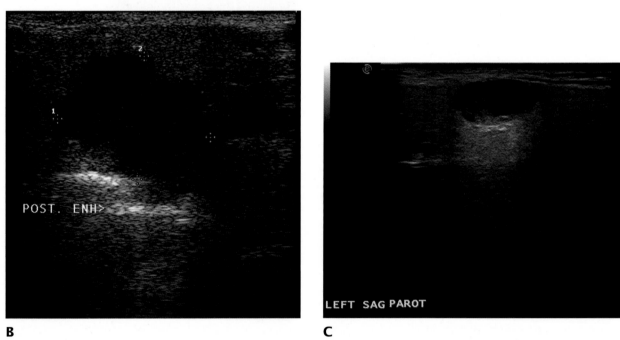

B

C

Fig 7–13. Pleomorphic adenoma of the parotid gland. Note lobulation and posterior acoustic enhancement; tumors may be homogeneous or heterogeneous. **A.** Left sagittal tail of parotid tumor; **B.** Left sagittal parotid with homogeneous tumor; **C.** Left sagittal view of a somewhat heterogeneous tumor that is well circumscribed.

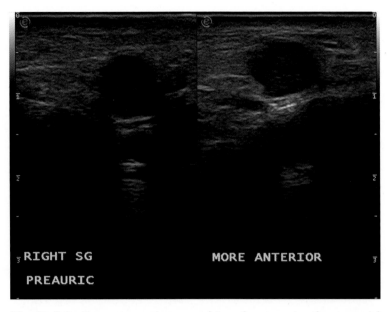

Fig 7–14. Recurrent pleomorphic adenoma in the parotid bed. Note multiple small hypoechoic nodules (*right sagittal views*).

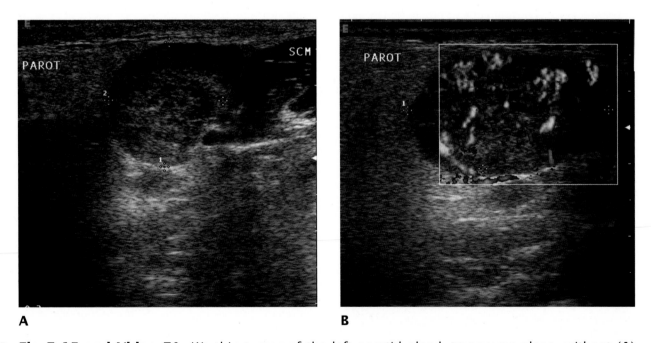

A
B

Fig 7–15 and Video 7A. Warthin tumor of the left parotid gland, transverse plane, without (**A**) and with (**B**) color Doppler. This particular tumor is heterogeneous and shows posterior acoustic enhancement. **Video 7A** shows another heterogeneous Warthin tumor on transverse ascending view through the left parotid.

Other Benign Tumors

Other rare benign tumors can arise from the salivary gland parenchyma (eg, oncocytoma, basal cell adenoma), but they do not have any specific or distinctive US features (Fig 7–16). Nonsalivary tumors can manifest within the major salivary glands (especially the parotids), and these include lipomas, schwannomas, hemangiomas, and other vascular malformations.[67-72]

Lipomas can occur anywhere in the body, and as with other locations, lipomas in the salivary glands appear on US as oval or elongated masses with sharp margins and a "feathered" or striated pattern of hyperechoic streaks throughout the lesion[15,73] (Fig 7–17 and Video 7B). Lipomas are typically hypovascular, and resemble somewhat the sonographic appearance of striated muscle. Clinically they are soft and somewhat compressible. Hemangiomas are the most common benign tumors in infants, and within the salivary glands they appear as heterogeneous lesions with sinusoidal spaces and calcifications that correspond with phleboliths.[69] They may be lobulated and septated, and their key sonographic feature is prominent vascularity by Doppler

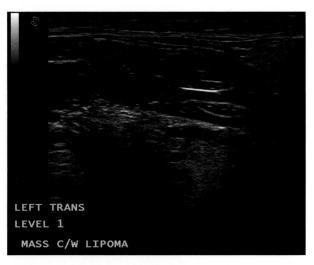

LEFT TRANS
LEVEL 1
MASS C/W LIPOMA

Fig 7–17 and Video 7B. Lipoma of the left submandibular gland, transverse plane. Transverse ascending **Video 7B** demonstrates separation of the left submandibular mass from the tongue by the thin hypoechoic mylohyoid muscle.

imaging (Fig 7–18). Other vascular lesions may manifest in the cheek and parotid of adults.[69] Neurogenic tumors tend to appear as fusiform lesions with anechoic areas.[72]

Malignant Neoplasms

Malignant neoplasms account for approximately 20% of all salivary gland tumors. The smaller the salivary gland in which a tumor arises, the greater its malignant potential; benign tumors of the minor salivary glands are relatively rare, and in the major salivary glands, a tumor of the sublingual or submandibular gland is much more likely to be malignant than is a tumor in the parotid gland. Classic US features of advanced malignant neoplasms of the salivary glands are like those in other organs, and include an irregular shape, irregular borders, hypoechogenicity, and heterogeneity.[12,19,74-77] However, malignant tumors may also be homogeneous, well-defined, cystic, and even lobulated similar to pleomorphic adenomas.[58,77-79] Even with malignant-appearing characteristics, it is not possible to distinguish between different histologic types of malignancy by US (Fig 7–19). Similarly, Doppler

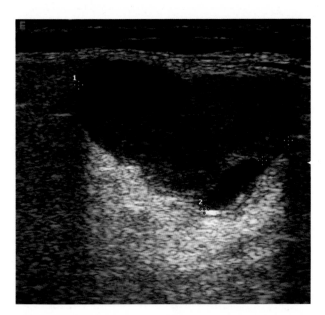

Fig 7–16. Benign basal cell adenoma of the right parotid, sagittal view. Tumor is well circumscribed and shows posterior acoustic enhancement.

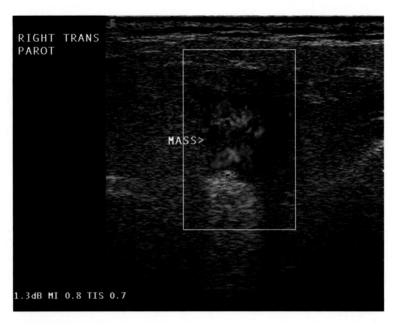

Fig 7–18. Vascular malformation of the right parotid, transverse plane.

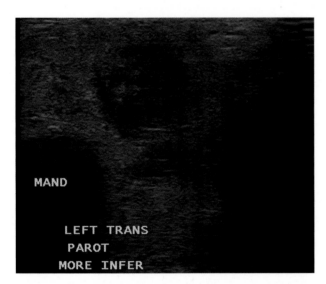

Fig 7–19. Invasive multifocal tumor in the left inferior parotid gland, seen on transverse view. Although the tumor is poorly circumscribed and heterogeneous, there are no pathognomonic features by US that can distinguish histologic type.

US does not allow reliable differentiation between benign and malignant salivary gland tumors.[60] Some malignant lesions show high vascularity and high systolic peak flow velocity[60] whereas others show increased intratumoral vascular resistance.[80] Hemorrhage into a tumor may create heterogeneous cystic and solid-appearing areas.

Malignant salivary gland tumors may grow rapidly, be fixed to the skin or the underlying soft tissues or bone, be painful or tender to palpation, be associated with lymph node mestastases, and cause facial nerve paralysis or paresis.[13,54]

The most common salivary gland malignancies are mucoepidermoid carcinoma and adenoid cystic carcinoma. Acinic cell carcinoma, squamous cell carcinoma, adenocarcinoma, and metastases from local (skin; squamous cell carcinoma, and melanoma) or distant (eg, breast, lung) primary tumors are also seen but are less common (Figs 7–20A, 7–20B, and 7–20C). The presence of abnormal-appearing lymph nodes or nodules within the parotid, even when small, should prompt a thorough head and neck exam with particular attention to the skin of the scalp and ears.

Mucoepidermoid carcinoma ranges from low-grade to high-grade with corresponding aggressiveness; it arises mostly in the parotid gland, and can occur at any age but its peak incidence is between 30 and 50 years of age[13] (Fig 7–21).

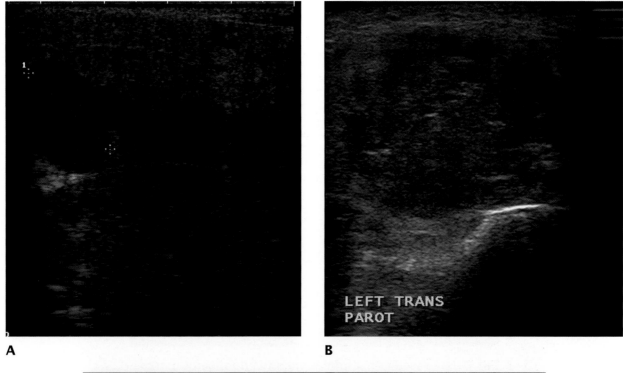

A   B

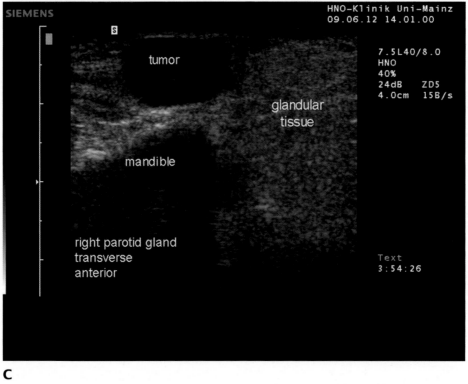

C

Fig 7–20. Malignant tumors in the parotid gland do not have pathognomonic features. **A.** Acinic cell carcinoma of the deep left parotid gland (*sagittal view*). This patient presented with severe facial pain and tenderness and US-guided FNA of this mass was exquisitely painful. **B.** Squamous cell carcinoma of the left parotid, (*transverse plane*). Note irregular margins and solid heterogeneous mass. This tumor was also painful and rapidly progressive. **C.** Adenocarcinoma of the left parotid gland. A tumor capsule is not detectable, there is no posterior acoustic enhancement, and subtle infiltration of the glandular tissue is apparent.

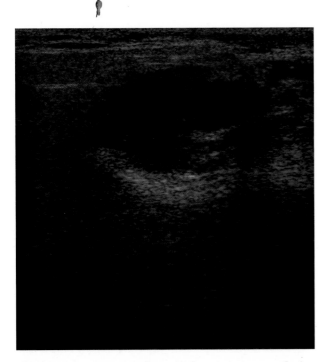

Fig 7–21. Mucoepidermoid carcinoma of the right parotid gland (*transverse view*). Although the tumor shows posterior acoustic enhancement and it is partially cystic, it is incompletely circumscribed and on final histology it proved to be a low-grade mucoepidermoid carcinoma.

Adenoid cystic carcinoma accounts for about 5% of parotid tumors but up to 20% of submandibular gland tumors (Figs 7–22A and 7–22B). Adenoid cystic carcinoma can also affect the minor salivary glands throughout the head and neck. This malignancy is neurotrophic and has a high incidence of late, especially pulmonary, metastases.

US examination of all salivary gland masses should include assessment of the contralateral glands as well as the intraglandular and cervical lymph nodes. CT or MRI scanning may also be beneficial for assessing local infiltration, facial nerve involvement, and deep cervical lymphadenopathy. As with US, CT and MRI have similar limitations in differentiating between histologic types of salivary gland tumors.[55]

US is often helpful in evaluating tumors of minor salivary gland origin, such as those arising from the base of tongue (Fig 7–23 and Video 7C). As with other head and neck malignancies, US is an invaluable tool in the evaluation of metastatic cervical lymphadenopathy as well (Fig 7–24). US is similarly useful in the follow-up surveillance of treated patients with salivary gland malignancies (Fig 7–25).

Lymphoma may arise within the lymph nodes of the parotid, or even within the salivary gland

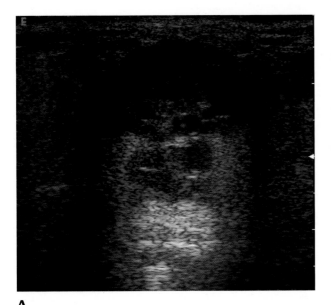

A

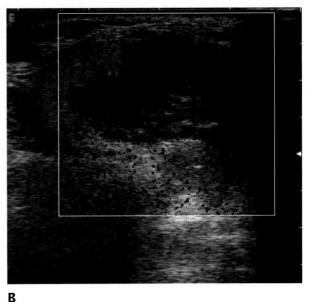

B

Fig 7–22. Adenoid cystic carcinoma of the left parotid. **A.** B-mode, sagittal plane showing heterogeneous poorly defined tumor with cystic component and posterior enhancement. **B.** Color Doppler, transverse view shows fine, punctuate vessels but relative hypovascularity.

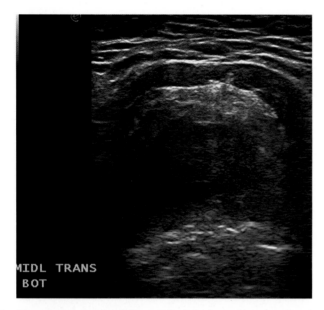

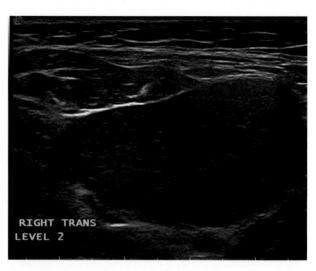

Fig 7–23 and Video 7C. Minor salivary gland malignancy. Midline transverse view of a primary adenocarcinoma arising in the base of tongue. **Video 7C**: Midline transverse ascending view through the base of tongue.

Fig 7–24. Metastatic lymphadenopathy from adenocarcinoma of the base of tongue (minor salivary gland, same patient whose primary tumor is shown in Fig 7–23). Image is a transverse view from right level 2.

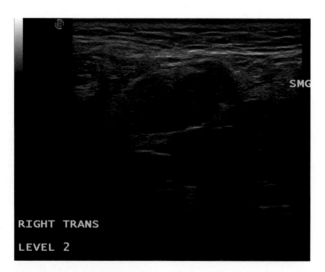

Fig 7–25. Surveillance US following surgery and radiation therapy for adenoid cystic carcinoma of the maxillary sinus reveals a lymph node metastasis in the right level 2 (*transverse view*).

parenchyma as extranodal disease. Multiple nodes are typically seen, including within the neck, and these nodes tend to be hypoechoic to anechoic and show diffuse, increased vascularity.[26,81] Patients with Sjögren's syndrome are at increased risk for developing salivary gland lymphoma.

Miscellaneous Salivary Gland Lesions

Cysts

Simple cysts are uncommon within the salivary glands. Cystic lesions may arise due to obstruction of the salivary ducts by tumor, calculi, inflammation, or following surgical or traumatic transection or ligation.[54] As with cysts elsewhere, US features include well-defined margins, anechoic interior, posterior acoustic enhancement, and absent internal blood flow by Doppler imaging[16] (Fig 7–26).

Benign lymphoepithelial lesions, frequently but not always associated with HIV infection, on the other hand are relatively common.[27] US features include multiple hypoechoic rounded areas of varying sizes scattered throughout the salivary gland parenchyma[27] (Figs 7–27A and 7–27B).

Ranula is a mucocele or pseudocyst of the small ducts of the the sublingual gland. Ranulas typically arise in the submucosa of the floor of the mouth, but plunging ranulas may present as submandibular

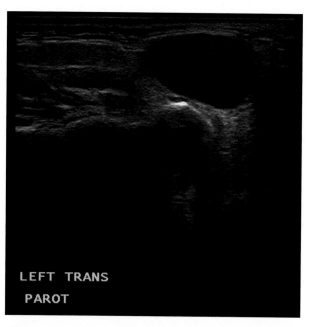

Fig 7–26. Benign parotid cyst, left transverse plane. Note reverberation echoes within the superficial aspect of the cyst, and posterior enhancement deep to the cyst and overlying the mandibular angle.

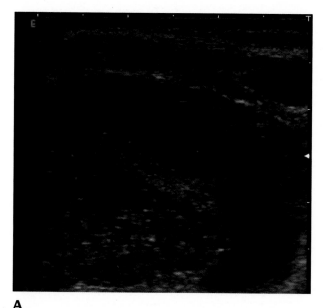

A

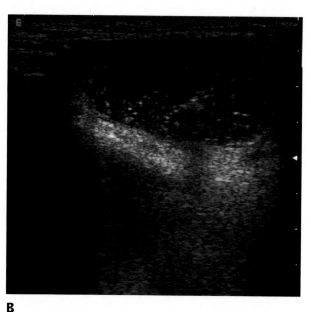

B

Fig 7–27. Benign lymphoepithelial lesions of the parotid gland. **A.** Large, debris-filled lymphoepithelial lesion in a patient with HIV infection and a history of Burkitts lymphoma (*right sagittal view*). **B.** Solitary lymphoepithelial cystic lesion in an 80-year-old woman without HIV infection (*left sagittal view*).

neck masses. Ranulas appear as hypoechoic to anechoic, avascular, sonocompressible lesions with posterior acoustic enhancement directly medial to the mandible (Fig 7–28).

Sialosis refers to recurrent, noninflammatory, painless swelling of the salivary glands, especially the parotid glands. Sialosis is associated with certain systemic diseases including malnutrition, cirrhosis, bulimia, and endocrine diseases.[13] US reveals enlarged and somewhat hyperechoic but otherwise homogeneous salivary glands.[15]

The semblance of parotid gland enlargement can actually be due to fatty "jowls," or to masseter muscle hypertrophy, both of which can easily be distinguished from parotid gland pathology by US.

On the other hand, shrinkage or atrophy and fibrosis of the salivary glands is commonly seen following radiation therapy for head and neck neoplasms. The well-known symptoms of xerostomia and loss of taste sensation are related to functional and structural impairment of salivary gland parenchyma, and the corresponding sonographic appearance is one of small, heterogeneous, hypovascular, and somewhat indistinct glands. Radioactive[131] Iodine ablation for thyroid cancer is also associated with salivary gland inflammation and injury. In the acute phase there is often gland enlargement associated with pain; in the chronic phase there may be ductal obstruction and the appearance of chronic sialadenitis, or gland shrinkage and atrophy (Fig 7–29).

A number of conditions, including amyotrophic lateral sclerosis (ALS), Parkinson's disease, and cerebral palsy, are associated with normal salivary gland anatomy but relative hypersecretion or inability to handle normal salivary flow. In such conditions, US examination of the salivary glands may be a component of evaluation and localization in preparation for therapeutic intervention (see Chapter 12).

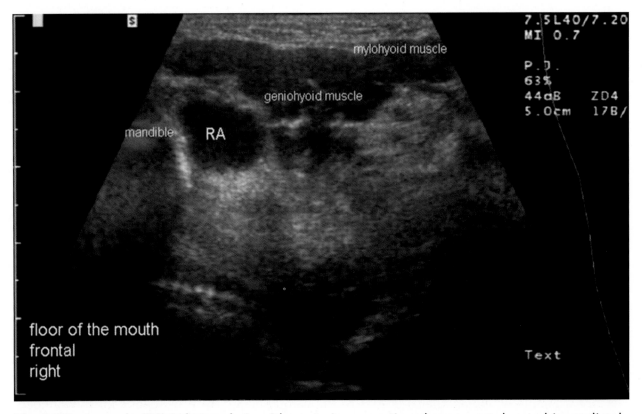

Fig 7–28. A ranula (*RA*) is hypoechoic with posterior acoustic enhancement, located immediately adjacent to the mandible in the floor of the mouth or submandibular region (*right paramedian sagittal view*).

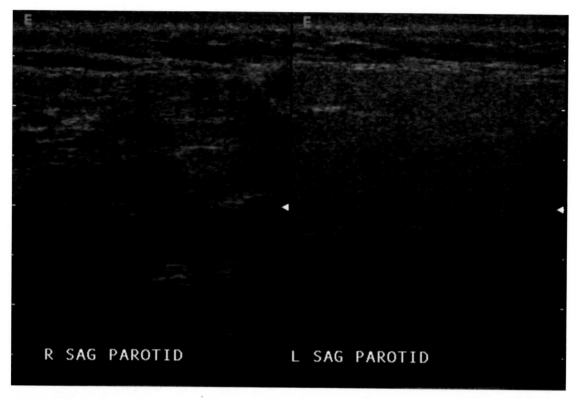

Fig 7–29. Unilateral atrophic chronic sialadenitis following [131]Iodine therapy for thyroid cancer. Note volume loss and fibrosis of the right parotid gland compared to a relatively normal-sized and homogeneous left parotid gland.

Summary

The salivary glands are highly accessible to ultrasonography for diagnostic examination as well as for guided interventions. Imaging information regarding the status of the salivary parenchyma, ductal system, mass lesions, and lymph nodes within the glands is readily available in the office setting, and can be integrated with the information obtained through examining the rest of the neck at the same interaction. Salivary US frequently eliminates the need for more costly and high-risk imaging studies.

Videos in This Chapter

Video 7A. See legend for Figure 7-15.

Video 7B. See legend for Figure 7-17.

Video 7C. See legend for Figure 7-23.

References

1. Yousem DM, Kraus MA, Chalian AA. Major salivary gland imaging. *Radiology*. 2000;216:19–29.
2. Alyas F, Lewis K, Williams M, et al. Diseases of the submandibular gland as demonstrated using high resolution ultrasound. *Br J Radiol*. 2005,78: 362–369.
3. Ridder GJ, Richter B, Disko U, Sander A. Gray-scale sonographic evaluation of cervical lymphadenopathy in cat-scratch disease. *J Clin Ultrasound*. 2001; 29:140–145.
4. Ying M, Ahuja A, Metreweli C. Diagnositic accuracy of sonographic criteria for evaluation of cervical

lymphadenopathy. *J Ultrasound Med*. 1998;17: 437–445.

5. Ying M, Ahuja A. Sonography of neck lymph nodes. I. Normal lymph nodes. *Clin Radiol*. 2003;58: 351–358.

6. Candiani F, Martinoli C. Salivary glands. In: Solbiati L, Rizzatto G, eds. *Ultrasound of Superficial Structures*. Edinburgh, Scotland: Churchill Livingstone, 1995;125–139.

7. Tevesi LM, Kolin E, Lufkin RB, Hanafee WN. MR imaging of the intraparotid facial nerve: normal anatomy and pathology. *Am J Roentgenol*. 1987; 148:995–1000.

8. Mandelblatt SM, Braun IF, Davis PC, Fry SM, Jacobs LH, Hoffman JC. Parotid masses: MR imaging. *Radiology*. 1987;163:411–414.

9. Laing MR, McKerrow WS. Intraparotid anatomy of the facial nerve and retromandibular vein. *Br J Surg*. 1988;75(4):310–312.

10. El-Hakim H, Mountain R, Carter L, Nilssen EL, Wardrop P, Nimmo M. Anatomic landmarks for locating parotid lesions in relation to the facial nerve: cross-sectional radiologic study. *J Otolaryngol*. 2003;32(5):314–318.

11. Divi V, Fatt MA, Teknos TN, Mukherji SK. Use of cross-sectional imaging in predicting surgical location of parotid neoplasms. *J Comput Assist Tomogr*. 2005;29(3):315–319.

12. Bradley MJ. Salivary glands. In: Ahuja AT, Evans RM, eds. *Practical Head and Neck Ultrasound*. London, England: Greenwich Medical Media; 2000:19–33.

13. Sikorowa L, Meyza JW, Ackerman LW. *Salivary Gland Tumors*. New York, NY: Pergamon; 1982.

14. Brook I. Acute bacterial suppurative parotitis: microbiology and management. *J Craniofac Surg*. 2003;14:37–40.

15. Gritzmann N, Rettenbacher T, Hollwerweger A, Macheiner P, Hubner E. Sonography of the salivary glands. *Eur Radiol*. 2003;13:964–975.

16. Traxler M, Schurawitzki H, Ulm C, et al. Sonography of noneoplastic disorders of the salivary glands. *Int J Oral Maxillofac Surg*. 1993;21:360–363.

17. Ching AS, Ahuja AT, King AD, Tse GM, Metreweli C. Comparison of the sonographic features of acalcuolous and calculous submandibular sialadenitis. *J Clin Ultrasound*. 2001;29:332–338.

18. Garcia CJ, Flores PA, Arce JD, Chuaqui B, Schwartz DS. Ultrasonography in the study of salivary gland lesions in children. *Pediatr Radiol*. 1998;28: 418–425.

19. Shimizu M, Ussmuller J, Donath K, et al. Sonographic analysis of recurrent parotitis in children: a comparative study with sialographic findings. *Oral Surg Oral Amed Oral Pathol Oral Radiol Endod*. 1998;86:606–615.

20. Thiede O, Stoll W, Schmal F. Clinical aspects of abscess development in parotitis [in German]. *HNO*. 2002;50:332–338.

21. Yeow KM, Hao SP, Liao CT. US-guided percutaneous catheter drainage of parotid abscesses. *J Vasc Interv Radiol*. 2000;11:473–476.

22. Bhatty MA, Piggot TA, Soames JV, McLean NR. Chronic non-specific parotid sialadenitis. *Br J Plast Surg*. 1998;51:517–521.

23. Fischer T, Muhler M, Beyersdorff D, et al. Use of state-of-the-art ultrasound techniques in diagnosing sarcoidosis of the salivary glands (Heerfordt's syndrome) [in German]. *HNO*. 2003;51:394–399.

24. Steiner E, Graninger W, Hitzelhammer J, et al. Color-coded duplex sonography of the parotid gland in Sjogren's syndrome [in German]. *Rofo*. 1994;160:294–298.

25. Gnepp DR. Metastatic disease to the major salivary glands. In: Ellis GL, Auclair PL, Gnepp DR, eds. *Surgical Pathology of the Salivary Glands*. Philadelphia, Pa: Saunders; 1991:560.

26. Chiou HJ, Chou YH, Chiou SY, et al. High-resolution ultrasonography of primary peripheral soft tissue lymphoma. *J Ultrasound Med*. 2005;24:77–86.

27. Martinoli C, Pretolesi F, Del Bono V, Derchi LE, Mecca D, Chiaramondia M. Benign lymphoepithelial parotid lesions in HIV-positive patients: spectrum of findings at gray-scale and Doppler sonography. *AJR Am J Roentgenol*. 1995;165:975–979.

28. Ahuja AT, Richards PS, Wong KT, et al. Kuttner tumour (chronic sclerosing sialadenitis) of the submandibular gland: sonographic appearances. *Ultrasound Med Biol*. 2003;29:913–919.

29. Bialek EJ, Osmólski A, Karpinska G, et al. US-appearance of a Küttner tumor resembling a malignant lesion: US-histopathologic correlation. *Eur J Ultrasound*. 2001;14:167–170.

30. Siewert B, Kruskal JBA, Kelly D, Sosna J, Kane RA. Utility and safety of ultrasound-guided fine needle aspiration of salivary gland masses including a cytologist's review. *J Ultrasound Med*. 2004;23: 777–783.

31. Kaba S, Kojima M, Matsuda H, et al. Kuttner's tumor of the submandibular glands: report of five cases with fine-needle aspiration cytology. *Diag Cytopathol*. 2006;34(9):631–635.

32. Holmes S, Gleeson MJ, Cawson RA. Mycobacterial disease of the parotid gland. *Oral Surg Oral Med Oral Pathol Oral Radiol Endod*. 2000;90:292–298.

33. Chou YH, Tiu CM, Liu CY, et al. Tuberculosis of the parotid gland: sonographic manifestations and sonographically guided aspiration. *J Ultrasound Med.* 2004;23:1275-1281.

34. Sa'do B, Yoshiura K, Yuasa K, et al. Multimodality imaging of cervicofacial actinomycosis. *Oral Surg Oral Med Oral Pathol.* 1993;76:772-782.

35. Tschammler A, Ott G, Schang T, Seelbach-Goebel B, Schwager K, Hahn D. Lymphadenopathy: differentiation of benign from malignant disease—color Doppler assessment of intranodal angioarchitecture. *Radiology.* 1998;208:117-123.

36. Kumar V, Cotran RS, Robbins SL. Disorders of the immune system. In: *Basic Pathology.* 6th ed. Philadelphia, Pa. Saunders; 1997:111-112.

37. Niemela RK, Takalo R, Paakko E, et al. Ultrasonography of salivary glands in primary Sjogren's syndrome: a comparison with magnetic resonance imaging and magnetic resonance sialography of parotid glands. *Rheumatology* (Oxford). 2004;43:875-879.

38. McCurley TL, Collins RD, Ball E, Collins RD. Nodal and extranodal lymphoproliferative disorders in Sjogren's syndrome: a clinical and immunopathologic study. *Hum Pathol.* 1990;21:482-492.

39. Tonami H, Matoba M, Kuginuki Y, et al. Clincal and imaging findings of lymphoma in patients with Sjögren syndrome. *J Comput Assist Tomogr.* 2003; 27:517-524.

40. Masaki Y, Sugai S. Lymphoproliferative disorders in Sjögren's syndrome. *Autoiimun Rev.* 2004;3: 175-182.

41. Escudier MP, McGurk M. Symptomatic sialadenitis and sialolithiasis in the English population: an estimate of the cost of hospital treatment. *Br Dent J.* 1999;186:463-466.

42. Lustmann J, Regev E, Melamed Y. Sialolithiasis: a survey on 245 patients and a review of the literature. *Int J Oral Maxillofac Surg.* 1990;19:135-138.

43. Marchal F, Dulgerov P, Becker M, Barki G, Disant F, Lehmann W. Specificity of parotid sialendoscopy. *Laryngoscope.* 2001;111:264-271.

44. Marchal F, Dulgerov P, Becker M, Barki G, Disant F, Lehmann W. Submandibular diagnostic and interventional sialendoscopy: new procedure for ductal disorders. *Ann Otol Rhinol Laryngol.* 2002; 111:27-35.

45. Zenk J, Constantinidis J, Kydles S, Hornung J, Iro H. Clinical and diagnostic findings of sialolithiasis [in German]. *HNO.* 1999;47:963-969.

46. Rauch S, Gorlin RJ. Disease of the salivary glands. In: Gorlin RJ, Goldmann HM, eds. *Thomas' Oral Pathology.* St. Louis, Mo: Mosby; 1970:997-103.

47. Avrahami E, Englender M, Chen E, Shabaty D, Katz R, Harell M. CT of submandibular gland sialolithiasis. *Neuroradiology.* 1996;38:287-290.

48. Jäger L, Menauer F, Holzknecht N, Scholz V, Grevers G, Reiser M. Sialolithiasis: MR sialography of the submandibular duct—an alternative to conventional sialography and US? *Radiology.* 2000;216: 665-671.

49. Becker M, Marchal F, Becker CD, et al. Sialolithiasis and salivary ductal stenosis: diagnostic accuracy of MR sialography with a three-dimensional extended-phase conjugate-symmetry rapid spin-echo sequence. *Radiology.* 2000;217:347-358.

50. Gritzmann N. Sonography of the salivary glands. *Am J Roentgenol.* 1989;53:161-166.

51. Diederich S, Wernecke K, Peters PE. Sialographic and sonographic diagnosis of diseases of the salivary gland [in German]. *Radiologe.* 1987;27:255-261.

52. Rinast E, Gmelin E, Hollands-Thorn B. Digital subtraction sialography, conventional sialography, high-resolution ultrasonography and computed tomography in the diagnosis of salivary gland diseases. *Eur J Radiol.* 1989;9:224-230.

53. Bialek EJ, Jakubowski W, Zajkowski P, Szopinski KT, Osmolski A. US of the major salivary glands: anatomy and spatial relationships, pathologic conditions, and pitfalls. *RadioGraphics.* 2006;26: 745-763.

54. Silvers AR, Som PM. Salivary glands. *Radiol Clin North Am.* 1998;36:941-966.

55. Renehan A, Gleave EN, Hancock BD, Smith P, McGurk M. Long-term follow-up of over 1000 patients with salivary gland tumours treated in a single centre. *Br J Surg.* 1996;83:1750-1754.

56. Klijanienko J, El-Naggar AK, Servois V, Rodriguez J, Validire P, Vielh P. Clinically aggressive metastasizing pleomorphic adenoma: report of two cases. *Head Neck.* 1997;19:629-633.

57. Laskawi R, Schott T, Schröder M. Recurrent pleomorphic adenomas of the parotid gland: clinical evaluation and long-term follow-up. *Br J Oral Maxillofac Surg.* 1998;36:48-51.

58. Shimizu M, Ussmüller J, Hartwein J, Donath K, Kinukawa N. Statistical study for sonographic differential diagnosis of tumorous lesions in the parotid gland. *Oral Surg Oral Med Oral Pathol Oral Radiol Endod.* 1999;88:226-233.

59. Bialek EJ, Jakubowski W, Karpinska G. Role of Ultrasonography in diagnosis and differentiation of pleomorphic adenomas: work in progress. *Arch Otolaryngol Head Neck Surg.* 2003;129: 929-933.

60. Schick S, Steiner E, Gahleitner A, et al. Differentiation of benign and malignant tumors of the parotid gland: value of pulsed Doppler and color Doppler sonography. *Eur Radiol.* 1998;8:1462-1467.

61. Zajkowski P, Jakuboski W, Bialek EJ, Wysocki M, Osmólski A, Serafin-Król M. Pleomorphic adenoma and adenolymphoma in ultrasonography. *Eur J Ultrasound.* 2000;12:23-29.

62. Yoo GH, Eisele DW, Askin FB, Driben JS, Johns ME. Warthin's tumor: a 40-year experience at the Johns Hopkins Hospital. *Laryngoscope.* 1994;104:799-803.

63. Gritzmann N, Türk R, Wittich G, Karnel F, Schurawitzki H, Brunner E. High-resolution sonography after surgery of cystadenoma lymphomatosum of the parotid gland [in German]. *Rofo.* 1986;145:648-651.

64. Yu GY, Ma DQ, Zhang Y, et al. Multiple primary tumours of the parotid gland. *Int J Oral Maxillofac Surg.* 2004;33:531-534.

65. Kim J, Kim EK, Park CS, Choi YS, Kim YH, Choi EC. Characteristic sonographic findings of Warthin's tumor in the parotid gland. *J Clin Ultrasound.* 2004;32:78-81.

66. Martinoli C, Derchi LE, Solbiati L, Rizzatto G, Silvestri E, Giannoni M. Color Doppler sonography of salivary glands. *AJR Am J Roentgenol.* 1994;163:933-941.

67. Koischwitz D, Gritzmann N. Ultrasound of the neck. *Radiol Clin North Am.* 2000;38;1029-1045.

68. Gritzmann N, Macheiner P. Lipoma in the parotid gland: typical US and CT morphology [in German]. *Ultraschall Med.* 2003;24:295-296.

69. Wong KT, Ahuja AT, King AD, Yuen EH, Yu SC. Vascular lesions of the parotid gland in adult patients: diagnosis with high-resolution ultrasound and MRI. *Br J Radiol.* 2004;77:600-606.

70. Chong KW, Chung YF, Khoo ML, Lim DT, Hong GS, Soo KC. Management of intraparotid facial nerve schwannomas. *Aust N Z J Surg.* 2000;70:732-734.

71. Hehar SS, Dugar J, Sharp J. The changing faces of a parotid mass. *J Laryngol Otol.* 1999;113:938-941.

72. Oncel S, Onal K, Ermete M, Uluc E. Schwannoma (neurilemmoma) of the facial nerve presenting as a parotid mass. *J Laryngol Otol.* 2002;116:642-643.

73. Chikui T, Yonetsu K, Yoshiura K, et al. Imaging findings of lipomas in the orofacial region with CT, US, and MRI. *Oral Surg Oral Med Oral Pathol Oral Radiol Endod.* 1997;84:88-95.

74. Howlett DC, Kesse KW, Hughes DV, Sallomi DF. The role of imaging in the evaluation of parotid disease. *Clin Radiol.* 2002;57:692-701.

75. Howlett DC. High resolution ultrasound assessment of the parotid gland. *Br J Radiol.* 2003;76:271-277.

76. Goto TK, Yoshiura K, Nakayama E, et al. The combined use of US and MR imaging for the diagnosis of masses in the parotid region. *Acta Radiol.* 2001;42:88-95.

77. Hardee PS, Carter JL, Piper KM, Ng SY. Metachronous bilateral primary adenocarcinoma of the submandibular glands. *Oral Surg Oral Med Oral Pathol Oral Radiol Endod.* 2001;91:455-461.

78. Yoshihara T, Suzuki S, Nagao K. Mucoepidermoid carcinoma arising in the accessory parotid gland. *Int J Pediatr Otorhinolaryngol.* 1999;48:47-52.

79. Suh SI, Seol HY, Kim TK, et al. Acinic cell carcinoma of the head and neck: radiologic-pathologic correlation. *J Comput Assist Tomogr.* 2005;29:121-126.

80. Bradley MJ, Durham LH, Lancer JM. The role of colour flow Doppler in the investigation of the salivary gland tumour. *Clin Radiol.* 2000;55:759-762.

81. Yasumoto M, Yoshimura R, Sunuba K, Shibuya H. Sonographic appearances of malignant lymphoma of the salivary glands. *J Clin Ultrasound.* 2001;29:491-498.

Chapter 8

ULTRASONOGRAPHY OF OTHER NECK MASSES

Hans J. Welkoborsky

Introduction

The advantages of ultrasonography (US) of the head and neck have been described throughout this textbook. This chapter aims to address the application of US to the differential diagnosis of neck masses not elsewhere discussed. The anatomy of the neck is ideally suited to ultrasound imaging because:

■ nearly all anatomic structures of interest are located relatively superficially, so that they are easily accessible to ultrasound scans,

■ soft tissues including adipose, muscle, and parenchymatous organs (ie, thyroid gland, salivary glands) create great impedance differences, and

■ many pathologic lesions have characteristic echotexture and sonomorphology.

In addition to being useful in the differential diagnosis of cervical lymphadenopathy, US is very helpful in the diagnosis of most neck masses. Many masses have distinctive ultrasound morphology, and combined with a patient's history can be highly suggestive of a particular diagnosis. It is important to note, however, that all sonographic characteristics are nonspecific. Therefore, definitive diagnosis can be made in most cases only by cytologic examination

of cellular smears obtained by fine needle aspiration or by histologic examination of operative specimens.

Commonly occurring neck masses include:

1. Lymph nodes (inflammatory nodes, malignant lymphoma, lymph node metastases)
2. Congenital masses and cysts
3. Benign lesions (eg, paraganglioma, neurinoma, lipoma)
4. Primary malignant neck masses (eg, sarcomas).

In this chapter the clinical, histologic, and sonomorphologic characteristics that aid in the differential diagnosis of these lesions are described.

Congenital Masses and Neck Cysts

Neck cysts are common congenital masses. According to their origin, medial cervical cysts (thyroglossal cyst) and lateral branchial cysts can be distinguished.

Thyroglossal Duct Cyst

Thyroglossal duct cysts (medial cervical cysts) develop from the thyroglossal duct in the embryonic pathway of the thyroid from the foramen caecum at the base of the tongue via the hyoid bone to the low anterior midline of the neck. Clinically these cysts appear as solitarily rounded clearly defined masses in the midline of the neck superior to the thyroid cartilage of the larynx, with a fistula to the skin in rare cases. Thyroglossal duct cysts usually present in children and young adults, often with an episode of acute infection and expansion. Sonographically the thyroglossal duct cyst is characterized by a hypoechoic well-defined round or oval mass with sharp borders and posterior enhancement (Fig 8-1). It is located close to the floor of mouth muscles. Inside the lesion some fine echoes may be present, origi-

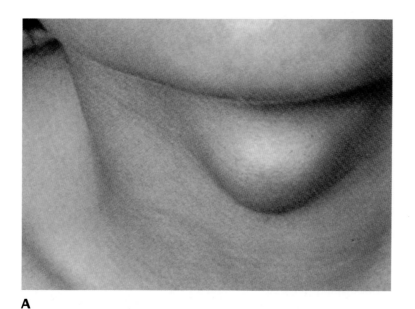

A

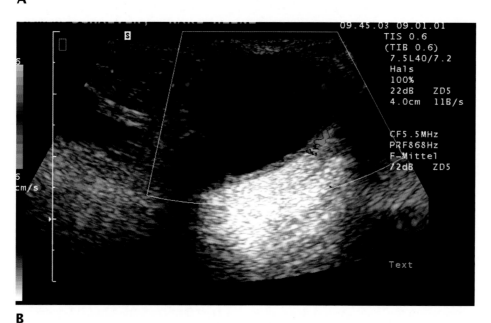

B

Fig 8–1. Thyroglossal duct cyst. Clinically (**A**), the lesion appears as a solitary roundish mass in the midline of the neck above the thyroid cartilage. Sonographically (**B**), it is characterized by a hypoechoic, clearly defined, compressible mass with sharp borders and typical posterior enhancement.

nating from the protein molecules in the cyst fluid. The lesion itself is compressible, and often movable, meaning the shape of the entire mass shifts from round to more oval and the location may shift when compressed by the ultrasound transducer, which is a characteristic sonographic finding in cysts.

US has proved useful in the intraoperative setting for localization and confirmation where patients who have presented with acutely enlarged or inflamed thyroglossal duct cysts no longer have a palpable mass by the time they arrive for scheduled surgery and the inflammation has subsided.

Branchial Cleft Cyst

Lateral branchial cysts or branchial cleft cysts originate from the second or third branchial arch. They are located in the lateral neck inferior to the angle of the mandible along the anterior border of the sternocleidomastoid muscle. Clinically patients present either with a slowly enlarging painless oval mass in this region of the neck, or in the event of acute inflammation, with a rapid appearance of a tender and fluctuant lesion with overlying erythema.

Sonographically the branchial cleft cyst is characterized as an oval or rounded, well-defined hypoechoic mass with posterior enhancement and some fine and homogeneous echoes inside the lesion originating, like in thyroglossal duct cysts, from the protein molecules of the cystic fluid (Fig 8–2). The lesion is compressible and shows no signs of infiltration into the surrounding tissue and no close relation to the large blood vessels. Small reactive-appearing lymph nodes can frequently be observed in the neighborhood of a branchial cleft cyst.[1] Color Doppler sonography reveals some blood vessels in the capsule of the cyst, especially during acute inflammation, but no vessels appear inside the lesion, which is of differential diagnostic importance.

Lateral neck fistulas have a common origin with branchial cleft cysts from the branchial arches.[2]

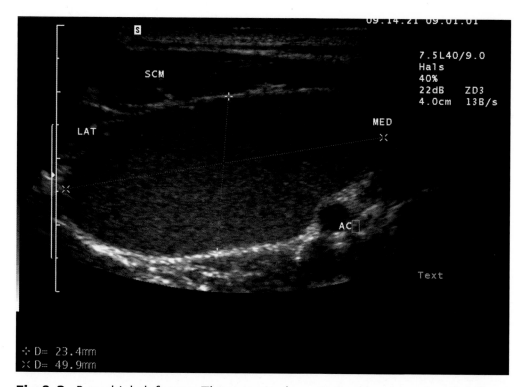

Fig 8–2. Branchial cleft cyst. The mass is characterized by an oval well-defined hypoechoic lesion with posterior enhancement, located along or deep to the anterior border of the sternocleidomastoid muscle. Fine and homogeneous echoes inside originate from protein molecules within the cystic fluid.

A fistula is only visible by US when it is dilated and the cavity contains cystic fluid. In such cases, the fistula opening and the fistula itself appear iso- or hyperechoic compared to the surrounding tissue and sometimes open into a cystic structure medially.

Lymph Nodes

Cervical lymph nodes are universally grouped into six different topographic anatomic regions according to the American Joint Committee on Cancer (AJCC) classification,[3,4] with further subdivisions of some of the levels. Each lymph node level drains distinct anatomic structures. The anterior floor of mouth, for example, is drained by the submental lymph nodes (level IA); the scalp and part of the auricle are drained by the occipital nodes (level V). Additional lymphatic drainage to the intraparotid and retroesophageal lymph nodes also occurs. As the density, water content, and acoustic impedance of lymph nodes is quite similar to that of the surrounding soft tissue, healthy lymph nodes cannot be visualized by US. Thus, only pathologic lymph nodes can be identified. With modern ultrasound units nodes of 3 mm in diameter can be detected.

In general, lymph nodes are assessed for their size, shape, internal architecture, hilum structure, echogenicity, nodal border, posterior enhancement, and ancillary features (ie, adjacent soft tissue edema.)[5] In many cases additional color-coded Doppler sonography helps in differentiating different causes of cervical lymphadenopathy. Metastatic malignant cervical lymphadenopathy is discussed further in Chapters 5 and 15.

Inflammatory Nodes

Affected lymph nodes are usually located in the drainage basin of a portal of entry (ie, tonsils; teeth; skin infections). In most cases they are small (4 to 20 mm in diameter). Larger nodes are less common. Lymph nodes appear solitarily or in chains. Reactive lymph nodes are oval, with a typical length-to-width ration of 2:1 or greater (Solbiati index)[6] (Fig 8–3). It is a rare neck US examination that does not reveal at least a few reactive lymph nodes, as they are so plentiful and dynamic within the neck.

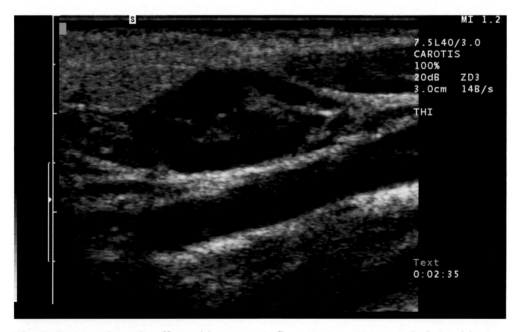

Fig 8–3. Lymph node affected by acute inflammation. Note oval-shaped lesion with posterior enhancement and a hilus structure, representing the central adipose and connective tissue in the node.

Acute Inflammation

Inflammatory nodes are hypoechoic and may or may not be sharply demarcated from the surrounding tissue. Spotted or more hyperechoic areas can sometimes be identified inside the nodes. In the majority of reactive nodes, a central hilar structure can be identified,[5] representing the central adipose and connective tissue within the node, in which small blood vessels appear (Fig 8–4). Using color Doppler sonography or power Doppler sonography, a hilar vascular pattern with central perfusion is a common finding[7-12] (Fig 8–5). Quantitative analysis of perfusion, that is, by estimating the vascular resistance

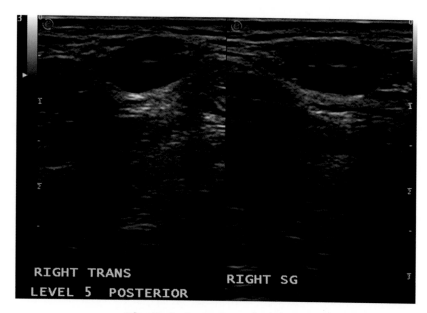

Fig 8–4. Lymph node hilum.

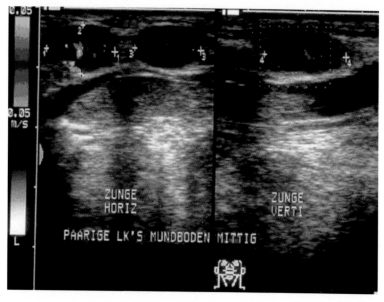

Fig 8–5. Lymph node affected by acute inflammation. Color-coded Doppler sonography reveals hilar vascular pattern and hilar perfusion.

(resistance index, RI, and/or pulsatility index, PI) reveals a lower pulsatility index for reactive lymph nodes compared with lymph node metastases, with an accuracy of nearly 90%.[9,12]

Abscess formation within lymph nodes is characterized by:

- peripheral increase of echotexture
- confluence of abutting lymph nodes, and
- change in the structure of the node with decrease of central echogenicity, coarse spotted echoes parallel to hypoechoic areas, intranodal necrosis, poorly defined nodal border, posterior acoustic enhancement, and sometimes perinodal soft tissue edema (Fig 8-6).

Chronic Inflammation

Lymph nodes associated with chronic inflammation can appear in any level of the neck. Typical examples are nodes affected by toxoplasmosis. Sonographically, these nodes fulfill the criteria demonstrated for acutely inflamed nodes. On the other hand, the borders and shape of the nodes are sometimes unsharp; the echogenicity is often increased with some echocomplex areas inside the node representing connective tissue membranes and septae. In most cases a hilar structure is present. Color-coded duplex sonography reveals hilar perfusion and central perfusion pattern, but the pulsatility is considerably lower than in acute inflammation (Fig 8-7).

Tuberculous lymph nodes often show higher echogenicity with calcification complexes inside.

Malignant Lymphoma

Lymph nodes in the neck can be affected by either Hodgkin's or non-Hodgkin's lymphoma. Malignant lymphoma can appear in all levels of the neck, in some cases bilaterally. Clinically, patients present with either unilateral or bilateral progressive lymphadenopathy in the neck which can occur in multiple levels including the nuchal region. The predominant age of the patients is the fourth through seventh decade. The nodes are of varying size and on palpation are soft or rubbery. Pain and tenderness are observed in only a minority of patients. Clinical signs for involvement of nerves due to nerve infiltration like hoarseness (recurrent laryngeal nerve infiltration) or facial palsy (facial nerve infiltration) are usually

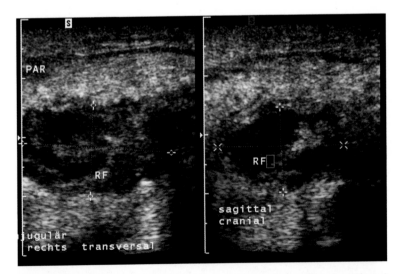

Fig 8–6. Abscess formation in a lymph node: perifocal increase of echotexture, change in the structure of the node with decrease of central echogenicity, coarse spotted echoes parallel to hypoechoic areas, intranodal necrosis, nonsharp border, and posterior enhancement.

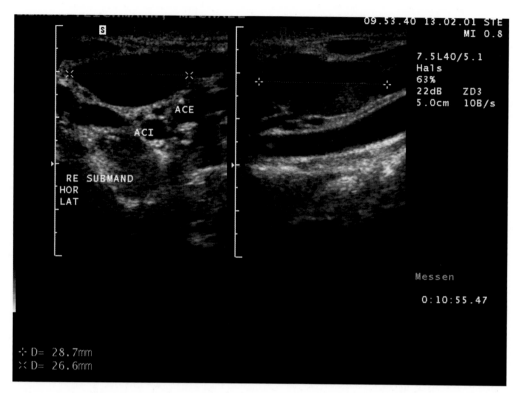

Fig 8–7. Lymph node affected by chronic inflammation. toxoplasmosis. US of a patient with toxoplasmosis shows nodes with slightly increased echogenicity with some septae and trabeculae inside representing connective tissue membranes.

absent. Some patients present with manifestations of malignant lymphoma in other regions, that is, thoracic, abdominal or pelvic region, or systemic symptoms such as fever, chills, night sweats, fatigue, pruritus, and weight loss. Thus careful staging examinations of the thorax and abdomen are required in cases of malignant lymphoma in the neck.

Histologically, Hodgkin's lymphoma is found in one-third of cases, with non-Hodgkin's lymphoma comprising two-thirds of cases and B-cell lymphomas being the most frequent tumor types.

Sonographically, affected lymph nodes are relatively round in shape with clear demarcation from the surrounding tissue and variable size. Signs of vessel or muscle infiltration are usually missing. The nodes appear either solitarily (less frequent) or are grouped in chains or in clusters. They are considerably hypoechoic and have been described as "empty" nodes (Fig 8–8 and Videos 8A, 8B, and 8C). Using modern ultrasound units, the nodes appear as hypoechoic masses with some homogeneous intralesional echoes, and sometimes with posterior enhancement. A clear hilum structure, as is found in lymph nodes affected by acute inflammation, is often missing. Nevertheless, in larger nodes some hilumlike structures can sometimes be identified, representing trabeculae of connective tissue.[13] Using color-coded duplex sonography several intranodal blood vessels can be visualized with a perfusion pattern that is predominantly peripheral. Nevertheless, the hilum structures in the center of the nodes represent blood vessels too, so that in most cases a mixed perfusion pattern, especially in larger nodes, is visible. In many cases vessels are arranged like a tree (Fig 8–9). Pulsatilty is variable to high and not as characteristic as in the differential diagnosis of inflamed versus metastatic nodes. The relatively homogeneous perfusion is the reason why central necrosis even in larger nodes is less frequent.

Some effort has been made in the past by investigators to determine the histologic subtype of lymphoma on the basis of sonographic characteristics.

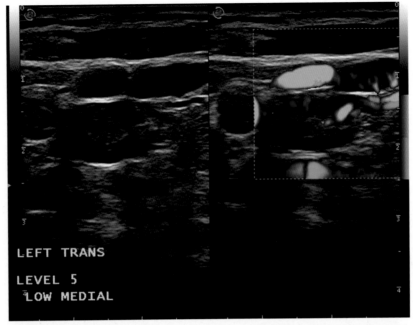

A

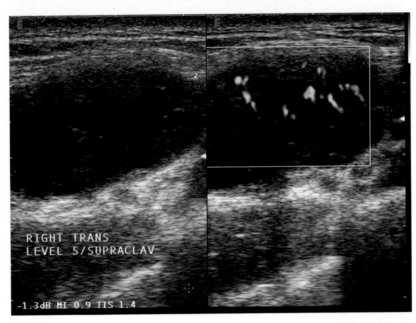

B

Fig 8–8 and Video Clips 8A, 8B, and 8C. Malignant lymphoma. Non-Hodgkin's lymphoma (**A**): Multiple hypoechoic nodes of different sizes with dorsal enhancement and hilus structures inside most of the nodes. Hodgkin's lymphoma (**B**): Enlarged node without visible hilum and with radiating vascular pattern. **Videos 8A, 8B**, and **8C** show multiple bilateral lymph nodes of varying sizes in chains as the ultrasound transducer is ascending through the left lateral neck (**8A**), ascending through the right lateral neck (**8B**) and sweeping from medial to lateral in the left neck (**8C**).

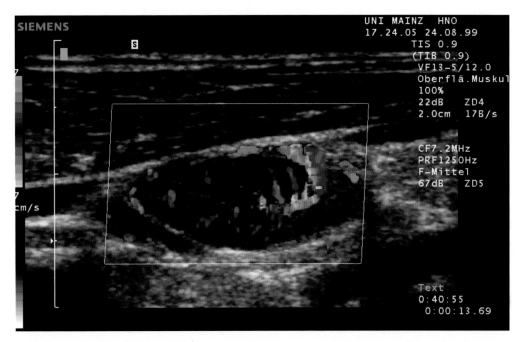

Fig 8–9. Color-coded duplex sonography of a lymph node affected by malignant non-Hodgkin's lymphoma. There is a hilus structure and blood vessels which are arranged like a "tree." The perfusion pattern is thus both peripheral and hilar.

Lymph nodes affected by Hodgkin's disease should have a contour with a lobular pattern, septumlike echoes, and tubular structures that correlate histopathologically with fibrous connective tissue surrounding lymph nodes and small vessels. B-cell lymphoma should have a tendency to lymph node fusion and spot- or line-echoes reflecting the replacement and destruction of lymph node architecture by proliferation of lymphocytes. T-cell lymphoma, finally, should be characterized by a prominent hilumlike echo, reflecting the prominent vascularization in these nodes with a dilated hilum area.[13] However, none of these characteristics is pathognomonic. By using modern ultrasound equipment with tissue harmonic imaging and/or contrast enhancers it is likely that more characteristics specific for particular tumor types will be described. Nevertheless, subtyping of lymphomas remains the domain of cytologic, histologic, and genetic studies. The sonographic characteristics of lymph nodes affected by acute or chronic inflammation and of malignant lymphoma nodes are summarized in Table 8–1.

Benign Lesions

Common benign lesions in the neck include paragangliomas, lipomas, neurinomas, and vascular malformations.

Paraganglioma

Paragangliomas originate from neuroendocrine precursor cells in the paragngliomatous tissue, which is widely distributed in the head and neck and has some function in the regulation of blood pH and carbon dioxide concentration.[14] According to their predominant tissue tumors can be grouped into paragangliomatous, angiomatous, and adenomatous subtypes.[15] Histologically, paragangliomas show tumor cells in a strandlike pattern, with cells separated by trabeculae of connective tissue with capillaries, imitating a paraganglion. The adenomatous subtype of tumors are characterized by few blood

Table 8–1. Sonographic Characteristics in Lymph Nodes Affected by Acute and Chronic Inflammation and Malignant Lymphoma, respectively

Sonographic Feature	Acute Inflammation	Chronic Inflammation	Malignant Lymphoma
Site	Drainage area of a portal of entrance	Drainage area of a portal of entrance	All levels of the entire neck
Size	Small or large	Small or large	Variable
Shape	Oval	Oval	Round or roundish
Intranodal architecture	Spotted areas	Echocomplex areas	Homogeneous; fine "granules"
Hilus structure	+++	++	+
Echogenicity	Hypoechoic	Hypoechoic; increased echogenicity compared to acute inflammation	Hypoechoic
Nodal border	Unsharp	Unsharp	Sharp
Posterior enhancement	+	+	(+)
Perfusion pattern	Hilar vascular pattern; central perfusion pattern	Hilar vascular pattern; central perfusion pattern	Mixed peripheral and central perfusion pattern
Pulsatility	Low	Low	High

vessels and capillaries between cell nests, whereas angiomatous tumors show numerous large blood vessels. Although paragangliomas are recognized as benign lesions, some of these (about 7%) show a biologic behavior similar to malignant tumors with a higher recurrence rate, invasive growth pattern, and development of metastatic disease. Criteria for determining the aggressive or malignant behavior of paragangliomas are: central necrosis, vascular invasion, nuclear polymorphism, number of mitoses per high-power field, percentage of sustentacular cells, and percentage of aneuploid cells and increased proliferation rate, respectively.[14-18] Nevertheless, these findings do not have consistent correlation with the histologic behavior of the lesion in all cases.

In the head and neck, paragangliomas of the carotid body and vagal paragangliomas are a most important differential diagnosis to cervical lymphadenopathy. They can be assessed sonographically with high diagnostic accuracy. For paragangliomas of other sites, such as in the jugulotympanic region or paranasal sinuses,[18,19] additional CT or MRI scans must be performed, as they usually extend underneath bony structures and are therefore not sufficiently accessible by sonography alone.

Clinically, paragangliomas of the carotid body are located in the superolateral neck, inferior or deep to the mandible. They are usually slowly growing, unilateral compact masses with a smooth surface, sometimes palpable pulsations and limited mobility with respect to the underlying tissue. They can usually be moved from side to side but have only limited movement in the vertical plane (Fontaine's sign)[20] (Fig 8-10). Occasionally they are associated with pain, hoarseness, dysphagia, or Horner's syndrome, a reflection of cranial or sympathetic nerve involvement.

Sonographically, paragangliomas of the carotid body appear as rounded or oval, hypoechoic, well-defined masses with some granules and hyperechoic areas inside the lesion, representing trabeculae of connective tissue (Fig 8-11). The echogenicity depends on the subtype of the tumor: Angiomatous subtype tumors are more hypoechoic due to the

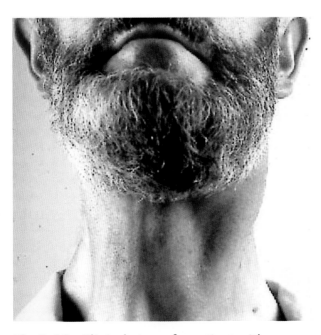

Fig 8–10. Clinical view of a patient with a paraganglioma of the carotid body. The mass is located in the lateral upper neck and extends underneath the mandible.

numerous and large vessels and decreased content of connective tissue. On the other hand, adenomatous tumors display a slightly higher echogenicity sometimes comparable to the echogenicity of salivary glands or thyroid gland. Other typical sonographic characteristics of carotid paragangliomas include:

1. Dissociation of the carotid bifurcation with a
2. Dorsolateral displacement of the internal carotid artery and
3. Ventromedial displacement of the external carotid artery.
4. Extremely increased perfusion of the tumor.
5. Numerous arterial and venous vessels and shunt vessels inside the lesion (Fig 8–12).

Power (pw) Doppler reveals a high pulsatility. With modern ultrasound units the connective tissue between the tumor and the adventitia and/or tunica muscularis of the vessel can be visualized, for determining a possible infiltration of the vessel wall, which is of great importance in the preoperative planning.

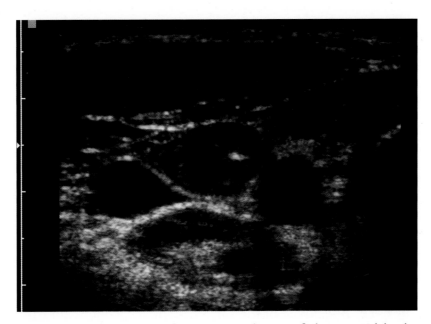

Fig 8–11. B-mode US of a paraganglioma of the carotid body. The tumor appears as a round or oval hypoechoic mass located at the carotid bifurcation, with some hyperechoic areas inside that represent trabeculae of connective tissue.

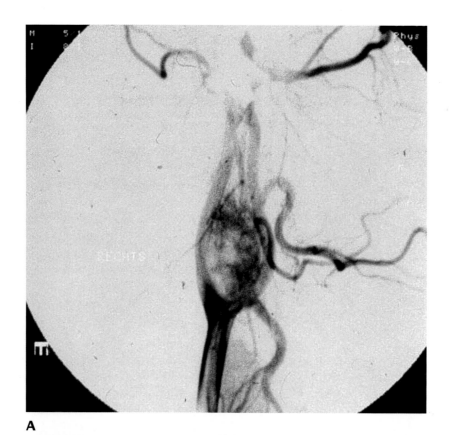

A

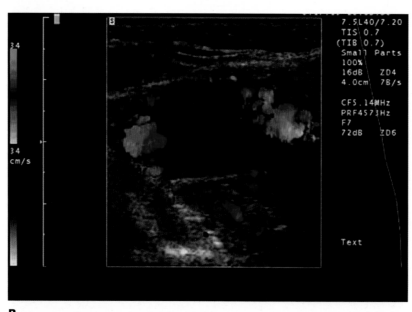

B

Fig 8–12. Angiogram of the same patient as in Figure 8–11 (**A**) and corresponding color-coded Doppler sonography (**B**). There is a dissociation of the carotid bifurcation with a dorsolateral displacement of the internal carotid artery and a ventromedial displacement of the external carotid artery.

With these clinical and sonographic characteristics in mind, the diagnosis of a paraganglioma of the carotid body can be made with high accuracy. A fine-needle aspiration biopsy is not necessary and is preferably avoided because of the risk of severe bleeding.

Other paragangliomas in the head and neck, which may be assessable by US are vagal paragangliomas or laryngeal paragangliomas. Vagal paragangliomas are localized in the rostral portion of the vagus nerve in the vicinity of the ganglion nodusum and in 5% of cases occur bilaterally. They are slowly growing, asymptomatic masses (unless advanced and associated with cranial neuropathies) deep to the angle of the mandible or in the parapharyngeal space. The sonographic characteristics are similar to those described for carotid body paragangliomas (Fig 8-13 and Video 8D).

Laryngeal paragangliomas are very rare. They usually occur in the supraglottic larynx and arise from the superior pair of the laryngeal paraganglia. They present as a long asymptomatic submucosal mass in the aryepiglottic fold, with hoarseness as the major symptom. Sonographically, this tumor can be visualized as a well-defined rounded or oval hypoechoic mass rising above the thyroid cartilage of the larynx which displays numerous vessels and high pulsatility.

Lipoma

Lipomas in the head and neck arise from adipose tissue. They can be distributed throughout the entire neck unilaterally and bilaterally with a higher frequency of occurrence in the sumandibular region, lateral neck, and nuchal area. In some cases, like in Madelung's disease, the adipose tissue of the entire neck, cheek, and nuchal region is affected.

Clinically these lesions occur as slowly growing masses. By palpation they are very soft and poorly demarcated from the surrounding tissue, with limited shift.

Sonographically, lipomas appear as masses with minimal demarcation from the surrounding tissue. In most cases, they occur in the subdermal adipose tissue, lateral to the fascia of the neck muscles. They appear as hypoechoic masses with unsharp borders. Inside the lesions there are hyperechoic featherlike areas, representing the trabculae of connective tissue inside the tumors (featherlike pattern of lipoma) (Fig 8-14 and Video 8E).

Usually there is no dorsal or posterior acoustic enhancement. Color-coded Doppler sonography reveals very few vessels and minimal perfusion.

Cervical Neurinoma

Neurinomas (neuromas, schwannomas) of the head and neck are benign tumors which originate either from the cranial nerves, cervical plexus, or cervical sympathetic trunk. Neurinomas of peripheral nerves are less frequent. On the other hand 25 to 45% of extracranial neurinomas occur in the head and neck region.[21] Histologically, they arise from the Schwann cells of the nerve sheaths. Another, similar group of neurogenic tumors are neurofibromas, that is, in patients with neurofibromatosis, which are rare in the neck. Malignant degeneration is uncommon.[22]

Clinically patients usually present with a unilateral, slowly growing mass in the lateral part of the neck or in the parotid gland. These tumors may be located within the parapharyngeal space. With palpation, many tumors can be shifted in an anterior/posterior direction but minimally in a cranio/caudal direction. Most patients are asymptomatic; hoarseness and/or dysphagia, however, may be present in cases of parapharyngeal space neurinoma or vagal neurinoma. Horner's syndrome may be present in cases of cervical sympathetic trunk tumors. Sonographically, there are no pathognomonic features. Usually, however, neurinomas appear as solitary hypoechoic solid tumors with posterior enhancement, slightly inhomogeneous echogenicity, and absence of an echogenic hilus structure. Some pseudocystic inclusions and regressive areas occur frequently.[23] They are rounded or oval masses and have a clear demarcation to the surrounding tissue. Nevertheless, the demarcation of the tumor is sometimes less clear toward the nerve of origin and the tumor may have a fusiform or tapering shape. Using high-resolution ultrasound transducers (7.5 to 15 MHz), it may be possible to visualize the nerves, hypoechoic

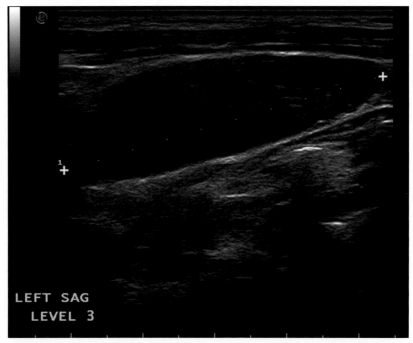

LEFT SAG
LEVEL 3

A

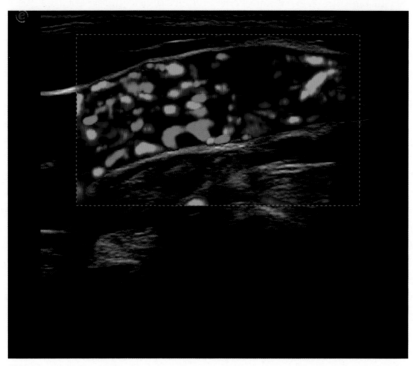

B

Fig 8–13 and Video 8D. Vagal paraganglioma. Asymptomatic superolateral neck mass that is well-defined, slightly heterogeneous internally (**A**, *left sagittal view)*, and quite hypervascular (**B**, *with color Doppler*), but does not splay the carotid artery bifurcation (**Video 8D**).

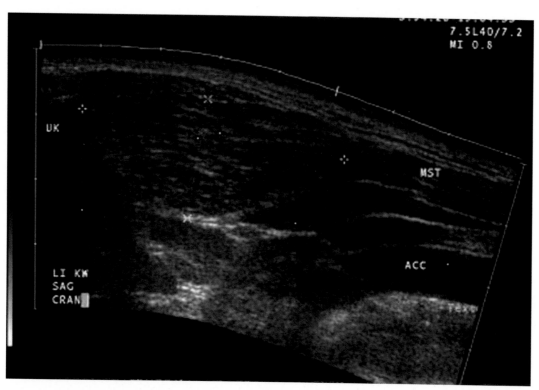

Fig 8–14 and Video 8E. Lipoma of the lateral neck. Poorly demarcated mass deep to the subdermal adipose tissue on US. Inside the lesion are hyperechoic featherlike areas, representing the trabeculae of connective tissue. **Video 8E** shows mobility of a right supraclavicular lipoma with respect to its surrounding soft tissues by sonopalpation

nerve fascicles and the relation of a schwannoma to the nerve of origin.[24-26] In cases of vagal neurinoma or neurinoma of the cervical sympathetic trunk, the carotid artery and the internal jugular vein may be displaced anterolaterally. Nevertheless, there is no relation of the tumor itself to the large vessels nor signs of vessel infiltration. Color-coded duplex sonography shows hypervascularization and blood vessels (Fig 8–15).[23,26,27]

In the rare cases of multiple schwannoma (schwannomatosis), intraoperative ultrasound examination has been shown to be valuable to localize and facilitate removal of even small tumors.[28]

Neurofibromas can be solitary or multifocal. Sonographically they appear as a concentric pattern of hypo- and hyperechoic areas ("target-sign") which represents the microanatomic structure of these lesions with fibrocollagenous tissue in the center and myxomatous tissue in the periphery. Thus, their echogenicity is usually more hyperechoic compared to the neurinoma.[26] Color coded Doppler sonography shows only few vessels and considerably poorer perfusion than in schwannomas (Fig 8–16).

Hemangioma

Hemangiomas are characterized by a proliferation of endothelial cells and pericytes. They appear anywhere in the neck with a predominance in the submandibular region, the lateral neck, and the salivary glands, in which they almost exclusively occur in the parotid gland. Clinically, these lesions are asymptomatic, soft, sometimes fluctuant swellings. They

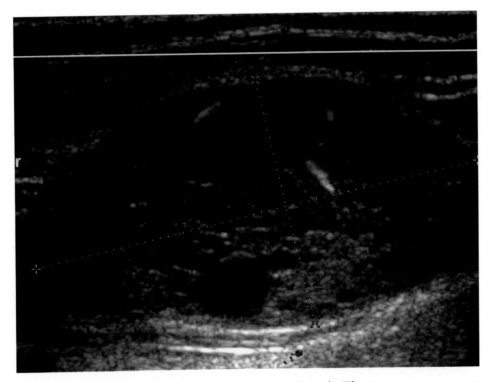

Fig 8–15. Cervical schwannoma of the lateral neck. The tumor appears as a hypoechoic solid mass with posterior enhancement and typical fusiform shape. There are some regressive areas and no hilar structure which is of importance for differential diagnosis. Color-coded Doppler sonography reveals some blood vessels inside the lesion.

usually appear during the first 6 months of life and most of them grow slowly; rapid growth is rarely observed.[29] These lesions are twice as common in females as in males. Histologically, hemangiomas are composed of varying sized and shaped vascular spaces. Juvenile variants comprise small round densely packed endothelial cells and clusters of pericytes. In the early stages, no vascular lumen might be present. These spaces develop with time, which creates the clinical impression of the rapidly "growing" hemangioma. The mature forms are capillary hemangiomas with endothelial cell linings without any atypia. Most juvenile hemangiomas involute in the first 7 years of age with no treatment required.[29]

Sonographically, the hemangioma appears as a hypoechoic poorly demarcated mass which often extends into the subcutaneous tissue and sternocleidomastoid muscle, the floor of mouth muscles, or the parotid gland. The lesion is penetrated by hyperechoic strands which represent trabeculae of connective tissue. Sometimes the trabeculae display like a "network" and pulsations inside the lesion are visible. Using color-coded duplex sonography dense congregations of blood vessels with different lumens are displayed (Fig 8–17A). The application of ultrasound contrast enhancers reveals an amplification especially of small vessels, which appear like a "thunderstorm" on the screen (Fig 8–17B). In cases of recurrent bleeding, functional deficits due to the tumor extension, or for cosmetic purposes, treatment consisting of percutanous or interstitial laser therapy, such as with a Nd:YAG laser, may be recommended. In these cases the laser fiber can be placed inside the lesion by ultrasound guidance and US can also be used for monitoring therapy progress.[30,31]

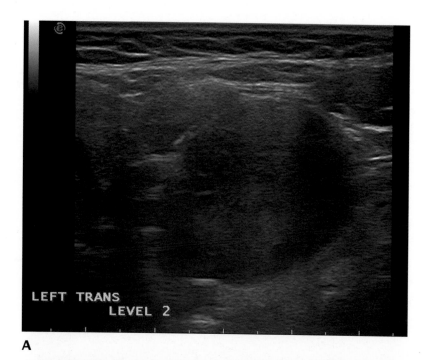

A

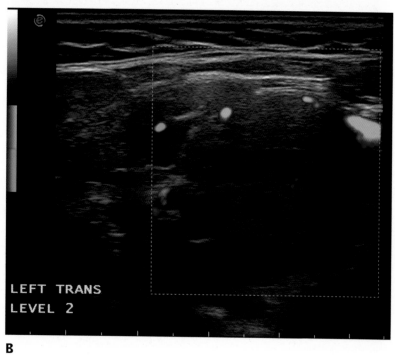

B

Fig 8–16. Neurofibroma. Note that this mass appears similar to a schwannoma such as seen in Figure 8–15A, but it is hypovascular on Doppler sonography (**B**).

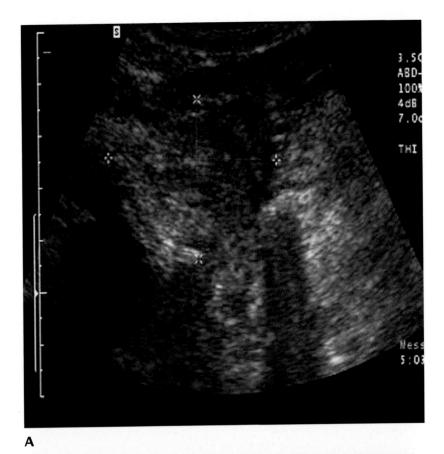

A

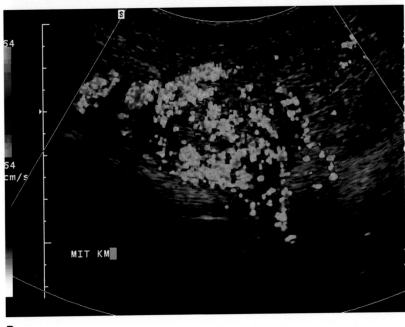

B

Fig 8-17. Hemangioma of the submental/submandibular region. Sonographically the lesion appears as a hypoechoic, poorly demarcated mass which is penetrated by hyperechoic strands, representing trabeculae of connective tissue (**A**). Application of a contrast enhancer (**B**) reveals numerous blood vessels.

Lymphangioma

Lymphangiomas are benign, slowly growing vascular lesions which are characterized by cystic and cavernous structures which have their origin in dilated lymph vessels and lymph channels.[32] They are probably developmental malformations rather than true neoplasms.[32,33] Lymphangiomas are common pediatric lesions that appear during the first years of life through adolescence. They are predominantly located in the head and neck area in general, with the lateral parts of the neck, the tongue, and the salivary glands (submandibular region; parotid gland) being the most frequent sites. Cystic lymphangioma of the neck is associated with Turner's syndrome.[34]

Clinically, lymphangiomas present as circumscribed, painless, soft and fluctuant swellings. Histologically, these lesions are characterized by thin dilated lymphatic vessels of different sizes which are covered with a thin endothelium. The lumina are either empty or contain watery, milky, or proteinaceous fluid and lymphocytes.[32] The lumina are seperated by trabeculae of connective tissue lined by a flat endothelium.

Sonographically, lymphangiomas may appear as poorly demarcated hypoechoic lesions which are penetrated by more hyperechoic strands that represent the trabeculae so that cavities of different size are formed. These cavities contain fine and homogeneous echoes, due to the protein molecules in their contents. In most cases there is a considerable dorsal or posterior acoustic enhancement (Fig 8–18). Usually there is no relation to the large blood vessels nor signs for infiltrative growth pattern. Color-coded duplex sonography reveals few if any blood vessels in the capsule but usually not inside the lesion.

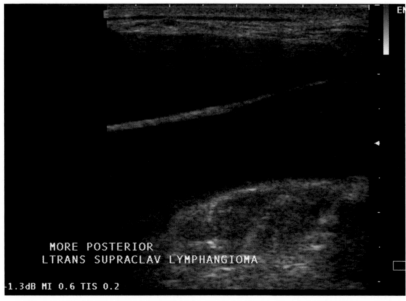

A

Fig 8–18. Lymphangioma of the lateral neck. The mass displays as a thin-walled, hypoechoic lesion with dorsal enhancement. It is penetrated by thin septae (**A**) which are vascularized (**B**) so that compartments of different size are formed. *continues*

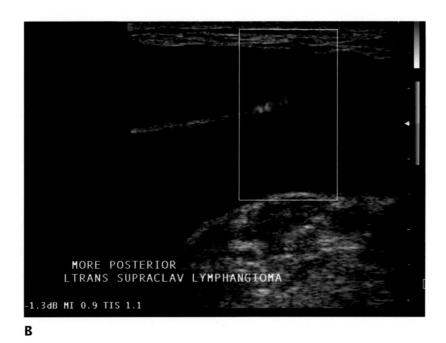

MORE POSTERIOR
LTRANS SUPRACLAV LYMPHANGIOMA

-1.3dB MI 0.9 TIS 1.1

B

Fig 8–18. *continued*

Miscellaneous Benign Neck Masses

A variety of additional benign space-occupying lesions in the head and neck can be visualized and characterized using real-time US.

Hypopharyngeal (Zenker's) diverticula are relatively common lesions in the region of the upper esophageal sphincter, in the inferior neck. They can often be seen by US in the paratracheal region, usually on the left side, inferior or posterolateral to the thyroid gland. Diverticula are easily confirmed by asking the patient to swallow while observing the distended lumen of the hypopharynx as saliva or debris shift with muscular contraction (Fig 8–19). Patients that have undergone endoscopic diverticulotomy may still have a visibly distended or relatively flaccid hypopharyngeal segment in spite of resolution of symptoms (Fig 8–20 and Video 8F).

Teratomas may be congenital or may represent residual masses following chemotherapy for germ-cell malignancies. These tumors are composed of cells derived from all three germ cell layers, and are accordingly often internally heterogeneous (Fig 8–21).[35]

Subcutaneous lesions such as cysts (epidermoid, dermoid, sebaceous), phleboliths, and other benign nodules are usually quite accessible to US examination. Such lesions are usually well demarcated but vary in their internal echogenicity according to their contents (Fig 8–22).

Other vascular lesions in the head and neck lend themselves to both B-mode and Doppler US. Internal jugular vein thrombosis is readily seen and may be a result of trauma (including surgery), coagulation disorders, or tumor invasion (Figs 8–23A and 8–23B and Videos 8G and 8H). Hematomas may vary in echogenicity depending on their age and location (Fig 8–24).

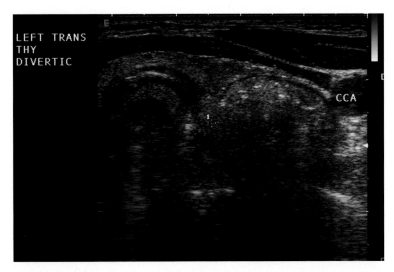

Fig 8–19. Zenker's diverticulum. The pouch is full of solid debris and is displacing the patient's left thyroid lobe anteriorly. Confirmation of its identity is facilitated by asking the patient to swallow during the US examination.

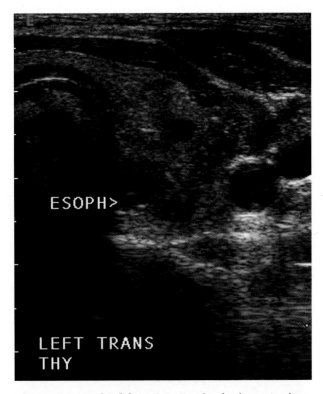

Fig 8–20 and Video 8F. Zenker's diverticulum following endoscopic diverticulotomy. Note slight residual evidence of retrothyroid pharynx, although the patient's symptoms had completely resolved. **Video 8F** shows residual, but asymptomatic, pharyngeal redundancy in a patient who had undergone successful diverticulotomy for a large Zenker's diverticulum.

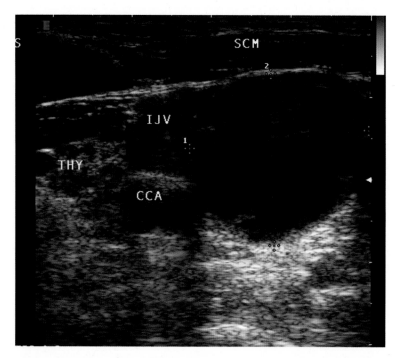

Fig 8–21. Teratoma. Supraclavicular mature teratoma following treatment of testicular carcinoma. This transverse image from the left level IV region shows a well-defined somewhat heterogeneous mass adjacent to the internal jugular vein, in the region of the thoracic duct.

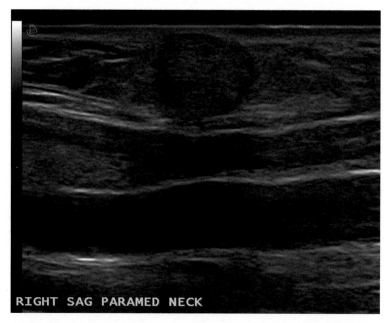

Fig 8–22. Benign subcutaneous nodules. This example shows a well-defined heterogeneous nodule within the subcutaneous plane that proved on excision to be a pilomatrixoma.

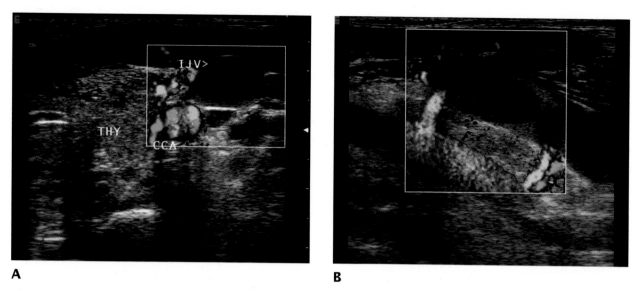

A

B

Fig 8–23 and Videos 8G and 8H. Internal jugular vein thrombosis. Left transverse (**A**) and sagittal (**B**) views of an incidentally noted partial thrombosis. **Videos 8G** (*transverse*) and **8H** (*sagittal*) show the turbulence and partial stasis of flow.

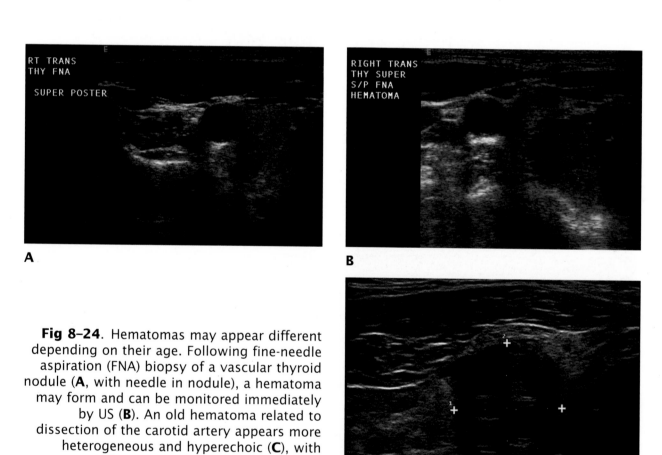

A

B

Fig 8–24. Hematomas may appear different depending on their age. Following fine-needle aspiration (FNA) biopsy of a vascular thyroid nodule (**A**, with needle in nodule), a hematoma may form and can be monitored immediately by US (**B**). An old hematoma related to dissection of the carotid artery appears more heterogeneous and hyperechoic (**C**), with carotid artery appearing in the midst of the hematoma.

C

Primary Malignant Neck Masses

Primary malignant neck masses are rare. In most cases they are histologically sarcomas (ie, rhabdomyosarcoma, angiosarcoma, chondrosarcoma, fibrosarcoma, leiomyosarcoma, radiation-induced sarcoma, and fibrous histiocytoma). They comprise less than 1% of all head and neck malignant tumors.[36]

Sarcomas

Sarcomas arise from mesenchymal tissue. The predominant tumor site is the neck and the parotid gland.[37-39] Clinically, they present as rapidly growing masses which are often fairly firm on palpation. Due to the frequently high aggressiveness of these lesions, early infiltration of neighboring tissue and/or overlying skin, large vessels in the neck, and nerve structures occur.

Sonographically, sarcomas present as poorly demarcated hypoechoic lesions with hyperechoic areas inside and signs of infiltration of surrounding tissue. Sometimes necrotic areas appear in the center of the lesion. Dynamic ultrasound palpation reveals decreased shifting of such tumors with respect to the underlying structures, including large vessels.

Lymph node metastases frequently occur. Color-coded duplex sonography in many cases reveals a peripheral perfusion pattern or areas with partial loss of perfusion. Diagnosis is based on the clinical and sonographic characteristics, and on cytologic examination of cell smears obtained by ultrasound-guided or free-hand fine-needle aspiration biopsies.

Chordomas are rare solid malignant tumors that are derived from the embryonic notochord, and in the head and neck region they arise at the skull base or along the cervical spine. Sonographically they share many of the features described for sarcomas, including heterogeneous hypoechoic infiltrative patterns (Fig 8–25).

"Branchiogenic" Carcinoma of the Neck

There is ongoing debate as to whether branchiogenic carcinomas, or branchial cleft cysts that have undergone malignant degeneration, exist or not. Some authors indicate that these lesions represent a cystic metastasis from a squamous cell carcinoma, rather than having anything to do with an original branchial cleft cyst,[40,41] whereas others are not convinced.[42] In a retrospective study of 136 cases of

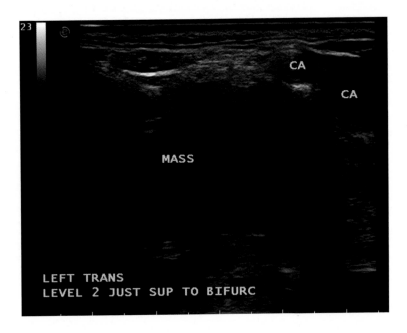

Fig 8–25. Primary malignancies of the neck are usually solid and infiltrative, such as this deep-seated chordoma.

cystic malignant lesions in the neck, Thompson et al.[43] found primary squamous cell carcinoma in the lingual or faucial tonsils and in the nasopharyngeal tonsillar tissue respectively in more than 72% of patients on the basis of histologic examination, so that the initial diagnosis of a branchiogenic carcinoma had to be revised. In a meta-analysis Goldenberg et al [44] conclude that some sites of squamous cell carcinoma are more likely to produce cystic metastases. Therefore, in most cases of reported malignant cystic lesions in the neck, these masses represent cystic lymph node metastases from clinically occult primary tumors of Waldeyer's ring. Thus,

the diagnosis of a branchiogenic carcinoma was often made erroneously in the past.

Clinically, these lesions present, like a branchial cleft cyst, as a painless progressive mass in the upper part of the neck anterior and deep to the sternocleidomastoid muscle. The majority of patients are adults, 35 years of age or older.

Sonographically, the mass is characterized, like a branchial cleft cyst, by an oval or roundish well-defined hypoechoic lesion with posterior enhancement and some fine and homogeneous echoes inside the lesion originating from protein molecules and cell debris in the cystic fluid (Fig 8-26). Due

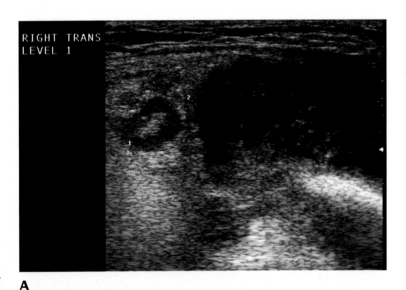

A

Fig 8–26. Lymph node metastases from head and neck squamous cell carcinoma can be cystic and/or necrotic, such as in these cases of known lip carcinoma (**A**, with adjacent solid node visible) and unknown but later identified primary carcinoma of the tonsil (**B**).

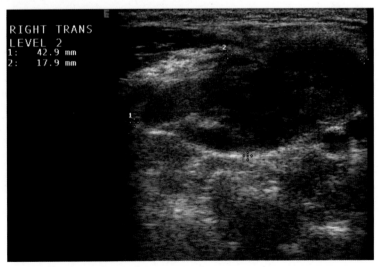

B

to the fact that most of the volume of these tumors is made up of a liquid center surrounded by a thin solid rim, the lesion is compressible. In cases of extracapsular spread, signs for infiltration into the surrounding tissue can be observed. There is sometimes a close relationship to the large blood vessels. In many cases, small lymph nodes can be identified in the neighborhood of the cystic lesion. Such lymph nodes might be reactive with a hilum structure or additional lymph node metastases. Color-coded duplex sonography reveals some blood vessels in the capsule of the cystic mass, but no vessels inside the lesion. Adult patients who initially present with a cystic mass in the upper lateral neck must be presumed to have a cystic metastasis until a benign histologic etiology is proven. Workup for metastatic carcinoma of unknown primary, including fine-needle aspiration biopsy, possible PET/CT scanning, and panendoscopy with histologic examination of appropriate biopsies of Waldeyer's ring is recommended in these cases.

Secondary Malignant Neck Masses

Metastatic lesions to the neck from infraclavicular primary malignancies take on the sonographic features of their tumors of origin. Such lesions are most often found in the supraclavicular region (Fig 8–27).

Primary Head and Neck Tumors Visible Through the Neck

In some instances, primary tumors of the upper aerodigestive tract can be visualized by transcervical US. Laryngeal and esophageal US are discussed in other chapters, and endoluminal US of the pharynx can be performed under certain circumstances and with specially adapted transducers that are not routinely available. Still, proximal aerodigestive tract sites of tumor origin such as the oropharynx and hypopharynx may reveal asymmetries or mass lesions using standard neck US probes that represent primary malignancies (Fig 8–28 and Video 8I).

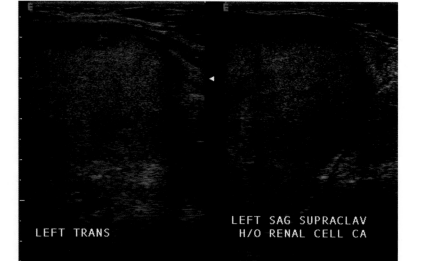

LEFT TRANS

LEFT SAG SUPRACLAV
H/O RENAL CELL CA

-1.3dB MI 0.6 TIS 0.2

Fig 8–27. Metastases from extracervical malignancies take on the characteristics of their primary tumors. This example of metastatic renal cell carcinoma was highly vascular on Dopper sonography.

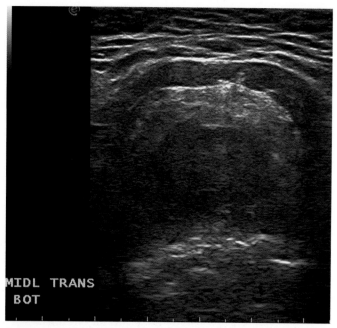

A

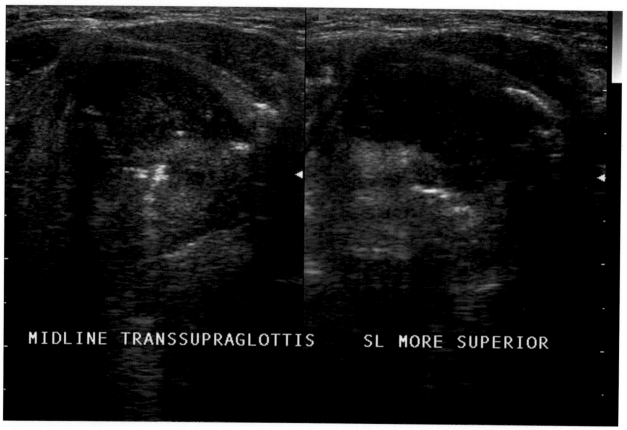

B

Fig 8–28 and Video 8I. Primary malignancies within the upper aerodigestive tract, such as in the base of tongue (**A**) and supraglottis (**B**) can often be visualized by transcervical US. Video 81 shows a transverse ascending US view of the same supraglottic tumor shown in **B**.

Videos in this Chapter

Video 8A. See legend for Figure 8–8.

Video 8B. See legend for Figure 8–8.

Video 8C. See legend for Figure 8–8.

Video 8D. See legend for Figure 8–13.

Video 8E. See legend for Figure 8–14.

Video 8F. See legend for Figure 8–20.

Video 8G. See legend for Figure 8–23.

Video 8H. See legend for Figure 8–23.

Video 8I. See legend for Figure 8–28.

References

1. Marsot-Dupuch K, Levret N, Pharaboz C, et al. Congenital neck masses. Embryonic origin and diagnosis. Report of the CIREOL. *J Radiol*. 1995;76: 405–415.

2. Nichollas R, Guelfucci B, Roman S, Triglia JM. Congenital cysts and fistulas of the neck. *Int J Pediatr Otorhinolaryngol*. 2000;55:117–124.

3. American Joint Committee on Cancer Staging. *American Joint Committee on Cancer Staging Manual*. 6th ed. New York, NY: Springer-Verlag; 2002.

4. Som PM, Curtin HD, Mancuso AA. An imaging-based classification for cervical nodes designed as an adjunct to recent clinically based nodal classifications. *Arch Otolaryngol Head Neck Surg*. 1999; 125:388–396.

5. Ahuja A, Ying M. Grey-scale sonography in assessment of cervical lymphadenopathy: review of sonographic appearances and features that may help a beginner. *Br J Oral Maxillofac Surg*. 2000; 38:451–459.

6. Görges R, Eising EG, Fotescu D, et al. Diagnostic value of high-resolution B-mode and power-mode sonography in the follow-up of thyroid cancer. *Eur J Ultrasound*. 2003;16:191–206.

7. Bandhauer F. Evaluation of cervical lymph nodes by ultrasound. *Schweiz Rundsch Med Prax*. 2005; 94:423–426.

8. Ahuja A, Ying M. Evaluation of cervical lymph node vascularity: a comparison of colour Doppler, power Doppler and 3-D power Doppler sonography. *Ultrasound Med Biol*. 2004;30:1557–1564.

9. Ying M, Ahuja A, Brook F. Accuracy of sonographic vascular features in differentiating different causes of cervical lymphadenopathy. *Ultrasound Med Biol*. 2004;30:441–447.

10. Ahuja A, Ying M, King A, Yuen HY. Lymph node hilus: gray scale and power Doppler sonography of cervical nodes. *J Ultrasound Med*. 2001;20:987–992.

11. Schade G. Experiences with using the ultrasound contrast medium levovist in differentiation of cervical lymphomas with colour-coded duplex ultrasound. *Laryngorhinootologie*. 2001;80:209–213.

12. Schreiber J, Mann W, Lieb W. Colour duplex ultrasound measurement of lymph node perfusion: a contribution to diagnosis of cervical metastases. *Laryngorhinootologie*. 1993;72:187–192.

13. Asai S, Miyachi H, Kawakami C, et al. Infiltration of cervical lymph nodes by B- and T-cell non-Hodgkin's lymphoma and Hodgkin's lymphoma: preliminary ultrasonic findings. *Am J Hematol*. 2001;67:234–239.

14. Lack EE, Cubilla AL, Woodruff JM, Farr HW. Paragangliomas of the head and neck region. *Hum Pathol*. 1979;10:191–217.

15. Kliewer KE, Cochran AJ. A review of the histology, ultrastructure, immunohistology, and molecular biology of extra-adrenal paragangliomas. *Arch Pathol Med*. 1989;113:1209–1218.

16. Linniola RI, Keiser HR, Steinberg SM, Lack EE. Histopathology of benign versus malignant sympathoadrenal paragangliomas. *Hum Pathol*. 1990;21: 1168–1180.

17. Welkoborsky HJ, Xiao Y, Mann WJ, Amedee RG, Dienes HP, Volk B. Studies for estimating the biologic behaviour and prognosis of paragangliomas in the head and neck. *Skull Base Surg*. 1995;5:149–156.

18. Gosepath J, Welkoborsky HJ, Mann WJ. Studies on the tumor biology and growth rate in jugulotympanic and carotid body glomus tumors. *Laryngorhinootologie*. 1998;77:429–433.

19. Welkoborsky HJ, Gosepath J, Mann WJ, Amedee RG. Biologic characteristics of paragangliomas of the nasal cavity and paranasal sinuses. *Am J Rhinol*. 2000;14:419–426.

20. Barnes L, Tse LLY, Hunt JL. Carotid body paraganglioma. In: Barnes L, ed. *Pathology and Genetics of Head and Neck Tumors*. Lyon: IARC Press; 2005:364–366.

21. Colreavy MP, Lacy PD, Hughes J, et al. Head and neck schwannomas. *J Laryngol Otol.* 2000;114: 119-124.

22. Bocciolini C, Dall'olio D, Cavazza S, Laudadio P. Schwannoma of cervical sympathetic chain: assessment and management. *Acta Otorhinolaryngol Ital.* 2005;25:191-194.

23. King AD, Ahuja AT, King W, Metreweli C. Sonography of peripheral nerve tumors of the neck. *AJR Am J Roentgenol.* 1997;169:1695-1698.

24. Giovagnorio F, Martinoli C. Sonography of the cervical vagus nerve: normal appearance and abnormal findings. *AJR Am J Roentgenol.* 2001;176: 745-749.

25. Kuo YL, Yao WJ, Chiu HY. Role of sonography in the preoperative assessment of neurilemmoma. *J Clin Ultrasound.* 2005;33:87-89.

26. Bendix N, Wolf C, Gruber H, Bodner G. Pictorial essay: ultrasound of tumors and tumor-like lesions of peripheral nerves. *Ultraschall Med.* 2005;26: 318-324.

27. Jecker P, Maurer J, Mann WJ. Ultrasound characteristics of lateral cervical space-occupying lesions. *Ultraschall Med.* 2001;22:130-135.

28. Senchenkov A, Kriegel A, Staren ED, Allison DC. Use of intraoperative ultrasound in excision of multiple schwannomas of the thigh. *J Clin Ultrasound.* 2005;33:360-363.

29. Odell, E. Haemangioma. In: Barnes L, ed. *Pathology and Genetics of Head and Neck Tumors.* Lyon: IARC Press; 2005:276.

30. Jacob R, Frommeld T, Maurer J, Mann WJ. Duplex ultrasonography-controlled Nd:YAG laser therapy of vascular malformations. *Ultrallschall Med.* 1999;20:191-196.

31. Offergeld C, Schellong S, Hackert I, Schmidt A, Hüttenbrink KB. Interstitial Nd:YAG laser therapy. Color-Doppler imaging guided (CDI)-laser therapy of hemangiomas and vascular malformations. *HNO.* 2003;51:46-51.

32. van der Waal, I. Lymphangioma. In: Barnes L, ed. *Pathology and Genetics of Head and Neck Tumors.* Lyon: IARC Press; 2005:195.

33. Chervenak FA, Isaacson G, Blakemore KJ, et al. Fetal cystic hygroma. *N Engl J Med.* 1983;309:822-825.

34. Bronshtein M, Zimmer EZ, Blazer S. A characteristic cluster of fetal sonographic markers that are predictive of fetal Turner syndrome in early pregnancy. *Am J Obstet Gynecol.* 2003;188(4): 1016-1020.

35. Brenner PC, Herr HW, Morse MJ, et al. Simultaneous retroperitoneal, thoracic, and cervical resection of postchemotherapy residual masses in patients with metastatic nonseminomatous germ cell tumors of the testis. *J Clin Oncol.* 1997;15(1): 1765-1769.

36. Simon JH, Paulino AC, Smith RB, Buatti, JM. Prognostic factors in head and neck rhabdomyosarcoma. *Head Neck.* 2002;24:468-473.

37. Koch BB, Karnell LH, Hoffman HT, et al. National cancer database report on chondrosarcoma of the head and neck. *Head Neck.* 2000;22:408-422.

38. Patel SG, See AC, Williamson PA, Archer DJ, Evans PH. Radiation induced sarcoma of the head and neck. *Head Neck.* 1999;21:346-354.

39. Wanebo HJ, Koness RJ, MacFarlane JK, et al. Head and neck sarcoma: report of the Head and Neck Sarcoma Registry. Society of Head and Neck Surgeons Committee on Research. *Head Neck.* 1992; 14:1-7.

40. Jereczek-Fossa BA, Casadio C, Jassem J, et al. Branchiogenic carcinoma—conceptual or true clinicopathological entity? *Cancer Treat Rev.* 2005;31: 106-114.

41. Huang CP, Wang HS, Kong YY, Wang J. Metastatic cystic squamous cell carcinoma in the neck mistaken as primary branchial cleft carcinoma: a report of 4 cases. *Zhonghua Zhiong Liu Za Zhi.* 2004; 26:634-637.

42. Girvigian MR, Rechdouni AK, Zeger GD, Segall H, Rice DH, Petrovich Z. Squamous cell carcinoma arising in a second branchial cleft cyst. *Am J Clin Oncol.* 2004;27:96-100.

43. Thompson LD, Heffner DK. The clinical importance of cystic squamous cell carcinomas in the neck: a study of 136 cases. *Cancer.* 1998;82:944-956.

44. Goldenberg D, Sciubba J, Koch WM. Cystic metastasis from head and neck squamous cell cancer: a distinct disease variant? *Head Neck.* 2006;28: 633-638.

Chapter 9

LARYNGEAL ULTRASONOGRAPHY

Timothy J. Beale
John S. Rubin

Laryngeal ultrasonography (US) is a useful skill for the head and neck radiologist and a valuable tool available to the otolaryngologist. It is complementary to CT and MRI, but due to the superficial location of the larynx actually offers images of higher resolution than either modality. In addition it is a real-time procedure with static image and video capture capability, can be combined with fine needle aspiration, is inexpensive, and does not involve ionizing radiation.

The aims of this chapter are four fold:

1. To offer the reader a brief history of laryngeal US;
2. To allow for an understanding of the techniques involved in laryngeal US;
3. To demonstrate the appearance of normal laryngeal anatomy on US;
4. To understand the uses of laryngeal US and to demonstrate the ultrasound appearances of common laryngeal pathology.

studies during that time period.[3-6] By 1973, echoes from the free margins of the true vocal folds could be "unequivocally identified."[7] By the late 1980s US was found to be useful for real-time evaluation, not only of the true vocal folds, but of the false vocal folds and of vocal fold movement.[8]

Due to its noninvasive nature, and as a natural outgrowth from fetal investigations in general, US has been used to investigate fetal human upper respiratory anatomy.[9] Its use has also been applied to normal and pathologic findings in infants and children[10] where, for example, it has been noted to allow for "easy subglottic examination" of cricoid hypertrophy, subglottic hemangiomas and laryngeal stenosis[10] and for laryngeal paralysis.[11] It has been used as an adjunct in cases of infantile laryngeal stridor, in one instance assisting in the diagnosis of a large (12-mm) congenital cyst arising from the aryepiglottic fold.[12] Over the last decade or so it has proven particularly useful for real-time evaluation of the true and false vocal folds and of vocal fold movement.[8]

A Brief History of Laryngeal Ultrasonography

Ultrasonography (US) has been posited to be a possible mode for investigation of the larynx since the 1960s.[1,2] The Japanese literature is replete with such

The Techniques Involved in Laryngeal Ultrasonography

US of the larynx is performed using a high-frequency (7 to 14 MHz) linear transducer which ensures high-resolution images. The patient typically lies supine

or recumbent, although the examination can also be performed in the sitting position. In order to understand the scanning routine line diagrams (Figs 9-1, 9-2, and 9-3) have been used in this chapter as an aid. The same diagrams have also been included in some of the later figures to help the reader understand the scanning plane used to obtain each image.

In each of the diagrams the hyoid bone and thyroid cartilage have been outlined, the position of the probe represented by a red rectangle, and the direction of movement of the probe represented with a black arrow.

The scanning routine that we utilize is as follows:

1. Starting in the transverse (axial) plane in the **midline** we scan from superior to inferior (see Fig 9-1). First identify the hyoid bone and then angle superiorly to assess the tongue base and floor of mouth. Then angle inferiorly to assess first the valleculae and then the thyrohyoid region for vallecular and thyroglossal duct cysts. Then angle inferiorly at the superior thyroid notch to assess the supraglottic larynx (pre-epiglottic and paraglottic spaces and the infrahyoid epiglottis).

   In the cricothyroid region, angle the probe both up and down to assess the true vocal folds, arytenoid cartilages, and Delphian node(s) (if present).

   Finally sweep the probe inferiorly to visualize the cricoid cartilage and subglottis.

2. Next scan again in the transverse (axial) plane sweeping the probe from superior to inferior in both a right and left **paramedian** position (see Figs 9-2A and 9-2B). Assess the following: (from superior to inferior): the faucial tonsil, lateral tongue base, and lateral valleculae; the thyrohyoid region, strap muscles, and thyroid laminae (and deep to the latter the paraglottic space and true vocal folds); the lateral cricoid cartilage and posteriorly the piriform fossae (sinuses) and cervical esophagus.

3. Next scan in the **sagittal** plane starting laterally (and therefore posteriorly), and sweep anteriorly to the midline (see Figs 9-3A and 9-3B). This scan plane is particularly useful for visualizing the pre-epiglottic fat, epiglottis, thyrohyoid, and cricothyroid regions.

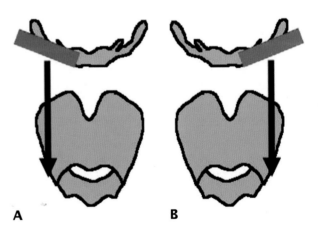

Fig 9–2. Scanning routine 2. Scanning in the right (**A**) and left (**B**) paramedian position with the probe in the transverse (axial) plane again starting just superior to the hyoid and extending inferiorly to the level of the cervical trachea. Remember to angle the probe inferiorly at the superior thyroid notch and superiorly in the cricothyroid region. This allows visualization of structures posterior to the thyroid cartilage, avoiding potential problems with thyroid cartilage calcification.

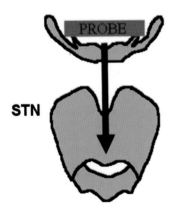

Fig 9–1. Scanning routine 1. Scanning in the midline with the probe in the transverse (axial) plane. The red rectangle indicates the linear probe positioned initially superior to the hyoid bone (*H*), then moved inferiorly in the direction of the black arrow and in addition angled inferiorly at the superior thyroid notch (*STN*).

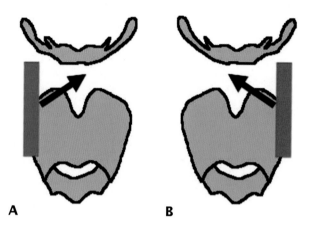

Fig 9–3. Scanning routine 3. **A.** and **B.** Scanning in the sagittal plane starting laterally (posteriorly) and sweeping to the midline.

The superior extension of the thyroarytenoid muscle into the paraglottic fat is best assessed in this plane.

Laterally part of the piriform fossae and postcricoid region can usually be visualized and inferior to this the cervical esophagus is nearly always clearly demonstrated.

4. Finally, to assess vocal fold movement scan through the cricothyroid region angling 30 degrees upward, viewing first on one side and then on the other. Identify the arytenoid cartilages first, then the true vocal folds. The vocal folds will abduct on inspiration and relax on expiration and are best assessed during quiet breathing (Videos 9A and 9B, midline transverse view). Assessment during phonation is difficult due to laryngeal movement.

Please note that although the superior supraglottis and tongue base are nearly always clearly demonstrated by angling the probe from the superior thyroid notch and the inferior supraglottis by angling the probe from the cricothyroid region, the true folds may be obscured if there is extensive calcification of the thyroid laminae.

Appearance of Normal Laryngeal Anatomy on Ultrasound

As with CT and MRI there is good soft tissue contrast between the normal laryngeal structures such as the laryngeal cartilages (thyroid, cricoid, and arytenoid), the fat within the pre-epiglottic and paraglottic spaces of the supraglottis, and muscle (thyroarytenoid and strap muscles) on US.

In addition there is usually good soft tissue contrast between these normal structures and pathology: the pre-epiglottic and paraglottic fat is bright (hyperechoic) and pathology (tumor and inflammation) is usually darker (hypoechoic).

The normal laryngeal anatomy on ultrasound is best understood by reviewing the annotated figures and legends.

Figs 9-4A through 9-4C demonstrate the **midline** laryngeal anatomy and Figures 9-5A through 9-5D the **paramedian** axial laryngeal anatomy from superior to inferior.

Figure 9-6 demonstrates the **sagittal** laryngeal anatomy.

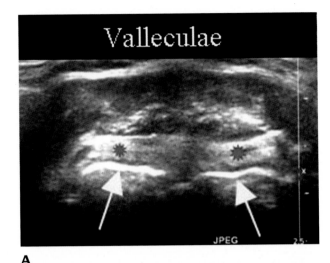

A

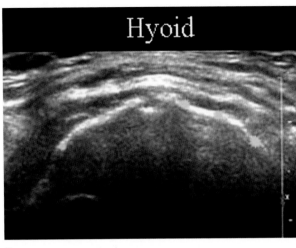

B

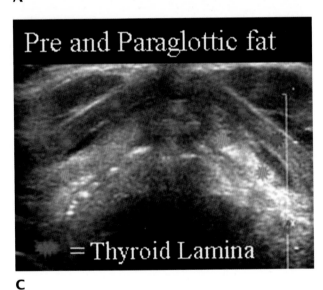

C

Fig 9–4. A–C. (superior to inferior). Midline transverse (axial) plane imaging is particularly useful for imaging structures and pathology involving the lingual tonsils, valleculae, pre-epiglottic and paraglottic fat. **A.** At the level of the valleculae (*red stars*), note the bright line of the posterior surface of the suprahyoid epiglottis (*white arrows*) indicating the air/mucosa interface. **B.** At the level of the hyoid bone (*yellow stars*), note the acoustic shadow deep to the hyoid bone. **C.** At the level of the supraglottis, note the thyroid laminae (*TL, red stars*) and the paraglottic fat (*pink stars*).The paraglottic fat is continuous anteriorly with the pre-epiglottic fat.

There are several important features to note:

1. The mucosa of the false vocal fold overlies fatty connective tissue that contains vessels, lymphatics, nerves, and the superior extension of the thyroarytenoid muscle. This fatty connective tissue within the paraglottic and pre-epiglottic spaces has a hyperechoic (bright) appearance on US (see Figs 9–4C and 9–5A).

2. The paraglottic and pre-epiglottic spaces are continuous anteriorly, a fact readily appreciated on US (see Fig 9–4C).[13]

3. The true vocal fold consists almost entirely of muscle (the more medial vocalis and the more lateral thyroarytenoid muscle) and is relatively hypoechoic (dark) (see Fig 9–5C).

4. The superior extension of the thyroarytenoid muscle is clearly seen against the contrasting hyperechoic paraglottic fat (see Figs 9–5B and 9–6).

5. The thyroid cartilage has a variable appearance depending on how much of the cartilage is calcified, ossified, or nonmineralized. However, even in patients with a completely calcified thyroid cartilage views of the larynx are possible by angling the probe inferiorly at the superior thyroid notch and superiorly in the cricothyroid region. The nonmineralized areas of cartilage,

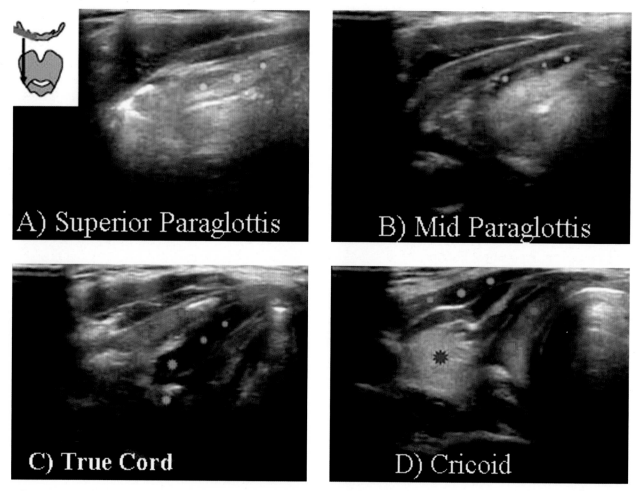

Fig 9–5. A-D (superior to inferior). Scanning in a right paramedian transverse (axial) plane as in Figure 9–2A. The following structures are clearly identified: **A.** At the level of the superior paraglottis, hyperechoic paraglottic fat (*yellow star*) and thyroid lamina (*TL, red star*). **B.** At the level of the mid paraglottis, superior slip of thyroarytenoid muscle *(turquoise star)*. **C.** At the level of the true cord, arytenoid cartilage (*orange star*) and true cord *(turquoise star)*. **D.** At the level of the cricoid cartilage, cricoid cartilage (*pink star*), right lobe thyroid (*blue star*), and strap muscle (*green star*).

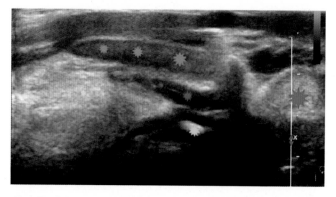

Fig 9–6. Parasagittal US. The following structures are clearly identified: thyroid lamina (*TL, green stars*), thyroarytenoid muscle (*red stars*), arytenoid cartilage (*yellow star*), and cricoid cartilage (*pink star*).

however, also allow good visualization of the internal anatomy of the larynx when the probe is placed directly over the cartilage as there is good transmission of the US beam whereas the heavily calcified or ossified segments of cartilage variably reflect a percentage of the US beam restricting visualization. Overall the laryngeal cartilages are more heavily calcified in males and increasingly calcify with age.

6. The arytenoid cartilages are hyperechoic (see Fig 9–5C) and in the younger patient may have a relatively hypoechoic interior.

7. The cervical esophagus is usually visualized on the left with the head in the midline, but may be seen on both sides as the pressure of the US probe or head turning displaces the esophagus. The various layers of the cervical esophagus can be identified (Fig 9–7).

The midline transverse view is of value in assessing vocal fold movement allowing for comparison of the two sides (Videos 9A and 9B).[13] However, the air-soft tissue interface at the level of the true vocal fold epithelium can cause inherent problems to US because air allows the beam to scatter. Thus, there are probably some minor reverberation artifacts in all cases. Although the edge of the vocal fold can generally be seen, Rubin et al[14] postulate that this reverberation effect makes it more difficult to visualize small solid lesions on the vocal fold edge.

One special feature is anisotrophy, whereby a perpendicular strike gives an echo dense signal, but any divergent angle causes the signal to drop rapidly. This may cause further confounding images when viewing the true vocal folds.

Uses of Laryngeal Ultrasound and Ultrasound Appearances of Common Laryngeal Pathology

Uses of laryngeal US include the following:

■ As an adjunct to CT/MRI, as well as indirect, direct, or fiberoptic laryngoscopy, for laryngeal squamous cell carcinoma (SCC) tumor staging.

■ In the assessment of other anterior cervical masses: query thyroid/thyroglossal/laryngeal in etiology?

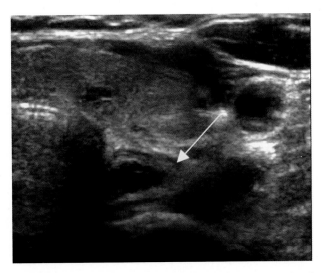

Fig 9–7. Transverse (axial) US image at level of thyroid. Note the cervical esophagus (*white arrow*) posterior to the left lobe of the thyroid.

- For the noninvasive real-time assessment of vocal fold function/paralysis/paresis/cysts.
- In the diagnosis of laryngoceles.
- For noninvasive assessment of laryngeal elevation, and thus as an aide in evaluating the dysphagic patient.
- In the evaluation of proximal tracheal stent insertion.
- As an adjunct in the diagnosis of epiglottitis.
- For visualizing the fetal airway.

Malignant Pathology

As an adjunct to CT/MRI in laryngeal SCC tumor staging: US is well established in the assessment of cervical nodes in patients with head and neck squamous cell carcinoma (SCC) and can be combined with fine needle aspiration (FNA). In conjunction with CT/MRI, US increases the accuracy of the nodal staging.[15,16]

We have found that knowledge obtained when assessing the primary laryngeal tumor on US increases the confidence when reporting the tumor extent on CT/MRI, in particular, when assessing possible involvement of the following sites: tongue base, superior thyroid notch, thyroid cartilage, and subtle extralaryngeal extension in the cricothyroid region. Furthermore it more easily picks up anterior cervical (level 6 cricothyroid or Delphian) nodal spread from a glotttic carcinoma.

SCC tends to be isoechoic or hypoechoic (darker) in comparison to muscle and markedly hypoechoic in comparison to fatty tissue as in the paraglottic and pre-epiglottic spaces.

Ultrasound is very good at delineating local tumor extension in the following manner:

A. Extralaryngeal spread:
- Tumor extension superiorly into the lingual tonsil and tongue base, areas very difficult to delineate on CT and MRI (Figs 9–8A and 9–8B).
- Subtle tumor extension through the superior thyroid notch (Figs 9–9A and 9–9B, and 9–10A and 9–10B).

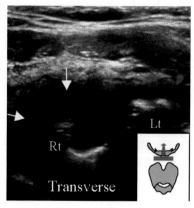
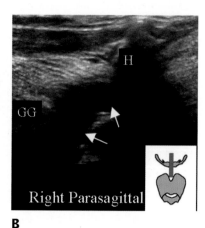

A   **B**

Fig 9–8. Extension of supraglottic SCC to the right lingual tonsil. Axial (**A**) and sagittal (**B**) US images of the lingual tonsil/tongue base. Note the markedly thickened and hypoechoic right lingual tonsil (*white arrows*) and compare to the left side. GG = genioglossus muscle, H = hyoid bone. The lingual tonsil and tongue base region are difficult to assess on MRI/CT and clinical inspection, but can usually be clearly visualised on US.

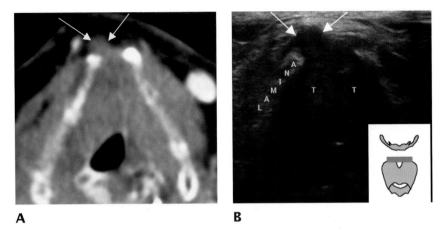

A

B

Fig 9–9. A. Axial CT and **B.** equivalent axial US image through the supraglottis at the level of the superior thyroid notch (*STN*). Note the fairly subtle right paramedian tumor extension through the STN (*white arrows*). The tumor extension is more clearly demonstrated on US. T = tumor in anterior true cords.

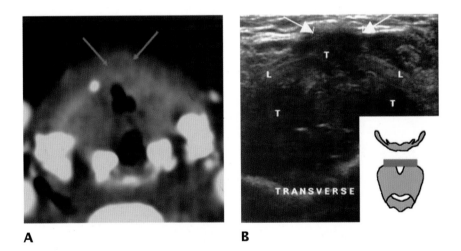

A

B

Fig 9–10. A. Axial CT and **B.** equivalent axial US image demonstrating tumor extension through the anterior thyroid laminae and STN (*red* (**A**) or *white* (**B**) *arrows*), which is difficult to identify on the CT image, but more obvious on the US image. T = tumor. L = thyroid lamina. CT/MRI image quality is sometimes suboptimal in head and neck cancer patients due to motion artefact as the irritating tumor may cause the patient to cough or swallow during image acquisition. US is not affected in the same way as the examination can be repeated until a clear view is obtained.

■ Tumor extension into the soft tissue of the cricothyroid region (Figs 9-11A, 9-12A, and 9-11B, 9-12B) and from there superiorly to involve the strap muscles.

■ Tumor extension through (eroded) thyroid laminae (Fig 9-13). Note also the large supraglottic tumor (Fig 9-14) where despite the tumor size there is preservation of a thin hyperechoic line (paraglottic fat)

between the tumor and thyroid cartilage indicating absence of cartilage involvement.

■ US is an excellent modality for imaging lateral spread of postcricoid carcinoma, that is, whether tumor is contained within or has extended through the muscle layers, and what is its relationship to the carotid sheath and thyroid gland (Figs 9-15A and 9-15B)?

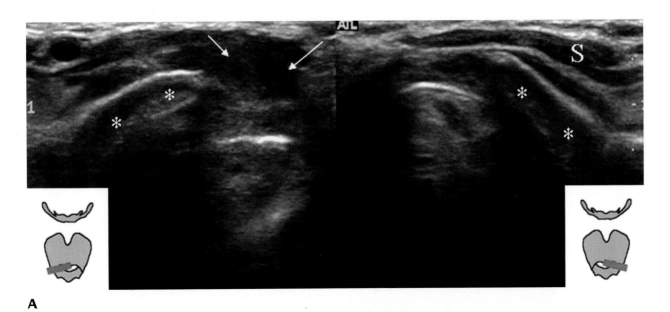

A

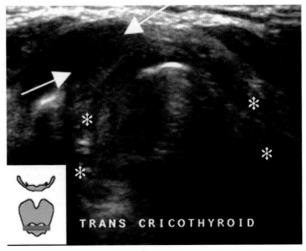

B

Fig 9-11. A. and **B.** Cricothyroid tumor extension: Note the subtle tumor extension (*arrows*) through the right cricothyroid membrane, making the tumor stage T4. Compare to the normal left side. * = cricoid ring, S = strap muscle.

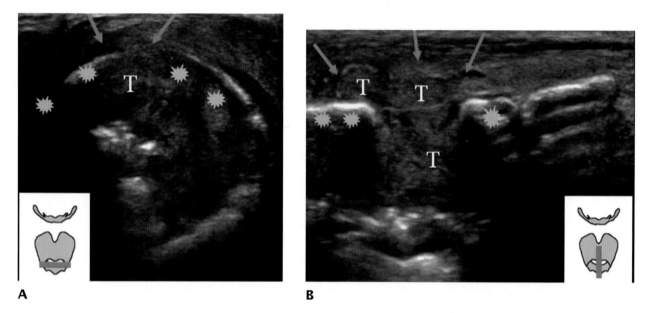

A   **B**

Fig 9–12. A. Sagittal and **B.** transverse US images of the subglottis showing extension of hypoechoic tumor (*T*), outlined by red arrows, extending anteriorly through the cricothyroid membrane and into the subglottis. T = tumor, green stars = thyroid lamina, pink stars = cricoid cartilage.

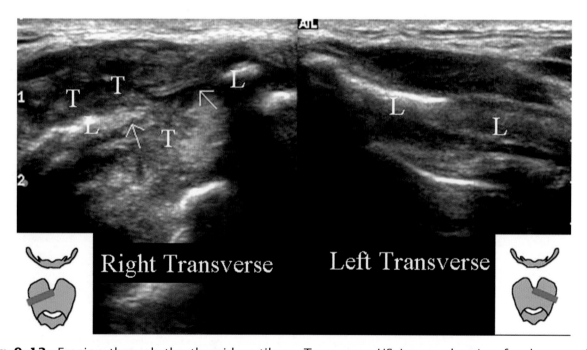

Fig 9–13. Erosion through the thyroid cartilage. Transverse US image showing focal tumor (*T*) extension through the right thyroid lamina (*L*). Compare to the normal left side. The arrows indicate the margin of the eroded cartilage.

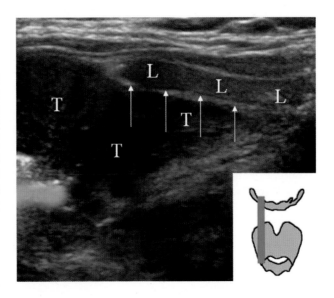

Fig 9–14. Thyroid cartilage invasion? Look for preservation of the hyperechoic line (*arrows*) representing residual paraglottic fat between the tumor (*T*) and thyroid lamina (*L*) to indicate absence of cartilage invasion in this patient with an extensive supraglottic tumor.

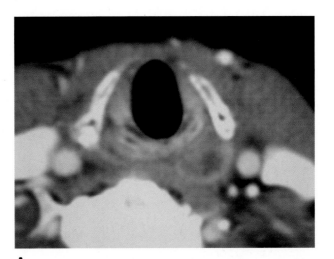

A

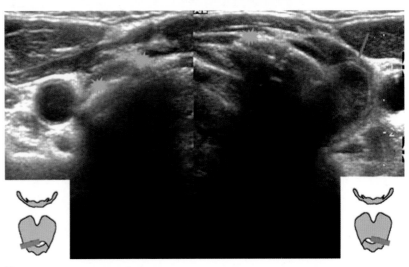

Fig 9–15. Postcricoid carcinoma. **A.** Axial CT and **B.** equivalent axial US images through the postcricoid region. Note the well-defined lateral margin of the tumor (*arrows*), which extends posterior to the left thyroid lamina (*green stars*).

B

B. Tumor extension within the larynx:

■ Within the larynx US can be used to demonstrate involvement of the true vocal fold (Figs 9-16A and 9-16B), the anterior commissure anteriorly (Fig 9-17), and arytenoids posteriorly (see Fig 9-16A).

■ Subtle involvement or invasion of the paraglottic fat can be shown (Figs 9-18 and 9-19).

C. Nodal disease:

■ US is better than CT for obtaining information on nodal disease. Micrometastases greater than 3 mm within lymph nodes may be seen on US and confirmed with US-guided FNA.

■ Delphian nodes which are difficult on CT to differentiate from adjacent strap muscle can be clearly imaged with US. (Fig 9-20).

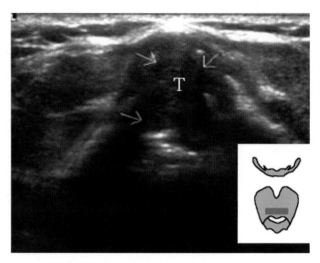

Fig 9–17. Transverse midline US demonstrating tumour (*T and arrows*) involving the anterior commissure and both anterior vocal folds.

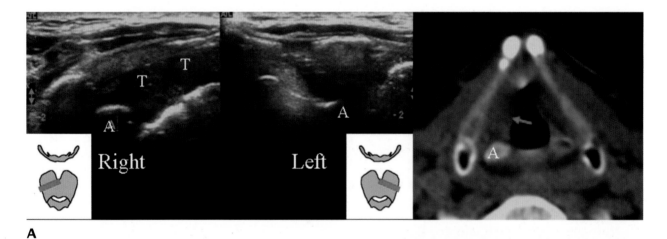

A

Fig 9–16. A. Transverse paramedian US at the level of the vocal folds demonstrating tumor thickening of the whole right vocal fold (T) and a relatively echogenic right arytenoid. Compare to the normal left side. Corresponding CT image (*right*) shows sclerosis of the right arytenoid and thickening of the right vocal fold (*arrow*). **B.** Transverse paramedian US on the left side in another patient showing involvement of posterior part of left vocal fold. T = tumor, L = thyroid lamina and arrows = paraglottic fat.

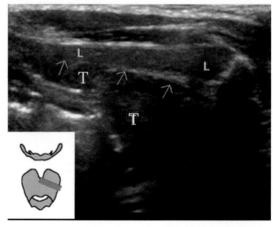

B

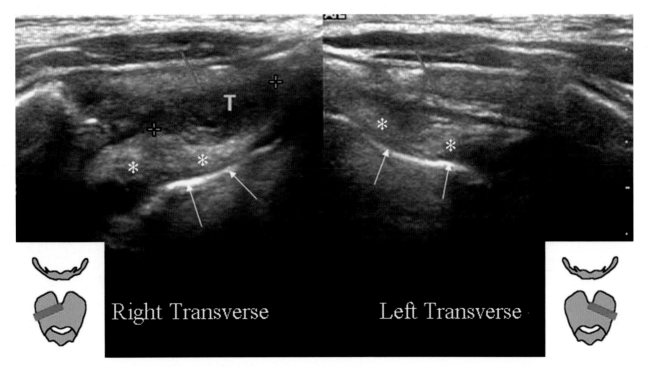

Fig 9–18. Transverse US demonstrating subtle submucosal extension of tumor (*T*) into the lateral paraglottic fat on the right, compared to normal anatomy on the left. Note the loss of the hyperechoic line (*red arrow*) between the tumor and thyroid lamina (*L*). White arrows = Free edge of false cord, stars = paraglottic fat.

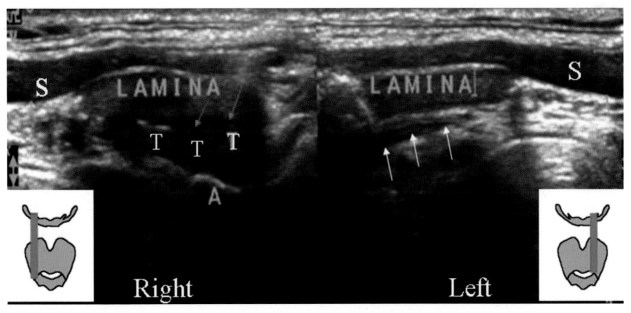

Fig 9–19. Supraglottic extension of glottic tumor. Parasagittal US scan. On the right, there is hypoechoic tumor (*T*) extending superiorly from the arytenoid (*A*) submucosally into the supraglottis (paraglottic fat). Note the superior slip of the normal thyroarytenoid muscle (*arrows on the patient's normal left side*). Note loss of the hyperechoic line between tumor and cartilage (*red arrows*). S = strap muscle.

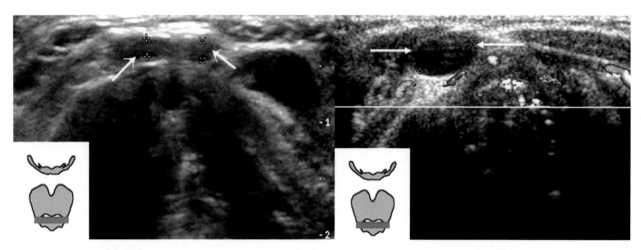

Fig 9–20. Nodal disease. Transverse US at the level of the cricothyroid membrane, demonstrating two cases of Delphian (Level 6) nodes indicated by arrows. These nodes are difficult to distinguish from the adjacent strap muscles on CT.

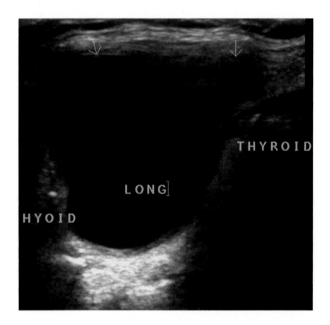

Fig 9–21. Thyroglossal duct cyst (TDC). Sagittal US image.

TDC Facts: Midline or paramedian cystic lesion, but often appear "solid" on US due to internal echoes.

Practical Tips:

Check the relationship of the swelling with the strap muscles.

Confirm that there is a normal thyroid gland.

Tap the cyst with a finger when scanning to move the internal echoes to confirm its cystic nature. Look for suprahyoid extension.

Benign Pathology

■ Thyroglossal duct cysts and thyroglossal tract remnants (Figs 9–21, and 9–22A and 9–22B) are clearly imaged and diagnosed with US. The characteristic location of the cyst within or just deep to the strap muscle is readily demonstrated. Due to internal echoes these cysts may appear to be "pseudo-solid," but tapping the cyst while scanning, or using power Doppler will confirm the cystic nature of the swelling.

■ The rare malignant papillary carcinoma within a thyroglossal remnant usually is seen as a solid echogenic mass

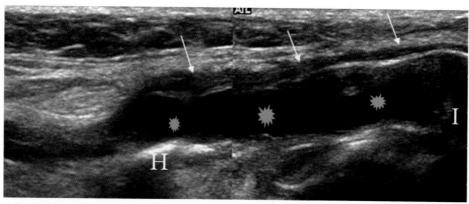

A

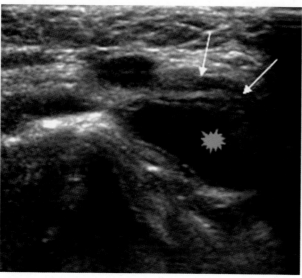

B

Fig 9–22. Thyroglossal tract remnant. **A.** Parasagittal and **B.** transverse paramedian US images. The thyroglossal tract cyst (*stars*) extends inferiorly from just superficial to the hyoid bone (*H*) to the superior thyroid isthmus (*I*). Note the strap muscle superficial to the cyst (*white arrows*).

occupying part of the cyst (Figs 9-23A through 9-23D).

- Vallecular cysts (Figs 9-24A and 9-24B) can clearly be identified and are usually unrelated to the patient's symptoms.
- True vocal fold cysts greater than 2 to 3 mm can be visualized as ovoid echo-poor areas (Fig 9-25). The superficial border tends not to be clear due to difficulty with

air/soft tissue interface. We[14] and others[17,18] have previously reported experience studying these types of lesions.

- Laryngeal mucoceles (Figs 9-26A, 9-26B, and 9-26C) are readily imaged and diagnosed. When a laryngeal mucocele is identified an attempt should be made to visualize the laryngeal ventricle to exclude an obstructing tumor.

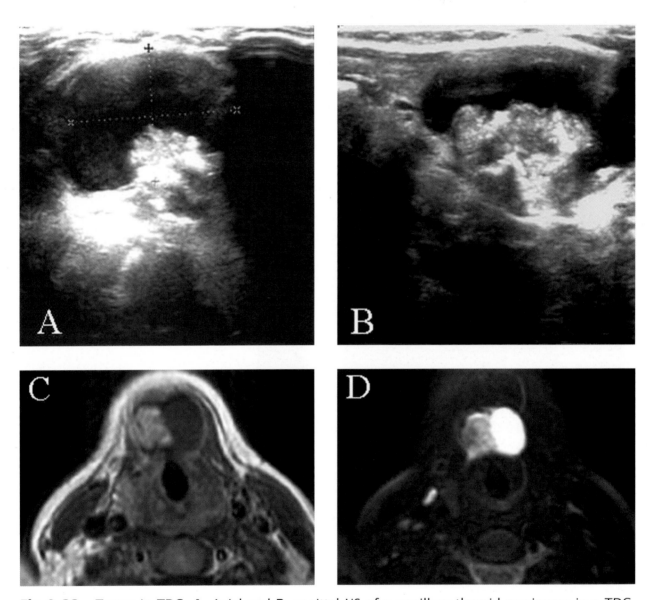

Fig 9–23. Tumor in TDC. **A.** Axial and **B.** sagittal US of a papillary thyroid carcinoma in a TDC. **C.** Axial T1 post-gadolinium and **D.** Axial STIR MRI image through same lesion.

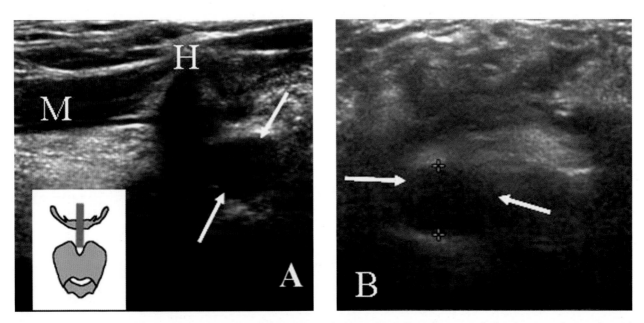

Fig 9–24. A. Sagittal and **B.** transverse US images showing a vallecular cyst (*white arrows*). H = hyoid bone, M = mylohyoid muscle.

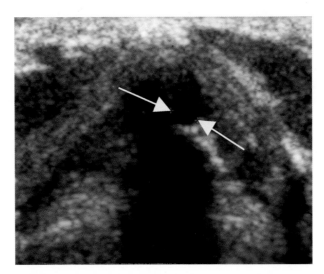

Fig 9–25. True vocal fold cysts. Vocal fold cysts of 2 to 4 mm can be identified on US as ovoid, echo-poor areas (*arrows*).

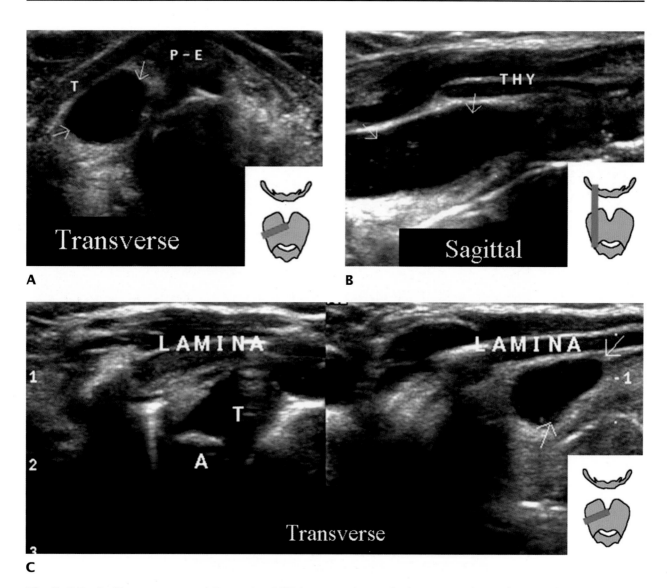

Fig 9–26. A. Transverse and **B.** sagittal US images through the supraglottic larynx demonstrating a laryngeal mucocele (*arrows*). P-E = pre-epiglottic space, T and THY = thyroid lamina. **C.** US images at the level of the right vocal fold (*left image*) and the right supraglottis (*right image*). In this patient the mucocele was discovered on US and shown to be secondary to a laryngeal tumor (*T*) extending into the laryngeal ventricle. A = arytenoid cartilage.

■ Assessment of tracheal stents. The suture used to fix the tracheal stent in situ can be clearly demonstrated on US. In patients with discomfort following placement of a tracheal stent, the suture and any surrounding inflammatory change/infection can readily be assessed (Figs 9–27A and 9–27B).

The authors do not have experience of assessing vocal fold function in children,[11] the diagnosis of epiglottitis,[19] or the assessment of the fetal airway using US[20] although these are all well described in the literature. Certainly in the course of performing head and neck US examinations, the dynamic assessment of vocal fold mobility is feasible and may be particularly pertinent in the setting of thy-

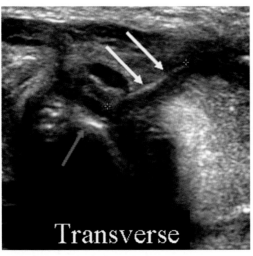
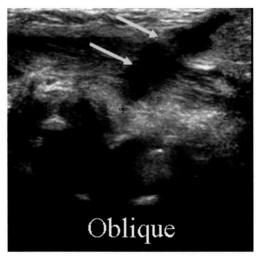

A   **B**

Fig 9–27. Tracheal stent. The pt complained of discomfort following tracheal stent and fixation suture insertion. **A.** Note the tracheal stent (*red arrow*) and suture (*white arrows*). **B.** Note the abnormal hypoechoic soft tissue surrounding the suture (*yellow arrows*) in keeping with inflammation and/or infection.

roid, parathyroid, and laryngeal disease. Furthermore, US has become a favored technique for the evaluation of the pharynx and larynx during swallowing (see Chapter 14). US guidance may also prove useful for performing therapeutic laryngeal injections.

Summary

The role of US in the larynx is expanding. It is a modality well suited to evaluate subtle changes in a real-time capacity. This chapter has provided an overview of our use of the modality in the larynx.

Videos in This Chapter

Videos 9A and 9B: Normal larynx midline transverse dynamic view of vocal fold movement in respiration and swallowing.

References

1. Mensch B, Analyse par exploration ultrasonique du mouvement des cordes vocales isolées. *C R Soc Biol.* 1964;158:2295-2296.
2. Hertz CH, Lindstrom K, Sonesson B. Ultrasonic recording of the vibrating vocal folds. *Acta Otolaryngol.* 1970;69:223-230.
3. Asano H. Application of the ultrasonic pulse-method on the larynx, *J Oto-Laryng Japan.* 1968; 71:108-109.
4. Asano H. Application of the ultrasonic pulse-method to the larynx [in Japanese]. *J Oto-Laryng Japan.* 1968;71:895-916.
5. Kitamura T, Kaneko T, Asano H, Miura T Ultrasonic diagnosis in oto-rhinolaryngology. *Eye Ear Nose Throat Monthly.* 1969;48:121-131.
6. Kitamura T, Kaneko T, Asano H, Ultrasonic diagnosis of laryngeal disease. *Jap Med Ultrason.* 1964;2:14-15.
7. Holmer NG, Kitzing P, Lindstrom K. Echo glottography. *Acta Otolaryngol.* 1973;75:454-463.
8. Raghavendra BN, Horii SC, Reede DL, Rumancik WM, Persky M, Bergeron RT. Sonographic anatomy of the larynx, with particular reference to the vocal cords. *J Ultrasound Med.* 1987;6:225-230.

9. Wolfson VP, Laitman JT. Ultrasound investigation of fetal upper respiratory anatomy. *Anat Rec.* 1990; 227:363–372.

10. Garel C, Contencin P, Polonvski JM, Hassan M, Narcy P. Laryngeal ultrasonography in infants and children: a new way of investigating. Normal and pathological findings. *Int J Ped Otorhinolaryngol.* 1992;23:107–117.

11. Friedman EM. Role of ultrasound in the assessment of vocal cord function in infants and children. *Ann Otol Rhinol Laryngol.* 1997;106:199–209.

12. Shita L, Rypens F, Hassid S, Vermeylan D, Struyven J. Sonographic demonstration of a congenital laryngeal cyst. *J Ultrasound Med.* 1999;18: 665–667.

13. Ahuja A, Evans R, eds. *Practical Head and Neck Ultrasound.* London: Greenwich Medical Media Limited; 2000.

14. Rubin JS, Lee S, McGuiness J, Hore I, Hill D, Berger L. The potential role of ultrasound in differentiating solid and cystic swellings of the true vocal fold. *J Voice.* 2004;18:231–235.

15. Sumi M, Ohki M, Nakamura T. Comparison of sonography and CT for differentiating benign from malignant cervical lymph nodes in patients with squamous cell carcinoma of the head and neck. *AJR Am J Roentgenol.* 2001;176(4):1019–1024.

16. Van den Brekel MW, Castelijns JA, Stel HV, Golding RP, Meyer CJ, Snow GB. Modern imaging techniques and ultrasound-guided aspiration cytology for the assessment of neck node metastases: a prospective comparative study. *Eur Arch Otorhinolaryngol.* 1993;250(1):11–17.

17. Chevallier P, Marcy PY, Padovani B, Raffaelli C, Coussement A, Bruneton JN. Aspect echographique et frequence des kystes larynges. *J. E. M. U.* 1998; 19:385–388.

18. Youssefzadeh S, Steiner E, Turetschek K, Gritzmann N, Kursten R, Franz P. Sonographie von larynxzysten. *Rofo Forstchr Geb Rontgenstr Neun Bildgeb Verfahr.* 1993;159:38–42.

19. Werner SL, Jones RA, Emerman CL. Sonographic assessment of the epiglottis. *Acad Emerg Med.* 2004;11:1358–1360.

20. Richards DS, Farah LA. Sonographic visualization of the fetal upper airway. *Ultrasound Obstet Gynecol.* 1994;4(1):21–23.

Chapter 10

TRANSESOPHAGEAL ENDOSONOGRAPHY

V. Raman Muthusamy
Janak Shah

Introduction

The development of the echoendoscope, resulting from the attachment of an ultrasound processor to the tip of a video endoscope, occurred in 1980. The procedure resulting from the use of this device became known as endoscopic ultrasound (EUS) or endosonography. This initial "radial" echoendoscope had a radially oriented transducer that produced images that were perpendicular to the axis of the scope. In the early 1990s, development of a linear array echoendoscope, in which the ultrasound image is parallel to the echoendoscope, allowed for real-time, endoscopic ultrasound-visualized fine needle aspiration (EUS-FNA). Over the past quarter century, EUS has been increasingly utilized as a diagnostic tool in the evaluation of the gastrointestinal wall and its adjacent structures. In this chapter, we discuss the use of transesophageal endosonography in diagnosing, staging, and even treating esophageal and periesophageal disease.

Transesophageal Endosonography Equipment and Technique

Transesophageal EUS is typically performed using forward or oblique viewing radial echoendoscopes or with a linear echoendoscope if EUS-FNA is necessary. When a mucosal lesion is being evaluated, a standard endoscope is used prior to endosonography if a forward viewing radial echoendoscope is not available. For evaluation of small mucosal lesions, a high-frequency (12 to 30 MHz) probe can be used through the biopsy channel of a standard endoscope in lieu of or in addition to a high-frequency (5 to 20 MHz) capable radial echoendoscope. Increased frequencies provide greater local (mucosal) resolution at the expense of impaired distant imaging. All current linear echoendoscopes and, increasingly, many radial echoendoscopes, use electronic processors, which allow for color flow and Doppler capabilities.

On insertion of the echoendoscope, the instrument is passed through the upper esophageal sphincter (UES), which is typically about 15 cm from the incisors. Customarily, a distal to proximal imaging technique is performed. Thus, the scope is typically advanced past the gastroesophageal junction (GEJ), located at about 40 cm from the incisors, into the stomach. From the proximal stomach, the celiac axis/celiac artery takeoff can be seen anterior to the aorta. The left adrenal gland, which is a frequent site of metastases in lung cancer, can be visualized just to the left of the celiac artery takeoff at this level. To the right of the celiac axis at this level, the left liver can be seen. Evaluation of the celiac axis and liver is an important part of the staging of esophageal malignancy.

If a radial EUS scope is used, the pullback technique is relatively straightforward, as a 360-degree view is obtained of the mediastinum on pullback technique. Initially, the right pleural space and the heart are seen from 30 to 40 cm from the incisors. The carina is typically located at 30 cm from the incisors, with the arch of the aorta typically located at 25 cm from the incisors. Subcarinal nodes are typically seen just below the carina at 30 cm and immediately superior to the left atrium, which lies adjacent to the esophagus between 30 to 35 cm from the incisors. The aortopulmonary (AP) window is seen between the aortic arch and the carina, typically at 25 to 30 cm from the incisors. As one approaches the UES on pullback, the trachea, hyoid bone, and thyroid gland may be seen.

If only linear imaging is being performed, the technique again consists of passing the scope into the stomach and evaluating the celiac axis, left adrenal, and left liver initially. The scope is then pulled back into the esophagus at the level of the GEJ and the descending aorta is found. The scope is then rotated 360 degrees until the aorta is again visualized. The instrument is then withdrawn 2 to 3 centimeters at a time and the process is repeated again, visualizing the structures at the same levels mentioned above for radial EUS imaging, until eventually the UES is reached. EUS-FNA, for which the technique is described in the next section, is then performed of any identified target lesions.

Endoscopic Ultrasound for Esophageal Cancer

At present, the most commonly performed indication for transesophageal EUS is for the evaluation and staging of esophageal malignancy. Initial treatment recommendations for patients with esophageal cancer are mainly dependent on the estimated preoperative tumor stage. For instance, patients with early localized disease are usually offered immediate surgery, whereas patients with locoregionally advanced disease may be candidates for preoperative chemoradiotherapy. For patients with early tumors that appear limited to the mucosa without regional lymphadenopathy, relatively newer and less invasive treatments such as endoscopic mucosal resection and endoscopic ablative therapies may be considered in select settings. Given that these varied management strategies are dependent on assessment of tumor extent, accurate image-based prediction of tumor stage is necessary to optimally guide the appropriate treatment for a particular patient. To that end, endoscopic ultrasound has become an important tool in evaluating patients with esophageal malignancy.

The histologic diagnosis of esophageal cancer is usually established on forceps biopsies obtained at diagnostic endoscopy. Once confirmed, the first step in evaluating a patient with esophageal malignancy is to exclude metastases. This is usually accomplished using noninvasive imaging procedures such as computerized tomography (CT) or positron emission tomography (PET). If metastases are present, further evaluation is rarely needed, and palliative measures may be considered.

If metastases are not present, EUS should be performed as a means to assess local tumor stage (Table 10–1). EUS can be performed, using small, through-the-scope catheter-based probes or echoendoscopes with built-in transducers at the instrument tip. By passing the instrument adjacent to the tumor, detailed images of the tumor extension through the esophageal wall can be obtained. The normal esophageal wall typically appears as an alternating, five-layer, targetlike pattern (Fig 10–1). The alternating patterns correspond to various histologic layers of the esophageal lumen. The initial superficial

Table 10–1. T and N Staging of Esophageal Cancer

Tis	Carcinoma in situ
T1	Tumor invades lamina propria or submucosa
T2	Tumor invades into (but not through) muscularis propria
T3	Tumor extends through muscularis propria into adventitia
T4	Tumor invades adjacent organs/structures
N0	No regional lymph node metastases
N1	Regional lymph node metastases

Source: Adapted from *AJCC Cancer Staging Manual,* 6th ed. New York, NY: Springer-Verlag; 2002.

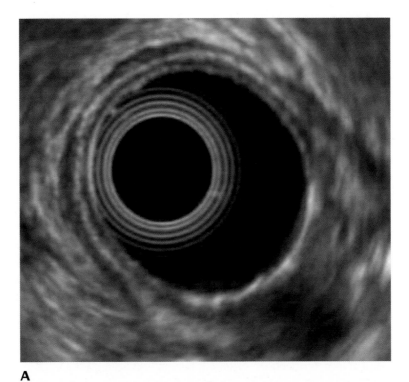

A

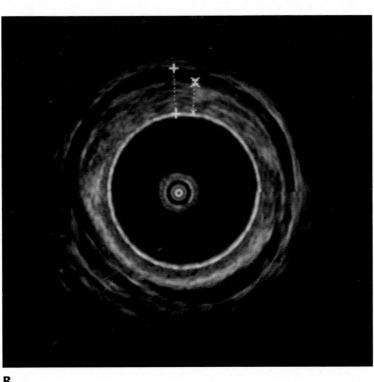

B

Fig 10–1. Normal EUS esophageal wall anatomy. **A.** Normal esophageal wall with five alternating hyperechoic (bright) and hypoechoic (dark) layers. The alternating layers correspond to separate histologic layers of the esophageal wall (eg, middle hyperechoic layer represents the submucosa). **B.** A full circumferential view of the distal esophagus using a 20-MHz catheter probe demonstrates the five esophageal wall layers at the 6 o'clock position and provides improved image resolution. Note at the 7 o'clock position, the fibrous sheath separating the inner circular and outer longitudinal muscle fibers of the muscularis propria (4th hypoechoic wall layer) is seen.

hyperechoic layer corresponds to the mucosal interface, or superficial mucosa. Subsequently, alternating hypoechoic and hyperechoic layers are seen as one proceeds radially outward. The hypoechoic second layer corresponds to the deep mucosal layer, which includes the muscularis mucosae and the lamina propria. The hyperechoic third layer corresponds to the submucosa. The hypoechoic fourth layer represents the muscularis propria, and with high-frequency imaging, this layer can be subdivided into inner circular and outer longitudinal layers, separated by a thin hyperechoic fibrous sheath. Finally, the hyperechoic fifth layer represents the end of the muscularis propria and its interface with the surrounding adventitia, as the esophagus does not contain a true serosal layer.

When an esophageal cancer is present, endosonographically it will appear as a hypoechoic, often irregular-shaped mass that disrupts the normal wall layer pattern. The depth of extension through the wall guides the endosonographer in estimating T stage (Figs 10–2 and 10–3 and Video 10A). In comparative studies, EUS seems superior to CT, magnetic resonance imaging (MRI), or PET scan for T staging,[1-3] with an overall reported accuracy of 85%.[3]

Tumor spread into local structures and organs (T4), such as the pericardium, lung, pleural space, and aorta can also be readily seen at EUS (Fig 10–4). Accuracy for EUS in confirming locally unresectable stage T4 disease is high (86%).[3] Given the morbidity and mortality rates associated with esophagectomy, EUS can be particularly valuable in identifying inappropriate candidates for surgical resection.

In an era in which nonsurgical methods to treat or ablate early esophageal tumors (especially with Barrett's esophagus) are emerging,[4,5] accurate pre-

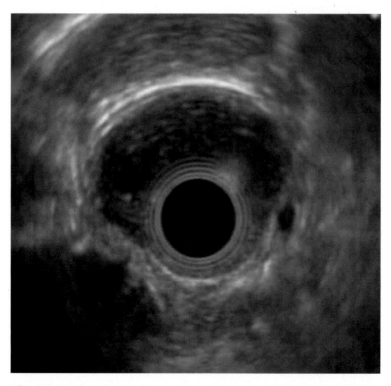

Fig 10–2. Esophageal cancer, tumor stage T2 by EUS. A hypoechoic mass extends from the 10 o'clock to 2 o'clock position (relative to the central EUS transducer). The lesion disrupts the normal alternating wall layer pattern, but does not extend into periesophageal tissue (adventitia) or into the trachea (hyperechoic stripe in the 12 o'clock position).

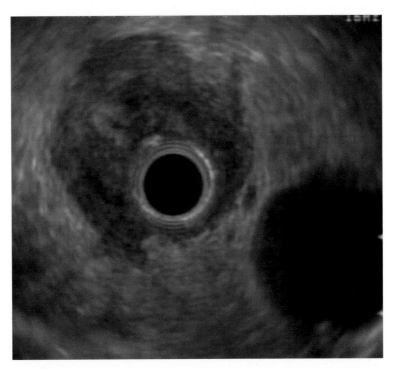

Fig 10–3. Esophageal cancer, tumor stage T3 by EUS. A hypoechoic mass extends from the 6 o'clock to 3 o'clock position. There is disruption of the outer esophageal wall layer (muscularis propria) with tumor extension into periesophageal soft tissue (at the 6 to 7 o'clock position). A clear plane between mass and aorta (at 4 o'clock) excludes aortic involvement.

diction of early T-stage tumors limited to the superficial wall layers is mandatory. High-frequency (12 to 30 MHz) EUS scanning using either catheter-based probes or newer model echoendoscopes with multirange frequencies plays an important role in this setting. Appropriate patients that are confirmed to have superficial tumors by EUS may immediately undergo endoscopic mucosal resection and/or endoscopic ablation. Various endoscopic resection techniques provide large tissue samples (can be used to remove a small tumor en bloc), and ablative therapies can be used to destroy residual neoplastic or preoplastic tissue. EUS is highly accurate in staging superficial tumors (85%),[4] and is thus critical in identifying tumors that may be amenable to nonoperative treatment.

EUS also provides valuable information on the presence or absence of local lymph nodes. For nodal staging, the echoendoscope is used to interrogate periesophageal tissue and the mediastinum the entire length of the esophagus. Examination of the celiac axis and hypopharyngeal region for lymphadenopathy is also a standard part of the exam. Depending on the location of the tumor, the finding of suspicious lymph nodes that are distant from the primary site (eg, celiac nodes with a proximal tumor, or proximal periesophageal nodes with a distal tumor) may significantly impact proposed management.

With the high resolution of EUS and the proximity of the probe to the area of interest, even smaller nodes (<10 mm) that are missed on other noninvasive imaging modalities are easily seen by EUS. In fact, lymph nodes as small as 2 to 3 mm can be identified using this technique. EUS appears more accurate than CT, MRI, or PET in N staging, with an overall accuracy of 77%.[3] Several sonographic criteria have been identified to help distinguish benign (Fig 10-5) from malignant peritumoral lymph nodes.

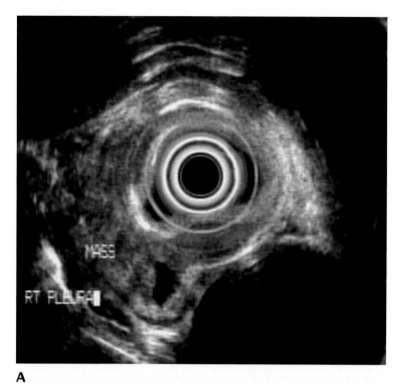

A

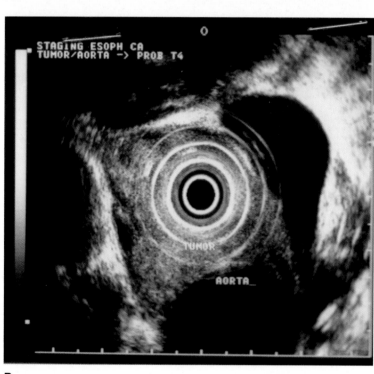

B

Fig 10–4. Locally invasive esophageal cancer (Stage T4) **A.** A hypoechoic mass extends from the 7 o'clock to 9 o'clock position. The mass penetrates through the esophageal wall, and involves the right pleura (bright echogenic plane representing pleura is penetrated). **B.** A circumferential, hypoechoic esophageal mass is seen in the mid-esophagus with a loss of the hyperechoic plane between the esophagus and the aorta at the arch (3 o'clock position) and the descending thoracic aorta (5 o'clock position). These findings represent T4 disease.

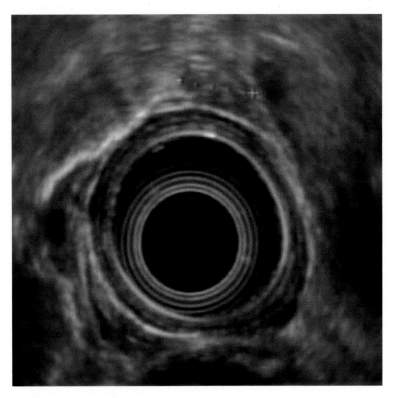

Fig 10–5. Benign appearing lymph node. Lymph node seen at 12 o'clock by EUS is heterogeneous, triangular-shaped, without smooth borders, and less than 1 cm (ie, no echofeatures suspicious for malignant involvement).

For N staging, the following characteristics are suggestive of malignant involvement (Fig 10–6 and see Fig 10–10): (1) homogeneous, hypoechoic pattern, (2) circular shape, (3) smooth borders, and (4) size greater than 1 cm.[6] EUS is highly accurate (>80%) in identifying malignant lymph nodes when all four sonographic findings are present, but this occurs in only 25% of cases.[7]

Endoscopic ultrasound guided fine needle aspiration (EUS-FNA) of suspicious lymph nodes can be performed, if needed, to cytologically confirm malignant spread. The technique involves the use of a linear-array echoendoscope that allows real-time visualization of the needle as it extends from the scope tip (Fig 10–7 and Video 10B). Under active ultrasonic guidance, the needle is advanced transesophageally into a lymph node, and an aspirated tissue sample is obtained. FNA biopsy needles come in a variety of sizes (19 to 25 gauge) and can be advanced up to 8 cm outside the gastrointestinal tract. Large bore instruments that provide a "core-biopsy" type specimen are available,[8] but there are no data to support these devices providing added utility over standard EUS-FNA for nodal sampling in esophageal cancer. If EUS-FNA is used, care should be taken to access the lymph node without traversing the primary tumor site. This will help avoid false positive contamination of the tissue sample, and decrease any potential risk of tumor seeding.

When performed, EUS-FNA improves assessment of nodal staging over EUS imaging alone, yielding high sensitivity, specificity, and accuracy (>90%) in several series.[9,10] The issue of whether to perform EUS-FNA over EUS alone depends on how the knowledge of nodal status would impact clinical management. For instance, EUS-FNA of a peritumoral lymph node would not likely alter the plan for preoperative, neoadjuvant treatment of a large tumor

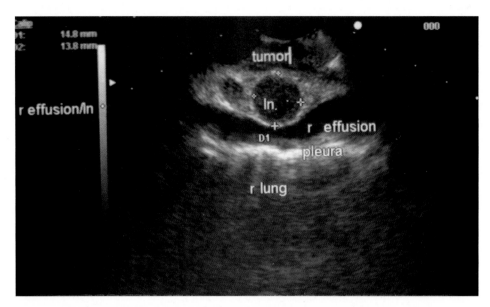

Fig 10–6. Appearance of malignant lymphadenopathy. This lymph node exhibits the characteristic features of malignant adenopathy. The lymph node is round, hypoechoic, has sharp (well-defined) borders, is greater than 1 cm in size, and is adjacent to the tumor (peritumoral location). EUS-FNA was not performed as the tumor would have to be traversed to access the lymph node.

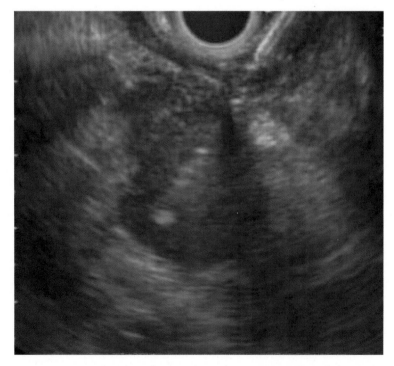

Fig 10–7. EUS-FNA of a suspicious periesophageal lymph node. A 22-gauge needle is advanced into a lymph node under active US guidance. On-site cytologic analysis confirmed poorly differentiated adenocarcinoma.

that extensively penetrates into periesophageal tissue (T3). On the other hand, EUS-FNA of a peritumoral lymph node in a patient with a superficial-appearing cancer (T1) may impact the clinical plan: (1) If negative, the patient may undergo immediate surgery, or possibly be considered for endoscopic resection or ablation. (2) If positive, the patient would be considered for preoperative chemoradiotherapy versus immediate surgery depending on institutional practice patterns. In general, EUS-FNA for nodal staging should be utilized when results would influence clinical management, with the understanding that false negative rates of up to 10 to 20% are reported.[9-11] To maximize sensitivity, 3 to 5 needle passes are made per lymph node to ensure adequate sampling. The needle is often "fanned" across the node in an attempt to obtain a broad sample of cells from the node. Suction may or may not be performed during EUS-FNA of lymph nodes. If the specimen is bloody, there may be a benefit to reducing or eliminating suction so as to achieve an improved specimen.

As most patients have undergone a noninvasive imaging test to exclude distant metastases prior to undergoing staging EUS, it has a limited role in M staging. That said, large portions of the hepatic parenchyma (especially left lobe) can be seen from transgastric and transduodenal approaches, and should be evaluated during the procedure. Published reports suggest that occult liver metastases are seen in up to 7% of patients with distal esophageal tumors[12] (Fig 10–8). In addition, EUS can detect malignant pleural effusions and celiac lymph nodes, the latter being considered M1a disease in patients without distal esophageal tumors (Figs 10–9 and 10–10). EUS-FNA can be used to confirm unsuspected metastatic spread identified at the time of EUS.

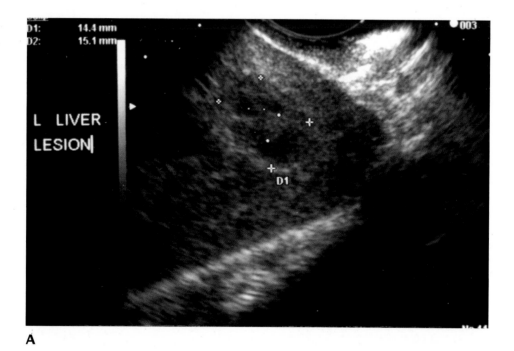

A

Fig 10–8. EUS detection of metastatic disease. **A.** This 1.5 × 1.4 cm hypoechoic irregular-shaped lesion was seen in the left liver of a patient with a previous negative CT in whom EUS was being performed prior to planned operative resection. *continues*

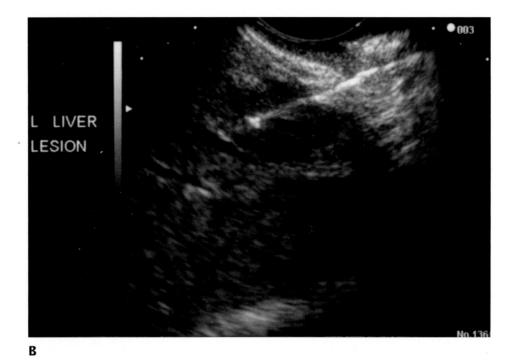

B

Fig 10–8. *continued* **B.** EUS-FNA of the lesion in (**A**) confirmed metastatic esophageal adenocarcinoma, leading to cancellation of the planned operative resection.

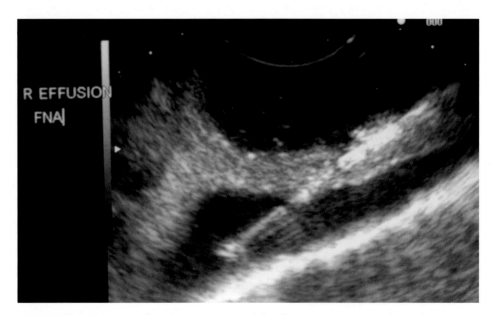

Fig 10–9. EUS-FNA of malignant pleural fluid. During EUS staging of a patient with esophageal adenocarcinoma that approached the right pleural space, a moderate amount of right pleural fluid was seen. EUS-FNA confirmed the diagnosis of a malignant effusion.

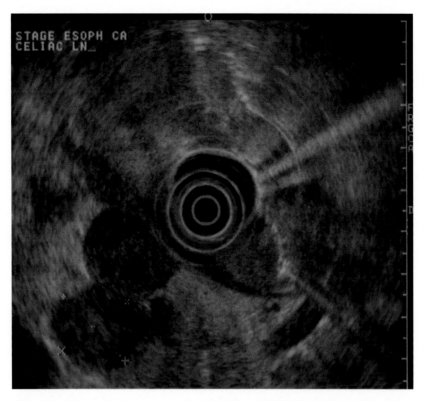

Fig 10–10. EUS detection of celiac lymphadenopathy. This radial EUS view obtained with the scope at the level of the gastro-esophageal junction shows two large, round, hypoechoic, >1 cm, peritumoral lymph nodes at the 7 o'clock position in a patient with distal esophageal adenocarcinoma. FNA was not performed as tumor would have needed to be traversed to achieve lymph node access, but the EUS morphology of these lymph nodes predicts malignant involvement with approximately 80% accuracy even in the absence of FNA.

EUS for Submucosal Lesions of the Esophagus

EUS examination of the esophagus is frequently performed for evaluation of a "submucosal" lesion seen on a prior endoscopy or, more infrequently, seen on cross-sectional imaging. These lesions are more appropriately referred to as subepithelial lesions, as many of them do not arise from the true submucosa of the esophagus. Lesions involving the first and second layers of the esophagus are typically mucosally based and can be diagnosed via surface mucosa sampling techniques such as biopsy or snare polypectomy. Lesions in the submucosa may represent hyperechoic lipomas, vessels such as varices, and cysts. The latter two structures typically appear anechoic on EUS. Hypoechoic lesions arising from the fourth layer of the esophagus, and occasionally the second layer, represent gastrointestinal stromal tumors (GIST) or leiomyomas (Figs 10–11A and 10–11B). Although these lesions have a characteristic hypoechoic appearance with a round to oval shape, differentiating between the two can be difficult. EUS-FNA

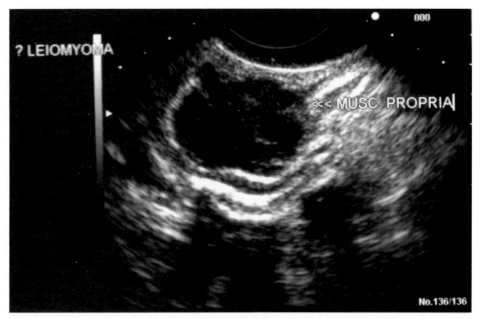

A

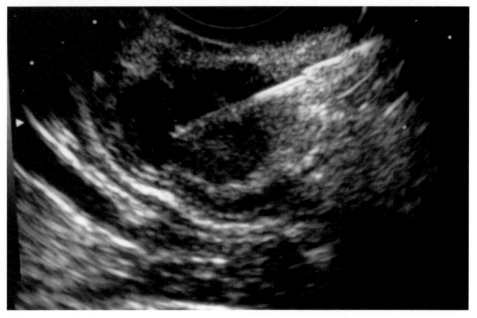

B

Fig 10–11. EUS evaluation of a gastrointestinal stromal tumor (GIST). **A.** Linear EUS examination reveals a hypoechoic, oval, intramural lesion in the distal esophagus. The lesion appears to arise from the first hypoechoic wall layer (deep mucosal layer) and does not appear to involve other esophageal wall layers. The hyperechoic submucosal layer and the hypoechoic muscularis propria (labeled) are clearly seen on the extraluminal side of the lesion. **B.** EUS-FNA of the lesion with a 22-g needle revealed spindle cells that stained positive for CD-117, consistent with a GIST likely arising from the muscularis mucosae. As the lesion was more than 3 cm in size and the patient was symptomatic with dysphagia, resection of the lesion was recommended.

can be used to obtain cellular material, which often reveals spindle cells (Fig 10–11B). This material can then be tested for expression of CD-117, which if present, suggests a GIST. Resection is typically based on size (greater than 3 cm) or the development of clinical symptoms such as dysphagia, as the echo characteristics of these lesions do not reliably predict their malignant potential. In addition, many "submucosal" lesions actually represent extrinsic compression of the esophagus by adjacent structures such as the aorta, heart, or mediastinal masses/adenopathy.

Recently, two publications regarding the diagnosis of mediastinal cysts via EUS-FNA have been reported.[13,14] Of note, 40% of patients had a CT that actually suggested a solid lesion. In total, 30 cysts were evaluated, with 22 undergoing EUS-FNA with antibiotic prophylaxis. Two malignancies and 20 benign cysts were diagnosed. All five patients who underwent both EUS-FNA and surgery had agreement between EUS obtained cytology and surgical pathology. Cysts were typically round or oval with a thin outer wall and typically located adjacent to the esophagus between the carina and the GE junction (Fig 10–12A). Some had a hypoechoic appearance with hyperechoic foci, consistent with some debris within the cyst. EUS-FNA revealed detached ciliary tufts in patients with foregut duplication cysts, and this finding may represent a useful marker for establishing this diagnosis (Fig 10–12B).[14]

EUS for Lung Cancer Staging

Although there are fewer than 15,000 new cases of esophageal cancer diagnosed each year in the United States, approximately 170,000 new cases of lung cancer will be diagnosed during the same interval. Thus, although transesophageal endosonography plays a central role in the evaluation of esophageal tumors, it may have a much greater impact in the evaluation of patients with lung cancer. Non-small cell lung cancer (NSCLC) accounts for 80% of new cases of lung cancer and surgery offers the best

hope of cure for patients with NSCLC. This treatment is recommended for patients with tumor confined to the lung (Stage I) and ipsilateral hilar lymph nodes (Stage II, given there is N1 disease). If mediastinal lymph nodes are present, Stage III disease is present. Patients with ipsilateral subcarinal or mediastinal lymph nodes have N2 disease (Stage IIIA), whereas patients with N3 disease (Stage IIIB) have contralateral mediastinal lymph nodes or any scalene or supraclavicular adenopathy. Patients with Stage IV disease have distant metastases and are not surgical candidates. Patients with Stage III disease typically undergo chemoradiation with possible surgery after treatment, but patients with Stage IIIA disease have a much improved prognosis compared to Stage IIIB patients who undergo surgery. For this reason, detection of mediastinal adenopathy and determining if malignancy is present in identified nodes is of paramount importance to obtain accurate staging, which, in turn, determines the treatment plan.

The currently used diagnostic and staging modalities for lung cancer include bronchoscopy with FNA, mediastinoscopy/thoracoscopy, CT, PET, and EUS with FNA. In addition, endobronchial ultrasound (EBUS) which allows for ultrasound-guided transbronchial FNA, has recently become available and is gaining popularity. However, as this chapter is focused on transesophageal EUS, we do not discuss the modality further other than to say the combination of EBUS and EUS, or "medical" mediastinoscopy, offers great promise due to the fact that transesophageal EUS has difficulty imaging the anterior mediastinal/paratracheal lymph nodes (levels 2 and 4), which are easily accessible with EBUS. Although transesophageal EUS is excellent at evaluating the aortopulmonary window (Fig 10–13), subcarinal space, and periesophageal tissues, other limitations of this technique do exist. Some lymph nodes cannot be sampled at level 6 due to intervening blood vessels between the esophagus and the lymph node.[15] Additionally, the criteria for malignant nodes mentioned previously do not predict lung cancer related malignant adenopathy as accurately, necessitating EUS-FNA for any suspicious adenopathy.

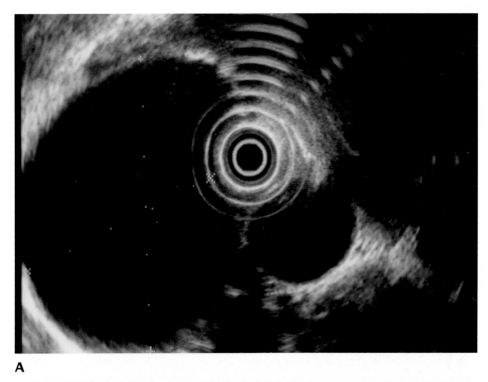

A

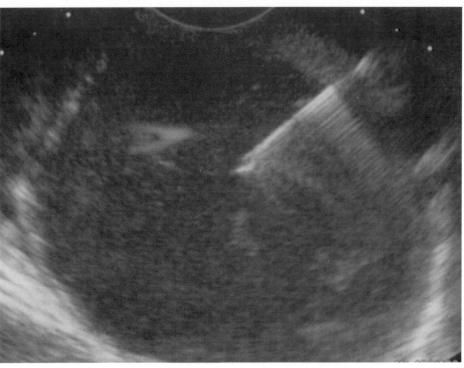

B

Fig 10–12. Esophageal duplication cyst diagnosed by EUS-FNA. **A.** A large right posterior anechoic lesion consistent with a cyst is seen intramurally in the distal esophagus from 6 o'clock to 12 o'clock on the radial EUS image. Note the lesion is much larger than the cross-section of the aorta, seen at 5 o'clock. Air artifact is also seen, represented by hyperechoic lines extending radially, at 12 o'clock and 1 o'clock. **B.** After administration of IV antibiotics, EUS-FNA with a 22-g needle revealed a thick light yellow mucoid liquid. On cytology, detached ciliary tufts were seen consistent with the diagnosis of an esophageal duplication cyst.

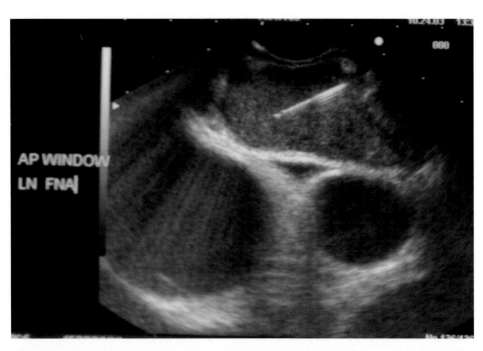

Fig 10–13. EUS-FNA of malignant aortopulmonary adenopathy. EUS-FNA of this large, oval shaped aortopulmonary window lymph node revealed NSCLC in this patient with a right lung primary lesion, resulting in Stage IIIB disease and cancellation of a planned operative resection. Note that unlike malignant adenopathy from an esophageal primary, this lymph node is neither hypoechoic nor circular, emphasizing the need to FNA any significant adenopathy during NSCLC staging.

Nodes as small as 4 mm can be sampled via EUS-FNA. Last, with the exception of tumor invading the mediastinum (Figs 10–14A and 10–14B) or esophagus, EUS also is frequently inaccurate at detecting or determining the T stage of the primary tumor, due to the intervening air within the lung between the tumor and the esophagus, precluding ultrasound visualization.

EUS-FNA is useful for both diagnosing malignancy as well as upstaging known malignant disease. In patients with a nondiagnostic bronchoscopy, EUS-FNA may establish a diagnosis (both malignant and benign conditions) in up to 97% of patients.[16] A comparison of simultaneous transbronchial biopsy and EUS-FNA showed that EUS-FNA had a higher diagnostic yield (86 to 65%).[17] EUS has also been compared to mediastinoscopy for staging of NSCLC. However, despite its consideration as the "gold standard" of NSCLC staging, mediastinoscopy has difficulty in detecting adenopathy in the aortopulmonary window and posterior mediastinum. In fact, 10 to 15% of patients undergoing surgery after a negative mediastinoscopy have inoperable disease.[18] A recent head to head comparison of mediastinoscopy and EUS-FNA showed sensitivities for paratracheal or subcarinal disease of 24 and 96%, respectively.[19] However, other data suggest that EUS and mediastinoscopy may be complementary studies. In patients undergoing surgery after a negative mediastinoscopy, this combination of studies identified unresectable disease in 36%, compared to 20% for mediastinoscopy alone and 28% for EUS-FNA alone.[20] When EUS was performed after negative CT imaging, as many as 25% of CT negative patients had advanced disease.[21] When compared to PET, multiple studies have shown that EUS is as sensitive and more specific (due to fewer false positives than PET), with an overall improved accuracy.[18]

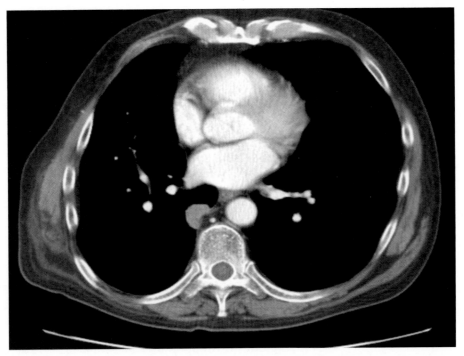

A

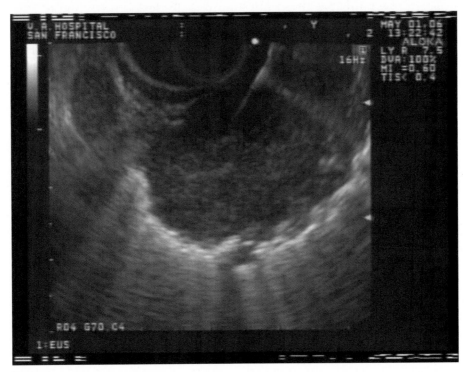

B

Fig 10–14. EUS evaluation of primary lung lesions. **A.** CT scan that reveals a periesophageal right pleural based mass. **B.** EUS-FNA of the lesion provided the initial diagnosis of non-small cell lung cancer.

Recent reviews of more than 50 studies, one of which was a meta-analysis of 18 studies, report overall EUS-FNA sensitivities of 61 to 100% (median 90%) and specificities of 71 to 100% (median 100%) in the detection of malignant adenopathy in patients with lung cancer.[18,22,23] The meta-analysis found that EUS-FNA identified 83% of patients with positive mediastinal nodes and 97% of patients with negative mediastinal adenopathy when histology or more than 6 month follow-up was used as the "gold standard." These numbers were improved in the subset of patients in whom adenopathy was also detected on CT scan.

In summary, transesophageal EUS appears to be an accurate staging modality in patients with potentially resectable lung cancer. It has the ability to detect nodes not seen on CT or PET and, conversely, it can determine whether PET positive nodes, in fact, are malignant via EUS-FNA. In addition, it is less invasive and less costly than mediastinoscopy, and allows for evaluation of the liver and left adrenal gland to detect distant metastases at the same time as the mediastinal exam. Finally, some recent data suggest that it may in fact be more accurate than surgical mediastinoscopy, which has traditionally been considered the gold standard. As its availability increases, the use of EUS and EUS-FNA should be considered in the preoperative evaluation of lung cancer patients.

EUS for the Evaluation of Head and Neck and Mediastinal Lesions

Although esophageal EUS has primarily been used to evaluate esophageal mucosal or submucosal lesions and for staging lung cancer, EUS has also been helpful in the evaluation of thyroid lesions, head and neck neoplasms, and in the classification of mediastinal masses in patients without known pulmonary malignancies. EUS has been used to determine the presence of esophagopharyngeal invasion in patients with thyroid cancer, the vast majority of whom underwent surgical resection. The accuracy of EUS in determining invasion into the muscularis propria of the esophagus was 82.7%, which was better than MRI (65.4%) or upper endoscopy (58.8%).[24]

In addition, it appeared that EUS was better at predicting esophageal invasion in mid to distal thyroid tumors compared to proximally located thyroid tumors. More recently, EUS-FNA has been shown to be capable of diagnosing previously undiagnosed thyroid disease. Dewitt and colleagues have reported on a patient with a long history of dysphagia, an unremarkable neck exam, and a neck CT scan with a calcified superior mediastinal mass behind the trachea.[25] The patient had a normal thyroid scintigraphy study and a normal upper endoscopy. The patient underwent EUS-FNA of the lesion, which was 5.7 × 3.9 cm in size and extended from 17 to 22 cm from the incisors. FNA diagnosed a benign nodular goiter.

EUS-FNA has also been helpful in the staging of a variety of head and neck tumors. Wildi and colleagues reported on a series of 32 patients with head and neck neoplasms undergoing 35 EUS examinations.[26] Examinations were done to evaluate for a suspicion of local esophageal invasion or for mediastinal adenopathy larger than 1 cm on CT scan. EUS was possible in all but one patient (benign esophageal stricture precluding scope passage). EUS demonstrated four cases of esophageal invasion and one case of pleural invasion out of 17 patients with suspected invasion. In the 17 examinations in 14 patients undergoing EUS for mediastinal adenopathy, EUS-FNA confirmed 8 cases of metastatic disease. EUS provided the first tissue diagnosis in two patients and diagnosed malignant adenopathy in one patient with a negative CT scan. EUS was found to change management of 71% of the patients with suspected esophageal invasion and 47% of those with suspected mediastinal adenopathy. Another study retrospectively analyzed 49 patients with non-lung cancer related mediastinal masses or lymphadenopathy.[27] EUS-FNA correctly diagnosed 46 out of 49 patients (94%), with nondiagnostic cytology in three patients (6%). Final diagnoses were based on long-term follow-up or surgical pathology. Overall, EUS-FNA diagnosed 22 malignancies and 24 benign conditions, and no complications were observed. Thus, in summary, EUS and EUS-FNA may also benefit patients with head and neck, upper mediastinal, or unknown mediastinal lesions by providing a less invasive diagnostic alternative (EUS-FNA) and improved staging accuracy.

Therapeutic Transesophageal Endosonography

In addition to the numerous diagnostic applications mentioned above, EUS-guided fine needle injection (EUS-FNI) may allow EUS to provide therapy in certain conditions. Previous studies have utilized EUS to guide injection of botulinum toxin into the lower esophageal sphincter as a treatment for achalasia.[28,29] The results of these studies have been somewhat equivocal when compared to results with non-EUS-guided techniques. In part, this is because after the initial injection of botulinum toxin, the injected fluid and associated air tends to track along the esophageal wall, making further discrimination of esophageal wall layers for subsequent injections quite difficult, if not impossible. Recently, an abstract was presented demonstrating benefit with the use of EUS-FNI of an adenovirus-based vector which incorporates tumor necrosis factor (TNF) alpha into its genome.[30] This vector is injected weekly via EUS-FNI intratumorally in patients with locally advanced esophageal cancer who are undergoing neoadjuvant therapy. The TNF-alpha is believed to act synergistically with chemoradiation in the treatment of these malignancies. Future studies with long-term follow-up are needed to substantiate these promising preliminary findings.

Complications and Precautions for Esophageal EUS

Given the overall larger diameter and limited tip flexibility of echoendoscopes as compared to standard endoscopes, perforation during EUS has been of greater theoretical concern than with standard esophagoscopy, and particularly in the region of the cervical esophagus. However, large series have reported procedural perforation rates similar to those seen with standard endoscopy (0.03–0.15%).[31,32] Iatrogenic perforations may be associated with older patient age, difficult esophageal intubation, and inexperience of the endosonographer.[33] Although unproven, the use of a partially inflated, water-filled balloon at the scope tip during esophageal entry has been advocated by some to minimize trauma.[14]

In the setting of esophageal cancer, dilation may be required to traverse a malignant stricture and complete a staging exam. Although some reports had suggested high perforation rates, subsequent studies revealed that dilation up to 14 to 16 mm was safe and provided important staging information that substantially impacted management.[12,35,36]

Transesophageal EUS-FNA has proven to be a very safe technique. Potential complications may include infection and hemorrhage. Infections related to EUS-FNA of solid targets are considered very uncommon. But, infectious complications following EUS-FNA of cystic lesions (eg, duplication cyst, bronchogenic cyst) have been reported, and prophylactic antibiotics should be administered when targeting cystic abnormalities.[13,37,38] Mild hemorrhage that required no specific therapy following EUS-FNA has been recognized in about 1% (slightly higher for cystic lesions).[39] Minimizing the number of FNA passes to that needed for diagnosis and using real-time Doppler flow imaging to avoid major vascular structures may help reduce bleeding risks.[40]

Summary

Esophageal endosonography has established itself as a useful and safe modality in the diagnosis of esophageal mucosal and intramural lesions, mediastinal lesions of unclear etiology, in the evaluation of mediastinal adenopathy, and even in the evaluation of head and neck masses. In addition, it is part of the routine staging workup of esophageal malignancies, and increasingly is being used in the staging of lung cancer. Although limited data exist currently, EUS may be used in a therapeutic role to provide antitumor therapy as well as in the treatment of benign conditions, such as achalasia. Improved echoendoscope and ultrasound processor technology, reduced equipment costs, increased awareness of the capabilities of this technique by medical professionals, and an expansion in the number of advanced EUS training programs should serve to improve utilization and accessibility to this valuable modality.

Videos in This Chapter

Video 10A. Electronic Radial Endoscopic Ultrasound Imaging of an Esophageal Cancer. This video shows an asymmetric, hypoechoic tumor on the left of the screen from the 7 to 12 o'clock position. The aorta is seen at 6 o'clock. The heart is seen beating to the left of the screen. Tumor area is measured and can be re-evaluated after neoadjuvant therapy in patients in whom this is performed to better predict curative resection. In this case, the tumor appears to involve the entire esophageal wall (T2), as the layers of the wall are no longer seen in the region of the tumor. However, the tumor does not invade through the wall, as the outer border of the tumor is smooth and circular. The fat plane between the tumor and aorta is preserved, as seen by a hyperechoic white line between the tumor and the lumen of the aorta. Color flow is used to clearly define the vasculature. The final portion of video shows a region of normal esophagus with a thin wall and evidence of the usual 5-layer echo pattern.

Video 10B. Fine Needle Aspiration of a Mediastinal Lymph Node. This video demonstrates endoscopic ultrasound guided fine needle aspiration (EUS-guided FNA) performed by a curved linear array echoendoscope. An oval hypoechoic mediastinal lymph node is seen from the 5 to 7 o'clock position. The lesion is adjacent to the heart, which is seen beating deep to the node. A 22-gauge needle, seen as a hyperechoic line entering the lymph node at the upper right of the screen, is inserted into the node via real time endoscopic ultrasound guidance. After the needle is inserted into the node, the stylet is used to clear any material that might have become trapped in the needle as it was advanced into the node. The stylet is then removed, and in most cases, suction is applied. The needle is then moved in a to and fro motion approximately 10 times within the node before suction is stopped and the needle is withdrawn from the node. The needle is then removed from the echoendoscope for specimen retrieval and cytologic analysis.

References

1. Kelly S, Harris K, Berry E, et al. A systematic review of the staging performance of endoscopic ultrasound in gastro-esophageal carcinoma. *Gut.* 2001;49:534-539.
2. Lowe VJ, Booya F, Fletcher JG, et al. Comparison of positron emission tomography, computed tomography, and endoscopic ultrasound in the initial staging of patients with esophageal cancer. *Mol Imaging Biol.* 2005;7:422-430.
3. Rosch T. Endosonographic staging of esophageal cancer: a review of literature results. *Gastrointest Endosc Clin North Am.* 1995;5:537-547.
4. Larghi A, Lightdale CJ, Memeo L, Bhagat G, Okpara N, Rotterdam H. EUS followed by EMR for staging of high-grade dysplasia and early cancer in Barrett's esophagus. *Gastrointest Endosc.* 2005;62:16-23.
5. Peters FP, Kara MA, Rosmolen WD, et al. Endoscopic treatment of high-grade dysplasia and early stage cancer in Barrett's esophagus. *Gastrointest Endosc.* 2005;61:506-514.
6. Catalano MF, Sivak MV, Rice T, et al. Endosonographic features predictive of lymph node metastasis. *Gastrointest Endosc.* 1994;40:442-446.
7. Bhutani MS, Hawes RH, Hoffman BJ. A comparison of the accuracy of echo features during endoscopic ultrasound (EUS) and EUS-guided fine needle aspiration for diagnosis of malignant lymph node invasion. *Gastrointest Endosc.* 1997;45:474-479.
8. Levy MJ, Jondal ML, Clain J, et al. Preliminary experience with an EUS-guided trucut biopsy needle compared with EUS-guided FNA. *Gastrointest Endosc.* 2003;57:101-106.
9. Eloubeidi MA, Wallace MB, Reed CE, et al. The utility of EUS and EUS-guided fine needle aspiration in detecting celiac lymph node metastasis in patients with esophageal cancer: a single center experience. *Gastrointest Endosc.* 2001;54:714-719.
10. Vazquez-Sequerios E, Norton ID, Clain JE, et al. Impact of EUS-guided fine needle aspiration on lymph node staging in patients with esophageal carcinoma. *Gastrointest Endosc.* 2001;53:751-757.

11. Vazquez-Sequeiros E, Wiersema MJ, Clain JE, et al. Impact of lymph node staging on therapy of esophageal carcinoma. *Gastroenterology*. 2003; 125:1626-1635.

12. McGrath K, Brody D, Luketich J, Khalid A. Detection of unsuspected left hepatic lobe metastases during EUS staging of cancer of the esophagus and cardia. *Am J Gastroenterol*. 2006;101:1742-1746.

13. Fazel A, Moezardalan K, Varadarajulu S, Drananov P, Eloubeidi MA. The utility and the safety of EUS-guided FNA in the evaluation of duplication cysts. *Gastrointest Endos*. 2005;62:4,575-580.

14. Eloubeidi MA, Cohn M, Cerfolio RJ, et al. Endoscopic ultrasound-guided fine-needle aspiration in the diagnosis of foregut duplication cysts: the value of demonstrating detached ciliary tufts in cyst fluid. *Cancer Cytopathol*. 2004;102:4,253-258.

15. Savoy AD, Ravenel JG, Hoffman BJ, Wallace MB. Endoscopic ultrasound for thoracic malignancy: a review. *Curr Prob Diag Radiol*. 2005;34(3): 106-115.

16. Annema JT, Veselic M, Rabe KF. EUS-guided FNA of centrally located lung tumours following a non-diagnostic bronchoscopy. *Lung Cancer*. 2005; 48(3):357-361.

17. Khoo KL, Ho KY, Nilsson B, Lim TK. EUS-guided FNA immediately after unrevealing transbronchial needle aspiration in the evaluation of mediastinal lymphadenopathy: a prospective study. *Gastrointest Endosc*. 2006;63(2):215-220.

18. Vilmann P, Herth F, Krasnik M. State of the art lecture: mediastinal EUS. *Endoscopy*. 2006;38(suppl 1): S84-S87.

19. Larsen SS, Vilmann P, Krasnik M, et al. Endoscopic ultrasound guided biopsy versus mediastinoscopy for analysis of paratracheal and subcarinal lymph nodes in lung cancer staging. *Lung Cancer*. 2005; 48(1):85-92.

20. Annema JT, Versteegh MI, Veselic M, et al. Endoscopic ultrasound added to mediastinoscopy for preoperative staging of patients with lung cancer. *JAMA*. 2005;294(8):931-936.

21. Wallace MB, Ravenel J, Block MI, et al. Endoscopic ultrasound in lung cancer patients with a normal mediastinum on computed tomography. *Ann Thorac Surg*. 2004;77(5):1763-1768.

22. Micames CG, McCrory DC, Pavey DA, Jowell PS, Gress FG. Endoscopic ultrasound-guided fine-needle aspiration for non-small cell lung cancer staging: a systematic review and metaanalysis. *Chest*. 2007;131(2):539-548.

23. Annema JT, Rabe KF. State of the art lecture: EUS and EBUS in pulmonary medicine. *Endoscopy*. 2006;38(suppl 1): S118-S122.

24. Koike E, Yamashita H, Noguchi S. Endoscopic ultrasonography in patients with thyroid cancer: its usefulness and limitations for evaluating esophagopharyngeal invasion. *Endoscopy*. 2002;34(6): 457-460.

25. Dewitt J, Youssef W, Leblanc J, et al. EUS-guided FNA of a thyroid mass. *Gastrointest Endosc*. 2004; 59(2):307-310.

26. Wildi SM, Fickling WE, Day TA, et al. Endoscopic ultrasonography in the diagnosis and staging of neoplasms of the head and neck. *Endoscopy*. 2004;36(7):624-630.

27. Devereaux BM, Leblanc JK, Yousif E, et al. Clinical utility of EUS-guided fine-needle aspiration of mediastinal masses in the absence of known pulmonary malignancy. *Gastrointest Endosc*. 2002; 56(3):397-401.

28. Hoffman BJ, Knapple WL, Bhutani MS, Verne GN, Hawes RH. Treatment of achalasia by injection of botulinum toxin under endoscopic ultrasound guidance. *Gastrointest Endosc*. 1997;45(1):77-79

29. Maiorana A, Fiorentino E, Genova EG, Murata Y, Suzuki S. Echo-guided injection of botulinum toxin in patients with achalasia: initial experience. *Endoscopy*. 1999;31(2):S3-S4.

30. Chang KJ, Senzer N, Swisher S, et al. Multi-center clinical trial using endoscopy (END) and endoscopic ultrasound (EUS) guided fine needle injection (FNI) of anti-tumor agent (TNFerade™) in patients with locally advanced esophageal cancer. *Gastrointes Endosc*. 2006;63(5):AB83.

31. Bournet B, Migueres I, Delacroix M, et al. Early morbidity of endoscopic ultrasound: 13 years' experience at a referral center. *Endoscopy*. 2006; 38:349-354.

32. Mortensen MB, Fristrup C, Holm FS, et al. Prospective evaluation of patient tolerability, satisfaction with patient information, and complications in endoscopic ultrasonography. *Endoscopy*. 2005;37: 146-153.

33. Das A, Sivak MV Jr, Chak A. Cervical esophageal perforation during EUS: a national survey. *Gastrointest Endosc*. 2002;53:599-602.

34. Sahai AV. Balloon-assisted esophageal intubation to prevent cervical perforation during EUS. *Gastrointest Endosc*. 2002;55:140-141.

35. Pfau PR, Ginsberg GG, Lew RJ, et al. Esophageal dilation for endosonographic evaluation of malig-

nant esophageal strictures is safe and effective. *Am J Gastroenterol.* 2000;95:2813-2815.

36. Wallace MB, Hawes RH, Sahai AV, et al. Dilation of malignant esophageal stenosis to allow EUS guided fine-needle aspiration: safety and effect on patient management. *Gastrointest Endosc.* 2000; 51:309-313.

37. Wildi SM, Hoda RS, Fickling W, et al. Diagnosis of benign cysts of the mediastinum: the role and risks of EUS and FNA. *Gastrointest Endosc.* 2003;58: 362-368.

38. Annema JT, Veselic M, Versteegh MI, et al. Mediastinitis caused by EUS-FNA of a bronchogenic cyst. *Endoscopy.* 2003;35:791-793.

39. Affi A, Vazquez-Sequeiros E, Norton ID, et al. Acute extraluminal hemorrhage associated with EUS-guided fine needle aspiration: frequency and clinical significance. *Gastrointest Endosc.* 2001;53: 221-225.

40. Shah JN, Muthusamy VR. Minimizing complications of endoscopic ultrasound and EUS-guided fine needle aspiration. *Gastrointest.* 2007;17:129-143.

Chapter 11

ULTRASONOGRAPHY OF THE FACE, PARANASAL SINUSES, AND EAR

Peter Jecker

Ultrasonography (US) of the face and the paranasal sinuses is quite feasible but is not commonly practiced for a variety of reasons. In contrast to the neck, the face is formed mainly by bony structures that reflect more than 90% of the ultrasound waves. Furthermore, the healthy sinuses are filled with air which does not reflect sufficient sound to create interpretable ultrasound images. Additionally, some of the paranasal sinuses, such as the posterior ethmoid and sphenoid sinuses, are located in the depth of the head and are not easily accessible for US. The temporal bone similarly prevents most of the ear structures from being well visualized by US.

Nevertheless, in certain situations US provides important information that contributes to the differential diagnosis of diseases in this region. In such circumstances, the healthy facial anatomy is often destroyed, such as by fracture in trauma, by bony destruction in malignant disease, or by filling with liquid or solid material in infectious or inflammatory conditions. Ironically, disruption of the normal anatomy can enable detection of structures and features that are normally invisible by US. Furthermore, the efficiency and affordability with which US can

be used to obtain first-line assessment of facial trauma or pathology in the emergency department or the outpatient clinic justifies a discussion of the potential applications of facial US.

Anatomy and Techniques

Bones of the face which are commonly accessible for US are the nasal bones, the zygoma, the frontal bone, the orbital rim, the maxilla, and the mandible. These bones are superficially located and thus, the examination should be performed using a high-frequency array, for example, 7.5 MHz. The focus and the depth of the image must be adjusted accordingly. For imaging of the paranasal sinuses, a lower frequency, for example, down to 5 MHz may be appropriate. The frontal sinus is flat in contrast to the maxillary sinus, but curved as well as linear-array transducers may be used. US imaging of the anterior ethmoid is essentially impossible with currently available equipment, due to its location behind the thick nasal and orbital bones. In contrast, the posterior ethmoid can be imaged with special maneuvers through the bulb from a lateral approach. The posterior ethmoid is separated from the orbit only by the thin lamina papyracea. Still, interpretation of sonographic findings in the sinuses is difficult and detailed anatomic sinus imaging is predominantly the domain of computed tomography at this time. Imaging of the facial bones is performed with the patient in a supine position as with neck US, whereas US of the sinuses should ideally be performed in an upright or sitting position with the head flexed forward if possible. This position ensures that in patients with fluid retention in the sinuses the fluid has contact to the anterior sinus wall which is essential for its detection (Figs 11–1A and 11–1B). US of the facial bones and sinuses is commonly performed using B-mode US, although A-mode (amplitude-modulated) US of the sinuses is historically a part of office-based sinus assessment, similar to transillumination. Doppler US of the sinuses is not necessary but can offer additional information for differential diagnosis of tumors. In such cases a very low PRF (pulse repetition frequency) is used to detect intratumoral blood vessels.

In contrast to the bony face, the bulb or eye, which is filled with fluid, and its surrounding muscles, which are solid soft tissues, can be identified very well by US. Tumor infiltration of the eye can be

detected in real-time imaging which of course is an advantage over other imaging modalities. The US transducer (7.5 to 12 MHz linear array) is applied directly to the eyelid with the patient in the supine position.

Specific Pathologies

Sinusitis

Using US it is possible to diagnose acute maxillary and occasionally frontal sinusitis. In most patients, acute maxillary or frontal sinusitis is a clinical diagnosis and US can offer support to this diagnosis. In the ICU setting where symptomatology may be less clear, US can be used at the bedside to detect maxillary and frontal sinus opacification. The sensitivity of US, performed in the supine position, for total maxillary sinus opacification has been reported at 100%, and when the bony sinus walls are visualized as well, the specificity is also 100%.[1] Another study of US diagnosis of ICU maxillary sinusitis, with CT correlation, described a good negative predictive value if the US was negative and a 100% positive predictive value if the US was strongly positive (termed "cupuliform echographia").[2] US of the sinuses is a rapid, painless, innocuous, and easily reproducible as well as low-cost imaging technique to support a clinical diagnosis, and is useful to follow such patients up. Similarly, US is a convenient technique to correlate with x-ray findings. For example, if sinus surgery is planned and a significant lag time has occurred since CT imaging, quick updated confirmation of pathology by US can confirm what has been previously delineated on prior CT imaging.

US is a helpful confirmatory study to the clinical diagnosis of outpatient sinusitis and it can aid in the selection of patients for surgical intervention.[3] US has also been used successfully to follow the resolution of residual sinus discharge following surgical maxillary sinus irrigation in children.

In healthy patients the echo of the anterior maxillary or frontal sinus wall can frequently be detected,

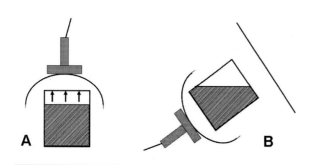

Fig 11–1. Fluid retention in the sinus is frequently overlooked in a supine position (**A**) because fluid has no contact to the anterior wall (*arrows*). Therefore, in cases of acute sinusitis, the ultrasound examination should preferably be done in an upright position with the chin on the sternum.

but the lumen of the air-filled sinus is not detectable. During acute sinusitis the lumen is filled with fluid, and in chronic sinusitis it can be completely filled with polyps or mucosal thickening which results in excellent conduction of the ultrasound wave. Therefore, in addition to the echo of the anterior sinus wall, a second echo from the posterior sinus wall can be detected (Fig 11–2). Detection of the posterior sinus wall is a characteristic of an obstructed sinus that is not air-filled, and this change can be detected in a transverse as well as in a sagittal plane.

Abscesses, Mucoceles, and Tumors

Abscesses of the face are commonly of dentogenic or sinugenic origin. Soft tissue abscesses are superficial to the bony structures and are therefore easily accessible to US. Their location is often adjacent to the mandible or to the maxilla or within the orbit. Like other fluid-filled processes, abscesses are characterized by a visible rim, by poor echogenicity, and by a distinct relative enhancement. The echo itself may be heterogeneous, depending on the suppurative area. Color Doppler can be applied but is not necessary. The region adjacent to the abscess shows hypervascularity, whereas the abscess interior is avascular. In doubtful cases, small abscesses can be aspirated using ultrasound guidance for needle insertion.

Orbital cellulitis and subperiosteal abscess are two distinct entities whose differentiation is important. Although abscess usually requires incision and drainage along with antibiotic therapy, cellulitis may be treated with antibiotics alone. Standardized orbital US has proven very useful, and in some cases more sensitive than CT, in the diagnosis of these orbital infections.[4]

Mucoceles are of sinugenic origin. Spontaneous mucoceles are very rare, and most patients have a

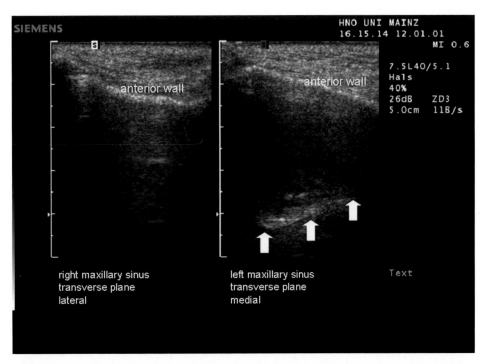

Fig 11–2. Acute sinusitis of the left maxillary sinus. The echo of the posterior wall can be seen on the left side (*arrows*) but not on the healthy right side.

history of prior head injury, often remote. In contrast to abscesses, it is typical to detect defects of the underlying bone at the base of mucoceles. The echo from mucoceles is homogeneous and like abscesses they are circumscribed, hypoechoic, and show a relative posterior acoustic enhancement (Fig 11–3). There is not hypervascularity as long as there is no infection.

B-mode US and color Doppler imaging have proven useful in the diagnosis of intraorbital and periorbital tumors in adults and especially in children, in whom a large spectrum of benign and malignant tumors may occur.[5] Pediatric orbital masses including hemangioma, dermoid, lymphangioma, rhabdomyosarcoma, encephalocele, and abscess have been well characterized by US,[5] and color Doppler sonography has enabled discrimination between vascular and avascular tumors. Whereas CT and MRI are invaluable in the evaluation of many orbital tumors, US is a less expensive initial option that is quick, noninvasive, devoid of radiation, does not require sedation, is easily repeated, and can be performed with the possibility of excluding malignancy in a patient's very first clinic visit. In some cases US can preclude the need for more expensive imaging. Still, CT and MRI are complementary in detecting bone erosion and intracranial extension when suspected, as well as the presence of blood products at various stages of breakdown. Ocular lesions are also detectable by US, and these include infection, trauma, foreign body, retinal detachment, and other intraocular structural abnormalities.[6]

In adults, inflammatory orbital conditions (such as diffuse pseudotumor or cellulitis), congestive conditions (such as dysthyroid exophthalmos), and hemorrhagic conditions have been distinguished from orbital tumors with a high degree of reliability. Accuracy of US for orbital tumor diagnosis, including localization, configuration, and extent, is as high as 94%[7,8] (Figs 11–4 and 11–5).

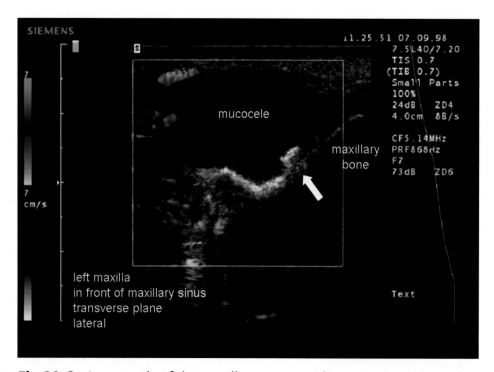

Fig 11–3. A mucocele of the maxillary antrum. The tumor is not vascularized and a bony defect to the maxillary sinus can be detected (*arrow*).

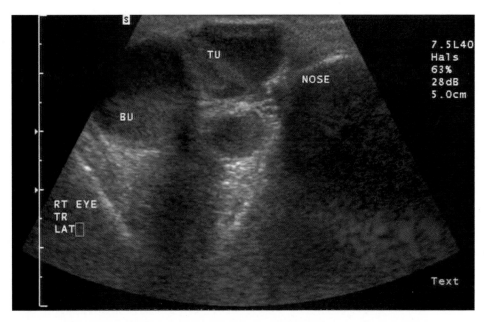

Fig 11–4. Transverse ultrasound image of the right orbit, showing well-defined tumor (*TU*) just medial to the bulb (*BU*).

Fractures

Displaced fractures of the superficial facial bones can be seen quite easily using US. Disruption of the normal bony contour leads to a strong echo at the site of a fracture suggesting loss of bony integrity. Small fractures without dislocation are often difficult to detect but these small fractures are usually without clinical consequence. The most common fracture is that of the nose (Fig 11–6). The diagnosis of nasal fracture with US is at least as sensitive as with conventional radiographs[9,10] and if US is performed as the first imaging study in cases of suspected nasal fracture, conventional radiography can usually be avoided. US provides various imaging planes without requiring positional change, and US carries no radiation which is especially advantageous in children. Equally important, US can provide information about the status of the cartilaginous septum, which is otherwise frequently unrecognized at the time of injury.[9] Sonographic findings of nasal fracture include disruption of bone continuity with or without separation of the fractured segment, displacement of the bone segments as being depressed or overriding, associated septal deviation or deformity, and separation of the piriform aperture of the maxilla and nasal bone. Soft-tissue edema and hypoechoic hematoma near the fracture lines are associated findings. Potential areas of difficulty for US imaging are the nasofrontal suture, the junction between the nasal bone and the piriform aperture of the maxilla, the vascular groove, and the distinction between an old fracture and an acute one. CT is quite useful in addition to sonography in cases of suspected complex facial trauma.

Fractures of the zygomatico-orbital complex are similarly amenable to US detection. An overall agreement of 85% between plain radiographs and US scans has been found,[11] and US is most reliable at the lateral wall of the maxillary sinus, where sensitivity is as high as 94% and specificity 100%.[11] Fractures of the zygomatic arch, the orbital rim, and the anterior wall of the frontal sinuses can be well visualized.[12] Furthermore, the success of closed reduction of such fractures can be immediately confirmed by postreduction or intraoperative US. The most significant shortcoming of US is its difficulty detecting nondisplaced fractures.

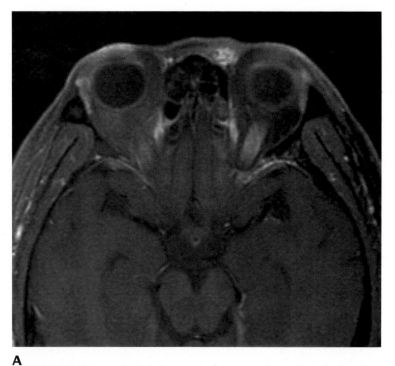

A

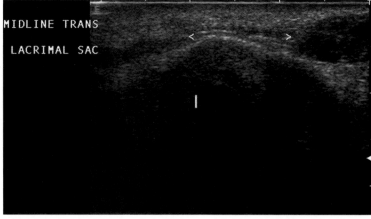

B

Fig 11–5. Left lacrimal sac tumor. The patient refused biopsy or excision but remained stable by MRI and US imaging for many years. **A**. Axial T1-weighted post-gadolinium image. **B**. Transverse midline orbital US showing hypoechoic ovoid nodule.

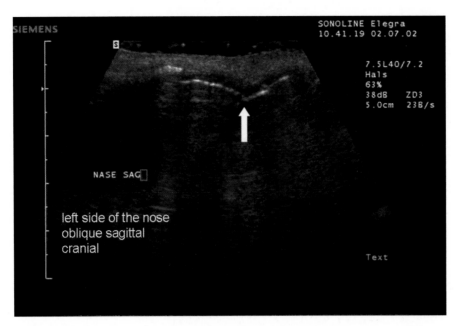

Fig 11–6. Fracture of the lateral nasal wall (*arrow*), seen on sagittal US. The bone is of high echogenicity.

US has been compared to plain radiographs in the detection of fractures of the mandibular condyle and ramus.[13] Whereas US is able to identify dislocated fractures of the ramus and the articular process in 67% of cases, US has poor sensitivity in detecting nondislocated fractures. As a result, US is not a favorable alternative to x-ray diagnosis of mandibular condyle and ramus fractures.

Orbital floor fractures are detected by US with an overall accuracy of 86% and a sensitivity of 85% or greater, compared with CT or direct surgical exploration[14] (Figs 11-7A and 11-7B). These numbers suggest that US is a useful adjunct to physical examination in the patient with facial trauma and suspected orbital floor fracture, including patients with associated cervical spine injuries or uncooperative patients in whom CT scanning may be impractical.

Subcutaneous Lesions

Subcutaneous lesions in the face include lesions of skin element origin, small abscesses as described above, as well as cysts, lipomas, neurofibromas, and other lesions. Solid masses can be differentiated from those filled with fluid. Cystic processes tend to be homogeneous and show posterior acoustic enhancement of the ultrasound signal. Solid processes may be homogeneous or heterogeneous (Figs 11-8 and 11-9A, 11-9B, and 11-9C). For example, a lipoma shows a typical feathered pattern (Fig 11-10). The neurofibroma is of medium echogenicity, similar to its surrounding muscles and soft tissues (Fig 11-11). In solid masses posterior acoustic enhancement is not typically seen (Figs 11-11 and 11-12). Depending on the origin and the composition of a mass, it may be compressible, such as if it is a lipoma or a cystic lesion.

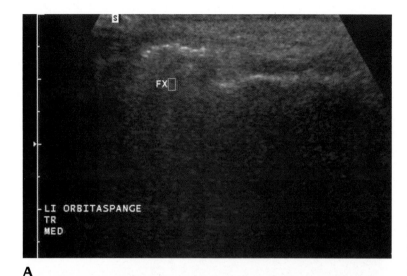

A

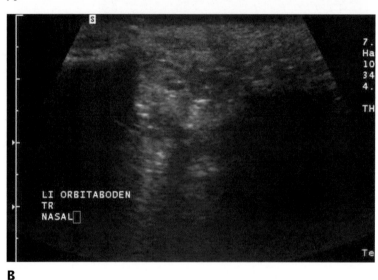

B

Fig 11–7. Orbital floor fractures. **A**. Transverse US view of left inferior orbital rim, showing bony stepoff. **B**. Transverse US view of left orbital floor, showing herniation of orbital contents into maxillary sinus.

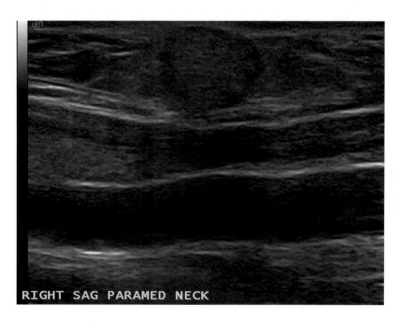

Fig 11–8. Well-circumscribed mildly heterogeneous subcutaneous nodule that proved to be a pilomatrixoma. Example here was located in the anterior neck but a similar appearance would be present in such a lesion of the face.

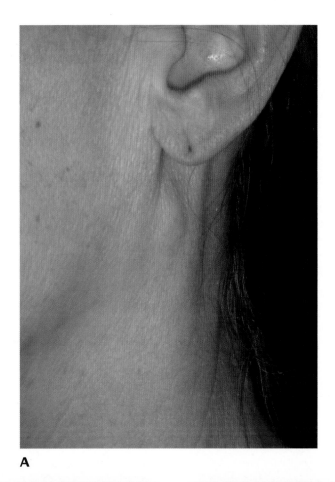

A

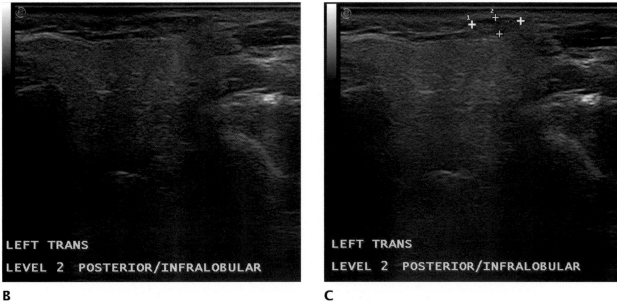

LEFT TRANS

LEVEL 2 POSTERIOR/INFRALOBULAR

B

LEFT TRANS

LEVEL 2 POSTERIOR/INFRALOBULAR

C

Fig 11–9. Clinical photograph (**A**) and transverse US image (**B** unlabeled, **C** labeled) of a benign subcutaneous dermatofibroma. The small size and superficial location would render this lesion difficult to see on cross-sectional imaging.

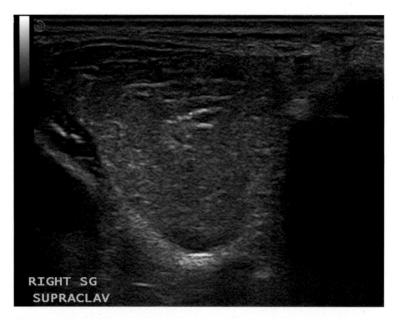

Fig 11–10. Right sagittal US view of a supraclavicular lipoma; note heterogeneous, feathered appearance to the interior of the lesion. Lipomas of the face have a similar sonographic appearance.

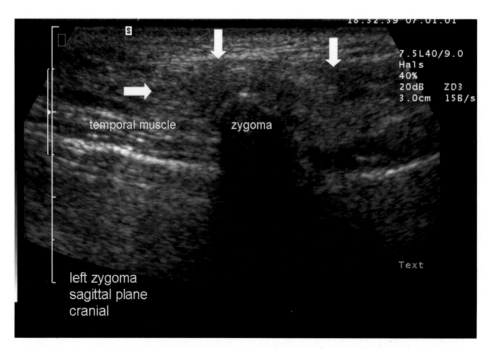

Fig 11–11. A solid tumor of medium echogenicity, similar to its soft tissue surroundings, located on the left zygoma. Note absence of posterior acoustic enhancement. Histologic examination revealed a neurofibroma.

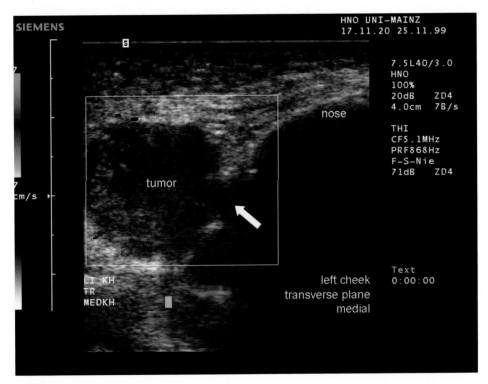

Fig 11–12. A patient with a history of malignant mucosal melanoma of the maxillary sinus developed a mass in the left cheek. The tumor is hypovascular and shows no relative posterior acoustic enhancement. Histologic examination revealed recurrent melanoma.

Vascular Lesions

Vascular lesions of the face are relatively rare (Figs 11-13 and 11-14). Vascular malformations including hemangioma, lymphangioma, and solid tumors which are highly vascularized must be considered. Using B-mode US hemangioma and lymphangioma are often compressible and hypoechoic; they are either heterogeneous or homogeneous. Sometimes very few blood vessels can be detected in spite of the vascular origin of these tumors (Fig 11-15). This apparent contradiction may confuse the examiner but it must be recalled that Doppler sonography detects the blood flow and not the vessels themselves. Therefore, in cases of low blood flow, as seen in low-flow hemangioma, little vascularity is detectable. This finding is in contrast to other imaging techniques, such as contrast-enhanced CT or MRI where the high amount of blood vessels are detected.

A hemangioma or lymphangioma must be differentiated from other, highly vascularized processes in the face, such as highly vascularized lymphoma or metastatic renal cell carcinoma (Fig 11-16).

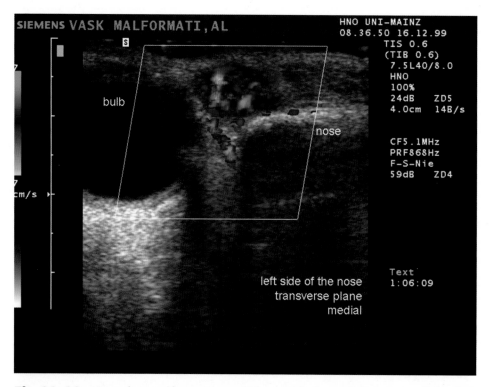

Fig 11–13. Vascular malformation of the medial canthal region of the left orbit.

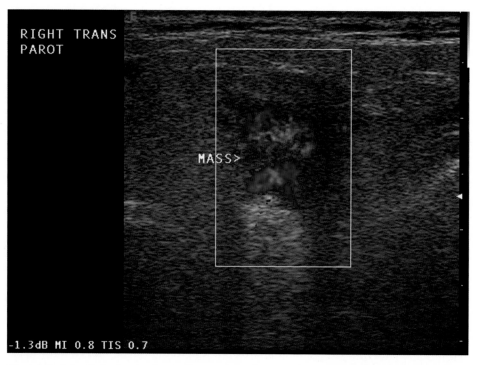

Fig 11–14. Relatively high-flow vascular malformation within the right parotid gland.

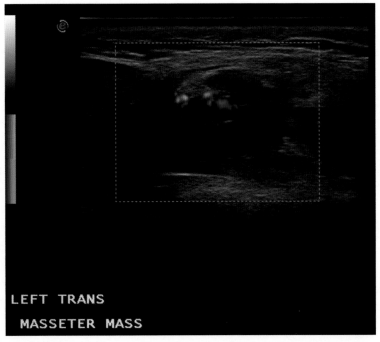

LEFT TRANS

MASSETER MASS

A

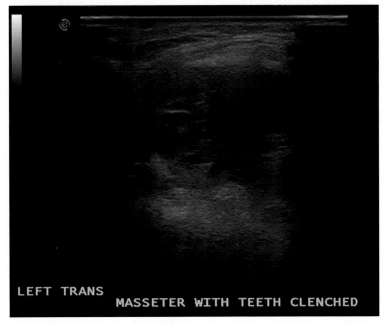

LEFT TRANS MASSETER WITH TEETH CLENCHED

B

Fig 11-15. Transverse US showing vascular malformation within the left masseter muscle. Note relatively low blood flow on color Doppler US (**A**) and enlargement of mass during teeth clenching and contraction of the masseter muscle (**B**).

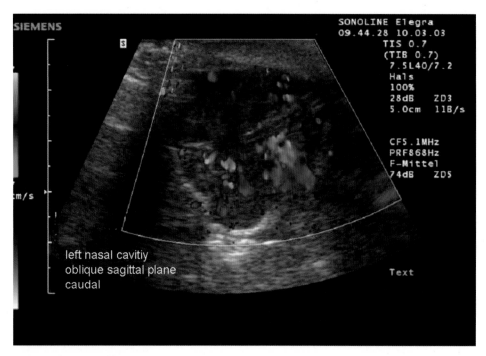

Fig 11-16. Endonasal growth of a highly vascularized tumor that was proven histologically to be a metastasis of renal cell carcinoma.

Middle Ear Lesions

Although US of the temporal bone itself is impractical, US can be useful in detecting a single but common entity within the middle ear, namely effusion. Application of A- and B-mode US to middle ear assessment has been limited by the availability of appropriate-sized transducers.[15-17] However, in a manner similar to detection of fluid or opacification of the maxillary sinus, endoluminal US via the external auditory canal can detect echoes from the tympanic membrane in healthy ears with an aerated middle ear space, while detecting echoes from both the tympanic membrane and the middle ear wall in the opacified middle ear. The amplitude of the echo from the middle ear wall is related to the viscosity of the effusion: the echo in serous otitis media is of high amplitude, whereas the echo from the middle ear with a mucoid effusion is lower.[18] Water or gel placed in the external auditory canal can serve as the transducing medium. With refinements in probe design, US of the middle ear could prove to be a more highly accurate method of determining the presence and characteristics of middle ear effusions than any noninvasive method currently in use. In fact, a commercially available ultrasonic "ear tester" (EarCheck, Innovia Medical LLC, Lenexa, Kans) is sold at retail stores to the public.

Prenatal Facial US

Although prenatal US is beyond the scope of this textbook, it bears mentioning that sonographic examination of the fetal face can provide information that may suggest congenital facial anomalies as well as syndromes involving other organs or systems.[19] Conventional facial imaging by two-dimensional (2-D) B-mode US has been enhanced by three-dimensional (3-D) fetal US. The incorporation of the temporal component to create so-called four-dimensional (4-D) US enables fetal facial expressions and movements to be observed and documented.

Antenatal diagnosis of cleft lip and cleft palate has proved challenging due to variable size and location of such defects, but 3-D US has enhanced the diagnostic process.[20] Other congenital lesions such as lymphangiomas[21,22] and teratomas[23] can be detected and their potential for causing airway obstruction recognized, resulting in adequate preparation and avoidance of unexpected airway emergencies at delivery.

Summary

In conclusion, although facial US has not been widely popularized, it has all of the advantages of US of the neck. In the hands of the clinician experienced in soft-tissue US of the neck, facial, sinus, orbital, and ear examinations are logical extensions of the application of US to head and neck disorders.

References

1. Lichtenstein D, Biderman P, Meziere G, Gepner A. The "sinusogram," a real-time ultrasound sign of maxillary sinusitis. *Intens Care Med.* 1998;24(10):1057–1061.

2. Puidupin M, Guiavarch M, Paris A, et al. B-mode ultrasound in the diagnosis of maxillary sinusitis in the intensive care unit. *Intens Care Med.* 1997;23(11):1174–1175.

3. Revonta M, Suonpaa J, Meurman OH. Ultrasound testing in the diagnosis and management of maxillary sinusitis in children [in German]. *HNO.* 1980;28(3):91–96.

4. Kaplan DM, Briscoe D, Gatot A, Niv A, Leiberman A, Fliss DM. The use of standardized orbital ultrasound in the diagnosis of sinus induced infections of the orbit in children: a preliminary report. *Int J Pediatr Otorhinolaryngol.* 1999;48(2):155–162.

5. Neudorfer M, Leibovitch I, Stolovitch C, et al. Intraorbital and periorbital tumors in children—value of ultrasound and color Doppler imaging in the differential diagnosis. *Am J Ophthalmol.* 2004;137(6):1065–1072.

6. Glasier CM, Brodsky MC, Leithiser RE, Seibert JJ. High resolution ultrasound with Doppler: a diagnostic adjunct in orbital and ocular lesions in children. *Pediatr Radiol.* 1992;22(3):174–178.

7. Dallow RL. Evaluation of unilateral exophthalmos with ultrasonography: analysis of 258 consecutive cases. *Laryngoscope.* 1975;85(11 pt 1):1905–1919.

8. Dallow RL. Reliability of orbital diagnostic tests: ultrasonography, computerized tomography, and radiography. *Ophthalmology.* 1978;85(11):1218–1228.

9. Hong HS, Cha JG, Paik SH, et al. High-resolution sonography for nasal fracture in children. *AJR Am J Roentgenol.* 2007;188(1):W86–W92.

10. Thiede O, Krömer JH, Rudack C, Stoll W, Osada N, Schmäl F. Comparison of ultrasonography and conventional radiography in the diagnosis of nasal fractures. *Arch Otolaryngol Head Neck Surg.* 2005;131:434–439.

11. McCann PJ, Brocklebank LM, Ayoub AF. Assessment of zygomatico-orbital complex fractures using ultrasonography. *Br J Oral Maxillofac Surg.* 2000;38:525–529.

12. Friedrich RE, Heiland M, Bartel-Friedrich S. Potentials of ultrasound in the diagnosis of midfacial fractures. *Clin Oral Invest.* 2003;7(4):226–229.

13. Friedrich RE, Plambeck K, Bartel-Friedrich S, Giese M, Schmelzle R. Limitations of B-scan ultrasound for diagnosing fractures of the mandibular condyle and ramus. *Clin Oral Invest.* 2001;5(1):11–16.

14. Jenkins CN, Thuau H. Ultrasound imaging in assessment of fractures of the orbital floor. *Clin Radiol.* 1997;52(9):708–711.

15. Alvord LS. Uses of ultrasound in audiology. *J Am Acad Audiol.* 1990;1(4):227–235.

16. Alvord LS, Fine PG. Real-time B-scan ultrasound in middle ear assessment. A preliminary report. *J Ultrasound Med.* 1990;9(2):91–94.

17. Wu CH, Hsu CJ, Hsieh FT. Preliminary use of endoluminal ultrasonography in assessment of middle ear with effusion. *J Ultrasound Med.* 1998;17(7):427–430.

18. Discolo CM, Byrd MC, Bates T, Hazony D, Lewandowski J, Koltai PJ. Ultrasonic detection of middle ear effusion. *Arch Otolaryngol Head Neck Surg.* 2004;130:1407–1410.

19. Kurjak A, Azumendi G, Andonotopo W, Salihagic-Kadic A. Three- and four-dimensional ultrasonography for the structural and functional evaluation of the fetal face. *Am J Obstet Gynecol.* 2007;196(1):16–28.

20. Platt LD, Devore GR, Pretorius DH. Improving cleft palate/cleft lip antenatal diagnosis by 3-dimensional sonography: the "flipped face" view. *J Ultrasound Med.* 2006;25(11):1423–1430.

21. Paladini D, Vassallo M, Sglavo G, Lapadula C, Longo M, Nappi C. Cavernous lymphangioma of the face and neck: prenatal diagnosis by three-dimensional ultrasound. *Ultrasound Obstet Gynecol.* 2005;26(3):300–302.

22. Rahbar R, Vogel A, Myers LB, et al. Fetal surgery in otolaryngology: a new era in the diagnosis and management of fetal airway obstruction because of advances in prenatal imaging. *Arch Otolaryngol Head Neck Surg*. 2005;131(5):393-398.

23. Morof D, Levine D, Grable I, et al. Oropharyngeal teratoma: prenatal diagnosis and assessment using sonography, MRI, and CT with management by ex utero intrapartum treatment procedure. *AJR Am J Roentgenol*. 2004;183(2):493-496.

Chapter 12

INTERVENTIONAL ULTRASONOGRAPHY

Kristin K. Egan
Lisa A. Orloff

Introduction

The widespread use of ultrasonography (US) in the clinical realm is a growing phenomenon, for good reason. In the head and neck region, US has applications well beyond diagnostic imaging, in the form of guiding interventional diagnostic and therapeutic procedures. The availability of ultrasound equipment and the cost-effectiveness of its use, especially in regions of limited medical resources, have contributed to the popularity of US. Once the sonographic anatomy of the head and neck region is understood, a logical extension is to use US to guide minimally invasive procedures with enhanced precision and insight yet without radiation exposure.

Ultrasound-Guided Fine Needle Aspiration

Fine-needle aspiration (FNA) biopsy is a commonly performed procedure in the cytologic evaluation of masses in the head and neck region. The acronym FNA has persisted, although this method would more accurately be called FNB or fine-needle biopsy,

as aspiration is not necessarily a part of the procedure. The most common and familiar indication is the evaluation of thyroid nodules (Fig 12–1 and Video 12A). Nonpalpable thyroid nodules present an obvious dilemma to the clinician when screening patients with suspected nodular thyroid disease or suspected recurrent thyroid cancer. In patients with thyroid nodules detected by US, FNA with ultrasound

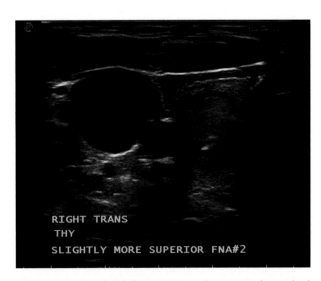

RIGHT TRANS
THY
SLIGHTLY MORE SUPERIOR FNA#2

Fig 12–1 and Video 12A. Ultrasound-guided FNA of a thyroid nodule (*short-axis technique*).

guidance has been shown to accurately assess and diagnose the majority of patients' lesions.[1] When FNA has been compared to coarse needle biopsy with ultrasound guidance to localize nodules in the thyroid, and surgical specimens later retrieved have been used to determine the results of detecting neoplasia, the diagnostic accuracy of the two methods has been shown to be equal.[2] Such a comparison supports the use of ultrasound-guided FNA (USG-FNA), with expected accuracy of 80%, sensitivity of 83%, and specificity of 77%.

After sampling, FNA specimens are reviewed by a cytopathologist or cytotechnologist. The use of USG-FNA with on-site evaluation of cytology specimens by a team composed of clinical physicians and pathologists has been shown to provide the most accurate and least uncomfortable results.[3] Patient discomfort, as measured by number of needle passes needed, and diagnostic errors, as measured by sample inadequacy rate, can be reduced through the use of ultrasound guidance and immediate examination of material obtained. Ultrasound guidance for FNA has even been proposed by some as a standard of care and its training has been advocated in residency programs. Nevertheless, for palpable thyroid masses, FNA without US guidance may still be preferable, due to its cost-effectiveness, expedience, and the related minimization of bleeding associated with swift needle passage and manual lesion stabilization.

Thyroid

At the time of FNA of thyroid lesions, certain preliminary findings can suggest specimen adequacy as well as diagnosis. The benign thyroid nodule yields visible colloid material, clusters of follicular cells often in a "honeycombed" pattern, round to oval nuclei with stippled chromatin, and foamy (degenerating) cells. Chronic lymphocytic thyroiditis (Hashimoto's thyroiditis) is typically characterized by a hypercellular aspirate dominated by a heterogeneous population of lymphocytes. Colloid is usually minimal or absent.[4]

Subacute thyroiditis (de Quervain's thyroiditis) frequently has cytologic features which include large multinucleated giant cells, a mixed inflammatory background, minimal or absent colloid, and occasionally a granulomatous reaction suggestive of fibrosis. Follicular neoplasm of the thyroid is a cytopathologic dilemma. Follicular adenoma cannot be differentiated from follicular carcinoma without surgical excision and determination of vascular or capsular invasion. On FNA, one will see a hypercellular specimen with microfollicular pattern and nuclear polymorphism and cellular atypia.[4] Furthermore, FNA of follicular neoplasms tends to be bloodier than FNA of other thyroid lesions.[4]

Thyroid carcinomas that are identifiable on FNA by cytopathologic analysis include papillary, medullary and anaplastic carcinomas. Papillary thyroid carcinoma shows large, round, irregular or grooved and often overlapping nuclei, pale nuclear chromatin, sheets of cells with papillary configuration, "pseudoinclusions," psammoma bodies, and viscous colloid. Medullary thyroid carcinoma shows hypercellularity, poor cell cohesion, spindle-shaped cells with elongated, eccentric nuclei, multinucleated cells, positive staining for calcitonin, and positive staining with Congo red if amyloid is present.[4]

Papillary thyroid cancer represents approximately 80% of all thyroid malignancies, and in addition to obtaining cytologic diagnosis, the aspirate obtained can be examined for genetic markers such as the BRAF mutation.[5] The identification of genetic mutations in thyroid carcinomas can assist in surgical planning as those papillary thyroid carcinomas with BRAF expressivity have a higher frequency of extrathyroidal invasion and a predisposition to metastasis.[6]

Aspirated material can also be tested for thyroglobulin or calcitonin levels. Such testing is especially useful in the evaluation of potential lymph node metastases or recurrent nodules in patients with known papillary or medullary carcinoma. These levels should be correlated with simultaneous serum levels. Serum thyroglobulin (TG) is frequently used as a marker for recurrent disease in patients with well-differentiated thyroid cancer who have undergone surgical thyroidectomy with or without radioactive iodine ablation. A shortcoming of serum TG measurement is that 12% or more of patients will have anti-TG antibodies that interfere with interpretation of the assay.[7] Furthermore, demonstration of an elevated TG level does not localize the recurrent or metastatic disease. Measurement of thyroglobulin or calcitonin in the aspirate from the FNA of any suspicious mass can confirm the presence and simultaneously localize recurrent disease.

Parathyroid

Ultrasound-guided FNA of parathyroid glands can prove especially useful in patients with hyperparathyroidism (HPT) undergoing reoperative neck surgery or with unusual or ectopic parathyroid glands. USG-FNA can be used to acquire cytology specimens and to obtain levels of parathyroid hormone (PTH) (Fig 12–2 and Video 12B). Parathyroid cytology is notoriously difficult to confirm, but the goal is primarily to distinguish suspected parathyroid lesions from lymph nodes or thyroid nodules, and to recognize malignant lesions when present. Although there is significant overlap in the cytomorphologic features of cells derived from parathyroid and thyroid glands, some distinguishing characteristics have been noted. The presence of stippled nuclear chromatin, prominent vascular proliferation with attached epithelial cells, and frequent occurrence of single cells and naked nuclei are useful clues that favor parathyroid origin. Cytology alone cannot differentiate between the different parathyroid lesions including hyperplasia, adenoma, and carcinoma.[8] But in addition to immediate cytologic assessment, the remaining contents from the sampling needle can be rinsed and diluted with 5 cc of normal saline and placed on ice for PTH analysis by immunoassay. A positive result in a study by Stephen et al using USG-FNA of parathyroid lesions was defined as an intact PTH level greater than 40 pg/mL in the sample from an enlarged parathyroid gland identified on US.[9] Although the results from this study were promising, drawbacks do exist with USG-FNA in hyperparathyroidism. Applying suction to the needle and syringe while aspirating can incorporate extraneous tissue or blood, and it can often be difficult to distinguish between thyroid and parathyroid cytology. Stephen et al did not correlate the results of the PTH level in the aspirate with serum PTH level. When questions arise in distinguishing thyroid and parathyroid cytology, the level of PTH can help in identification. However, when serum level of PTH is not taken, one can obtain a false positive result from simply having PTH in the blood of the aspirate taken from a nonparathyroid source. Therefore, it is preferable to send simultaneous PTH levels from serum and aspirate sample and classify as positive only those cases where the aspirated levels are higher than serum PTH levels.

Preoperative USG-FNA can be useful in patients with HPT and coexisting thyroid nodules, and helps to identify yet minimize the need for thyroidectomy when malignant thyroid disease is ruled in or ruled out preoperatively. Tc99 sestamibi scans and US are often complementary in patients with HPT. In one study of patients with primary HPT and negative sestamibi scans, US successfully localized 86% of parathyroid lesions.[10] On the other hand, US can better characterize and distinguish thyroid disease that confounds the interpretation of sestamibi parathyroid scans.[11]

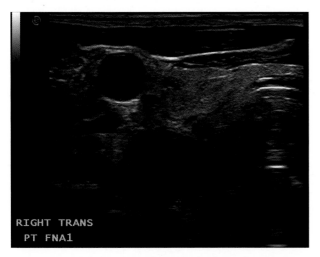

Fig 12–2 and Video 12B. Ultrasound-guided FNA of a parathyroid adenoma (*short-axis technique*). In the video, note that the needle traverses the thyroid gland to reach this deep parathyroid, and the sample was sent for cytology and PTH assay.

Other Neck Masses

USG-FNA can be used in the evaluation of other neck masses, such as those described in greater detail elsewhere in this textbook (Fig 12–3 and Video 12C).

Nonpalpable neck masses can be localized with US and sampled for cytologic diagnosis. Even palpable neck masses that have undergone nondiagnostic FNA without ultrasound guidance warrant repeat FNA with ultrasound guidance. The identification of squamous cell carcinoma in a neck mass can prompt the search for a primary source, or confirm recurrent or persistent disease in a previously diagnosed and treated patient. In cases of suspected lymphoma, flow cytometry can be performed on

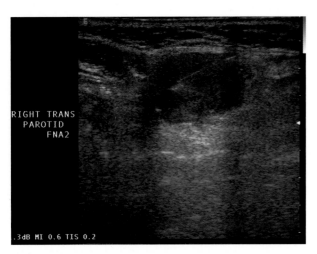

Fig 12–3 and Video 12C. Ultrasound-guided FNA of a parotid mass (*short-axis technique*).

aspirates in addition to cytopathology and immuno-cytochemistry analysis. The ease and rapidity with which USG-FNA can be done facilitates expedient evaluation and treatment of benign and malignant head and neck masses.

Technical Aspects of USGFNA

FNA techniques vary considerably between individuals and institutions. This chapter aims to evaluate the modifications that can be employed, including use of US, in order to improve the diagnostic success of FNA. US enables visualization of the needle tip within the target mass to ensure that the cells examined are indeed from the suspected area. The number of needle passes through the area of interest and the use of suction on a syringe attached to the needle have been heavily debated (Fig 12–4). If the needle is clearly visualized within the area of interest, one pass may be sufficient[10]; however, additional passes will allow more sample to be examined. A greater number of passes will also potentially cause more bleeding which may obscure the results. "Hunting" for the needle with US during the procedure may lead to more bleeding, but on the other hand US can also guide redirection of the needle to

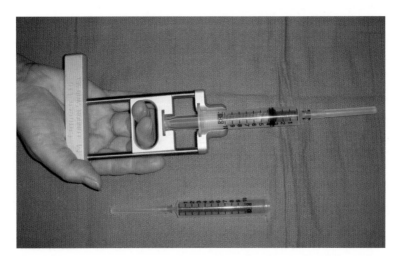

Fig 12–4. USG-FNA can be performed using a syringe in an aspirating device, or by the "capillary technique" using an open-barreled syringe into which the plunger can be reinserted to expel the sample after biopsy.

preferred sites within the target lesion. For example, the solid portion of a mixed cystic and solid lesion can be sampled by USG-FNA, or an area of initial hemorrhage from a first pass on USG-FNA can be avoided on subsequent passes (Fig 12–5 and Video 12D). Aspiration on the syringe while in the sample has been advocated to increase the amount of sample, but may also increase bleeding and may increase the amount of extraneous tissue and blood that is obtained. If suction is used, it is important to release suction before exiting the sample to avoid contamination by tissue or cells outside of the mass.

Needle size affects the sample obtained in FNA. Large-bore needles such as 14 to 19 gauge have historically been used in needle biopsy. However, finer needles carry a lesser risk of trauma such as hematoma, and a theoretical reduced risk of spreading malignancy. Successful USG-FNA using 25-gauge needles has been clearly demonstrated.[12] We tend to favor 23- to 25-gauge needles. Adequate sampling has been obtained in the first pass in 89% of liver lesions, and 87% of lung lesions. Needle lengths of 1.5 inches (38 mm) are usually sufficient for the head and neck region, but longer 40 to 50-mm length needles can be useful for deeper lesions, as they increase the angles and depths that can be accessed.[13] Orienting the bevel of the needle toward the ultrasound transducer improves visualization of the needle tip.

Many ultrasound devices have special features designed to facilitate USG-FNA. Attachable needle guides are available for some transducers, although these guides limit flexibility in biopsy direction and are discouraged by many experienced clinicians. Some US consoles have a biopsy function that adds a diagonal line on the monitor to facilitate directional aim of the needle. The positioning of both the patient and the individual performing the FNA can be adjusted to optimize access. The operator may stand or sit at the patient's side or at the head. Depending on the location of the lesion and the surrounding structures at risk, the transducer can be rotated 360 degrees to determine the safest or shortest line to the lesion. Although diagnostic US uses conventional transverse and sagittal planes for imaging, once a lesion has been characterized and targeted for FNA, the transducer can be oriented to any position that will facilitate the USG-FNA procedure. For example, to approach a lesion in the left lobe of thyroid, a right-handed operator may prefer to come

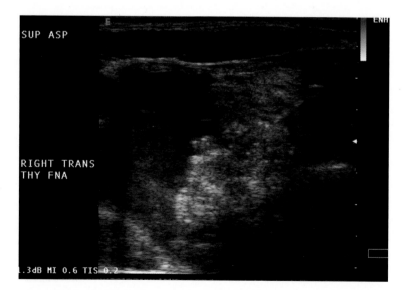

Fig 12–5 and Video 12D. USG-FNA of the solid component of a predominately cystic thyroid nodule that proved to be papillary carcinoma. **Video 12D.** USG-FNA showing redirection of the needle by steepening the angle of insertion to better target the intended lesion.

from medial to lateral, that is, trachea side rather than carotid side, and to stand at the patient's head and do the procedure "upside down."

The use of the short-axis or angled versus the long-axis or vertical approach to USG-FNA is determined by operator preference and accessibility of the target area or lesion. With the long-axis approach, the needle is inserted just adjacent to the midpoint of the long axis of the transducer and a nearly vertical trajectory is used. One will only see the tip of the needle as a bright spot within the target once the needle tip arrives at the plane of the image (Figs 12–6A and 12–6B, and Video 12E). Alternatively, the short-axis technique involves inserting

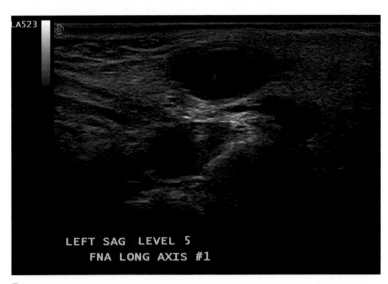

A

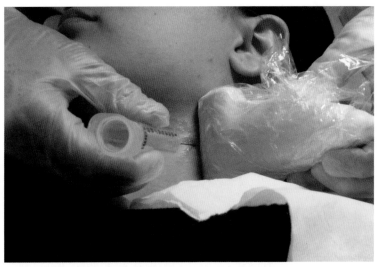

B

Fig 12–6 and Video 12E. USG-FNA by the long-axis technique. Needle is inserted at the mid-point of the long axis of the transducer after the lesion is centered deep to the transducer. **Video 12E.** USG-FNA of a level 2 lymph node with metastatic papillary thyroid cancer by the long-axis technique.

the needle just adjacent to the midpoint of the short axis of the transducer and exactly parallel to it at a 45-degree angle (or an angle ranging from about 30 to 70 degrees depending on the depth of the target and the length of the needle). This approach allows visualization of the entire length of the needle and its trajectory as it advances from just beneath the skin toward and into the lesion (Figs 12–7A and 12–7B, and Video 12F).

The impact of differing degrees of preparation and sterility during ultrasound-guided office-based procedures has also been debated. Preparation ranges

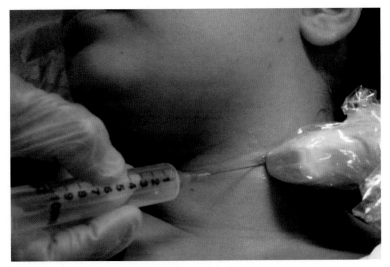

A

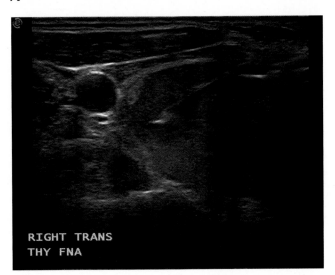

B

Fig 12–7 and Video 12F. USG-FNA by the short-axis technique. Needle is inserted at the mid-point of the short axis of the transducer and visualized as it enters the intended lesion. **Video 12F**. USG-FNA of a node harboring metastatic squamous cell carcinoma by the short-axis technique. The node is located between the internal and external carotid arteries in the left level 2 region.

from a simple skin disinfection procedure with an alcohol-based swab and no cover on the transducer to an iodine-based skin disinfectant, use of sterile aqueous jelly and a sterile transducer cover.[13] A reasonable compromise involves alcohol-based skin disinfection and nonsterile aqueous gel applied to the footprint of the transducer before and after its coverage with plastic wrap or with a disposable glove secured with a rubber band (Fig 12–8). These inexpensive techniques have been used extensively by the senior author and infectious complications have not been encountered. The use of local anesthetic, though not universal, is also favored for patient comfort and thereby to help minimize patient movement during sampling. Local anesthetic can be injected in the skin and subcutaneous plane at the intended needle entry site. Anesthetizing the pathway leading down to the target, especially if it traverses muscle, can reduce pain associated with the FNA procedure, although the risk of hematoma and a bloody biopsy specimen is greater with increased aggressiveness of anesthetic injection.

Ultrasound-Guided Abscess Drainage

Like USG-FNA for cytologic analysis, ultrasound-guided needle aspiration is applicable to a variety of head and neck abscesses. Transcervical US can be

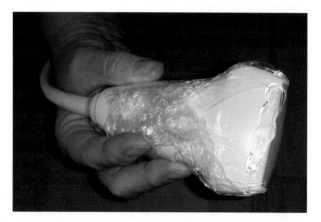

Fig 12–8. Ultrasound transducer covered with clear plastic wrap, with gel inside and outside of wrap, for interventional procedures.

diagnostic for peritonsillar abscesses, and can be combined with transoral needle aspiration, which is a minimally invasive option for such abscess management.[14] Ultrasound-guided needle aspiration of abscessed lymphadenitis in infants and young children may spare the need for imaging that uses ionizing radiation or general anesthesia required for imaging as well as more invasive procedures. Early odontogenic abscesses and orbital abscesses can be similarly diagnosed and managed. Ultrasound-guided aspiration can aid in the initial assessment and management of infected thyroglossal duct and branchial cleft cysts. US can also be utilized to confirm tuberculous abscesses of the cervical lymph nodes or the thyroid gland through simultaneous diagnostic imaging and guided fine-needle aspiration sampling.[15]

Ultrasound-Guided Injection

As with sampling , US can be used to guide targeted injections for head and neck disorders to enhance the precision of needle placement.

Botulinum Toxin

Botulinum toxin (BT) has been shown to reduce saliva secretion when injected directly into the salivary glands of patients with sialorrhea.[16] Treatment with BT can be an effective therapeutic alternative to surgery or systemic anticholinergic agents in patients with conditions including amyotrophic lateral sclerosis (ALS), cerebral palsy (CP), Parkinson's disease, and bulbar stroke. Ultrasound guidance has been incorporated for localizing the injection site in both the parotid and the submandibular glands. Its use has been advocated to guarantee precise and safe injection even in unfavorable anatomical conditions, to avoid unintended targets, and to maximize the delivery of BT into the desired target.[17] Ultrasound guidance in procedures involving the salivary glands decreases the risk of unintended chemodenervation of adjacent muscles, such as the masseter, digastric, geniohyoid, and others that may affect chewing and swallowing, as well as injury to major vessels which course in close proximity.

US-guided BT injection is quick, simple, minimally painful, and repeatable. With the patient in a reclining or supine position as tolerated, high-resolution (7.5 to 13-MHz) B-mode US is used to localize the submandibular and parotid salivary glands, which are injected percutaneously using aseptic technique and a 25- or 27-gauge needle (Fig 12–9 and Video 12G). Injections typically consist of about 25 units of BT per gland and are titrated up or down to patient response. Follow-up information regarding subjective changes in drooling, adjustments in systemic antisaliva therapy, and objective salivary flow help dictate future treatment.

When successful, BT injection is a much less invasive, temporary but easily repeatable alternative to surgical rerouting of the submandibular ducts.[18,19]

Salivary fistulae and sialoceles are other salivary gland disorders that are amenable to ultrasound-guided botulinum toxin treatment. These conditions usually occur following parotidectomy surgery or parotid gland trauma, where residual or injured parotid tissue secretes saliva into a cavity at the site of an excised parotid tumor, or saliva is secreted that leaks out through the skin incision or laceration and prevents healing. These conditions respond poorly to pressure dressings and systemic anticholinergic agents but in our experience and that of others[20] have responded dramatically to ultrasound-guided botulinum toxin injection of the parotid gland. Doses of 100 to 300 units of BT have been successful, with the most favorable response occurring when the BT is diluted in approximately 10 cc of saline and injected in a diffuse manner throughout the residual salivary parenchyma, to maximize the inhibition of salivary secretion (Figs 12–10A and 12–10B, and Video 12H).

Sclerotherapy

Sclerotherapy is a treatment option for a variety of disorders involving cysts, effusions, and vascular or lymphatic malformations. US facilitates localization of fluid collections and precise placement of needles or catheters for aspiration of fluid and/or instillation of sclerosing agents under direct visualization. Even solid hormonally active lesions can be treated by percutaneous sclerotherapy. Preferred sclerosing agents include doxycycline and 96% ethanol. The mechanism of action of ethanol is through cellular dehydration and protein denaturation followed by small vessel thrombosis, hemorrhagic infarction, coagulative necrosis, and reactive fibrosis.[21]

Patients with nonfunctioning cystic thyroid nodules with benign cytology are the most common and likely candidates for a minimally invasive percutaneous approach to cyst obliteration that avoids surgery. Simple ethanol instillation through the same needle after aspiration of fluid from a cystic thyroid nodule results in resolution of the cystic portion of the nodule in more than 90% of patients, confirmed by follow-up sonography.[21] Ideal candidates for this procedure are young, otherwise healthy patients with solitary cysts less than 3 cm in diameter. Ethanol therapy avoids external scarring, exposure to radiation or the heightened possibility of hypothyroidism which can follow surgery or [131]Iodine ablation.

Ethanol sclerotherapy of thyroid lesions can be performed on an outpatient basis, without or with

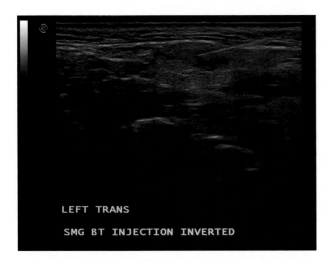

LEFT TRANS

SMG BT INJECTION INVERTED

Fig 12–9 and Video 12G. Ultrasound-guided botulinum toxin injection of the major salivary glands for treatment of sialorrhea (inverted transverse view of the left submandibular gland being injected from a position at the head of the bed looking toward the patient's feet). **Video 12G.** Ultrasound-guided botulinum toxin injection of the major salivary glands for treatment of sialorrhea associated with ALS (inverted transverse view of the left submandibular gland being injected).

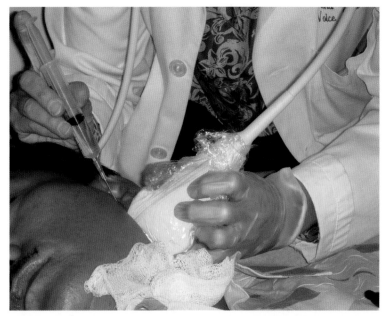

A

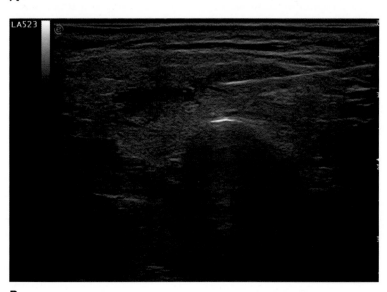

B

Fig 12–10 and Video 12H. Ultrasound-guided injection of a postparotidectomy sialocele with botulinum toxin. **Video 12H**. Ultrasound-guided injection of a postparotidectomy salivary fistula with botulinum toxin. Following accessory parotid lobectomy via an anterior approach, saliva was draining through the anterior cheek incision. This surgical approach is not recommended but this patient's fistula was cured with a single injection.

local anesthesia, and with the patient resuming normal activity following the procedure. A full examination should be completed prior to the procedure, including diagnostic thyroid US and FNA of the target lesion, to rule out malignancy. Other diseases such as Graves' disease or toxic multinodular goiter, for which ethanol sclerotherapy is not suitable, should also be ruled out. Coexisting nodules should also be fully evaluated with USG-FNA to minimize the risk of later need for thyroidectomy, with attendant fibrosis due to prior sclerotherapy as a potential added risk factor.[22,23]

European and Asian experience with ultrasound-guided sclerotherapy of thyroid nodules has been successful not only for nonfunctioning thyroid cysts but also in the treatment of autonomously functioning thyroid nodules and even solid cold thyroid nodules. Variability in outcomes has been attributed to technician experience, and reported complication rates have declined as experience with the procedure has grown.[23] Nevertheless, risks of the procedure include temporary or permanent vocal fold paralysis[22] due to ethanol seepage outside the thyroid capsule or to nerve compression by a sudden increase in intranodular pressure, neck pain, extraglandular fibrosis, worsening of thyrotoxicosis (which can be prevented in hyperthyroid patients by pretreatment with beta-blockers or methimazole), overlooked malignancy, hematomas and thrombosis, and fainting due to vasovagal response.[23] Even the most experienced and well-published of international practitioners of thyroid and parathyroid sclerotherapy have cautioned that ethanol injection has never been compared by prospective randomized trials to conventional surgical or medical treatments, and should be reserved for patients who cannot or will not undergo standard therapy.[24] Similarly, use of US-guided interstitial laser photocoagulation to treat autonomous thyroid nodules has shown promise and warrants further evaluation.[25]

Ethanol sclerotherapy of hyperfunctioning parathyroid glands is an effective, though still considered experimental, therapeutic option for hyperparathyroidism (HPT). Following USG-FNA confirmation of parathyroid lesions (by cytology and/or PTH assay), instillation of ethanol leads to a significant decrease in serum concentrations of ionized calcium, total calcium, and intact PTH.[22] Serial ethanol injections are usually necessary, up to a maximum of three treatments, preferably in close succession (daily or weekly as opposed to monthly). Success rates of 79% have been reported for treatment of primary HPT, but the treatment is recommended only for patients not fit for surgery. For those patients with persistent HPT after sclerotherapy that required surgery, 80% were found to have fibrosis surrounding their parathyroid tumors; vocal fold paralysis was also noted in at least 6% of sclerotherapy recipients. Horner's syndrome has been another reported complication.[26] Ethanol sclerotherapy has been studied somewhat more extensively in patients with renal HPT but medical management with surgical treatment of refractory HPT are still the mainstay of treatment.[27,28]

Various other lesions of the head and neck are amenable to treatment with percutaneous ethanol injection under ultrasound guidance. Postoperative lymphoceles have been treated with doxycycline or ethanol after aspiration of the fluid collection. Chylous fistulae and chylomas can be aspirated and sclerotherapy performed to prevent recurrence. Benign lymphoepithelial cysts of the parotid gland are associated with human immunodeficiency virus (HIV) in both children and adults. Ultrasound guided sclerotherapy with doxycycline or ethanol presents a viable alternative to surgery, and can be carried out in the office setting[29] (Fig 12–11 and Video 12I). Many craniofacial venous malformations also lend

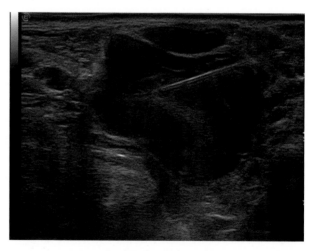

Fig 12–11 and Video 12I. Ultrasound-guided sclerotherapy of an HIV-related lymphoepithelial cyst of the parotid gland.

themselves to treatment with sclerotherapy. Both ethanol and sodium tetradecyl sulfate have been shown to be effective sclerosing agents, although serial injections may be necessary. For more extensive lesions, a combination of sclerotherapy and surgery may yield the best result.[30]

Laser

An even newer development in the minimally invasive treatment of thyroid masses involves interstitial laser thermal ablation (LTA) or photocoagulation under ultrasound visualization.[25,31] This technique has been applied to single autonomous hyperfunctioning thyroid nodules, compressive nodular goiters, and even anaplastic thyroid carcinoma, with success in decreasing the volume of such lesions.

Up to four 21-gauge spinal needles are inserted into the core of the target mass under ultrasound guidance. A sterile 300-micrometer quartz optical fiber is inserted through the sheath of the needle(s) and a continuous-wave neodymium: yttrium-aluminum-garnet (Nd:YAG) laser delivers energy of 1800 J per fiber (power output set at 3 to 5 watts) to induce tissue necrosis. Volume reduction varies with energy deposited and number of sessions; normalization of thyrotropin (TSH), free thyroxine (FT4), and free tri-iodothyronine (FT3) has been observed in hyperthyroid patients thus treated. Noted side effects have included mild burning pain and transient dysphonia. Ultrasound investigation 24 hours after the procedure has demonstrated a central hypoechoic area (zone of vaporization) at the site of laser insertion surrounded by a hyperechoic rim (zone of carbonization) and an outer hypoechoic layer (zone of coagulative necrosis).

Needle Localization for Excisional Procedures

The use of wire localization in the preoperative setting to facilitate identification and surgical removal of masses has been used extensively in the field of breast surgery in conjunction with mammography. This technique is now being exploited in the field of

head and neck surgery in conjunction with US. Schwannomas of the cervical sympathetic chain are often difficult to localize with displacement of the carotid artery and internal jugular vein and US can be used for localization.[32] The surgical excision of parapharyngeal space tumors can be facilitated by the use of preoperative ultrasound guidance in addition to the use of preoperative FNA to assist in diagnosis.[33]

In cases of recurrent adenopathy of the cervical region in a previously operated neck, the use of ultrasound guided needle localization can help to identify and guide the resection of suspicious cervical lymphadenopathy, such as in patients with thyroid as well as head and neck cancer.[34] This targeting can result in a precise surgical dissection and a reduction in operating time while minimizing patient risks.

The principle of ultrasound guided needle localization has also been used to assist in the removal of soft-tissue foreign bodies. Objects including wood, glass, stone, metal, and lead pencil, can be visualized sonographically and under ultrasound guidance a hemostat can be introduced to remove the object.[35] This principle can be extrapolated to gain surgical advantage in any setting where the target of resection is difficult to identify by direct vision, palpation, or dissection, but can be visualized sonographically.

Intraoperative Ultrasound

The management of thyroid malignancy has been enhanced by the use of US in the operating room. To complement the information obtained through preoperative US and ultrasound-guided FNA, intraoperative US can be performed after removal of the thyroid gland to further evaluate nonpalpable cervical lymph nodes, especially in the central neck and thyroid bed, and guide further surgery.[36] Preoperative US of this area is particularly prone to underestimating disease due to interference by the thyroid gland itself .

Intraoperative US also facilitates the performance of minimally invasive parathyroidectomy in patients with primary hyperparathyroidism, especially those who clearly demonstrate a solitary parathyroid adenoma and normal thyroid tissue. Ultrasound-guided parathyroidectomy uses a directed approach to incision planning and excision of sonographically enlarged parathyroid glands. Such a minimally invasive procedure can even facilitate the use of local anesthesia and result in decreased pain and recovery time, decreased hospital stay, and decreased cost associated with parathyroidectomy.[37] The use of preoperative US can identify those patients who are candidates for the use of intraoperative ultrasound guidance, similar to Tc99-MIBI dosage with radioguided surgical excision.[38]

Ultrasound-Guided Vascular Access

Ultrasound guidance for vascular access has become a common emergency department practice. Anesthesiologists are also becoming increasingly familiar with US-guided line placement. Findings from studies of US-guided internal jugular vein cannulation are instructive even for those clinicians who do not routinely perform central venous catheterization themselves. Both nonrandomized and randomized studies comparing US guidance to the traditional landmark approach to internal jugular vein access reported significant improvements in overall success rates (eg, 94-100% vs 79-88%) and complication rates (eg, 1.7-4.6% vs 8.3-16.9%).[39,40] Further studies have demonstrated through bedside US examination that there is overlap of the carotid artery by the internal jugular vein in more than 50% of patients,[41] and that head position has a significant influence on the degree of overlap.[42]

Summary

The use of US to guide interventional procedures in the head and neck region, as elsewhere in the body, provides precision with increased anatomic visualization and decreased guesswork. US also facilitates the use of minimally invasive approaches to diagnose and treat innumerable pathologic conditions.

Videos in This Chapter

Video 12A. See legend for Figure 12-1.

Video 12B. See legend for Figure 12-2.

Video 12C. See legend for Figure 12-3.

Video 12D. See legend for Figure 12-5.

Video 12E. See legend for Figure 12-6.

Video 12F. See legend for Figure 12-7.

Video 12G. See legend for Figure 12-9.

Video 12H. See legend for Figure 12-10.

Video 12I. See legend for Figure 12-11.

References

1. Marqusee E, Benson CB, Frates MC, et al. Usefulness of ultrasonography in the management of nodular thyroid disease. *Ann Intern Med*. 2000; 133:696-700.

2. Karstrup S, Balslev E, Juul N, Eskildsen PC, Baumbach L. US-guided fine needle aspiration versus coarse needle biopsy of the thyroid nodules. *Eur J Ultrasound*. 2001;13:1-5.

3. Redman R, Zalaznick H, Mazzaferri EL, Massoll NA. The impact of assessing specimen adequacy and number of needle passes for fine-needle aspiration biopsy of thyroid nodules. *Thyroid*. 2006;16:55-60.

4. Gharib H, Thyroid fine needle aspiration biopsy. In: HJ Baskin, ed. *Thyroid Ultrasound and Ultrasound-Guided FNA Biopsy*. Boston, Mass: Kluwer Academic Publ; 2000.

5. Groussin L, Fagin JA. Significance of BRAF mutations in papillary thyroid carcinoma: prognostic and therapeutic implications. *Nat Clin Pract Endocrinol Metab*. 2006;2(4):180-181.

6. Xing M, Westra WH, Tufano RP, et al. BRAF mutation predicts a poorer clinical prognosis for papillary thyroid carcinoma. *J Clin Endocrinol Metab*. 2006;90:6373-6379.

7. O'Leary PC, Feddema PH, Michelangeli VP, et al. Investigations of thyroid hormones and antibodies based on a community health survey: the Busselton thyroid study. *Clin Endocrinol*. 2006;64(1): 97-104.

Chapter 13

VASCULAR ULTRASOUND
CAROTID AND TRANSCRANIAL DOPPLER IMAGING

Michael Moussouttas
Samuel Trocio
Tatjana Rundek

Prologue

This chapter is meant to be of interest to:

■ Those who work on and around the carotid or vertebral arteries and its branches,

■ Those who wish to know how to recognize incidental carotid artery stenosis in varying degrees in their routine use of B-mode US in the neck,

■ Those who use Doppler for simple assessment of presence and relative quantity of blood flow and desire a better understanding of its physics and principles,

■ Those who may be interested in measuring intima-media thickness (IMT),

■ Those who manage patients that are at risk for stroke and cerebrovascular or peripheral vascular disease,

■ Those who might someday apply sonothrombolysis to thrombotic disorders,

■ Those who seek a concise and clinically relevant review of cerebrovascular anatomy and physiology.

Introduction

During the last decade, ultrasonography of the extracranial and intracranial arteries has become an established and indispensable noninvasive diagnostic and monitoring tool in patients with symptomatic cerebrovascular disease, and in asymptomatic individuals at increased risk for vascular disease. Technologic advances in the various modes utilized by ultrasound systems have enabled a precise real-time imaging of anatomy, physiology, and pathophysiology of the extracranial and intracranial circulations. Recent studies have confirmed the utility of ultrasonography (US) in the risk stratification of patients with active or latent cerebrovascular disease, and ongoing trials are assessing the correlation between US findings and clinical outcomes in patients undergoing medical treatment for risk factor modification.

ABCs of Ultrasound

Modern ultrasound systems combine several US modes or displays (Fig 13-1). They include:

A (Amplitude) mode: where echoes are displayed as vertical deflections.

B (Brightness) mode: where echoes are displayed in various levels of gray, depending on the intensity of reflected signals.

C (Color, Cine) mode: where Doppler signal of blood flow velocities is displayed in color.

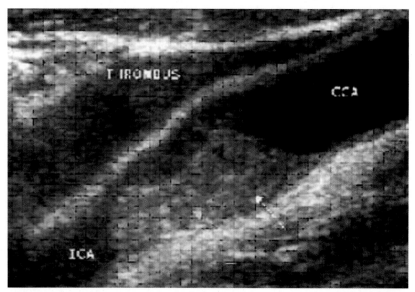

A

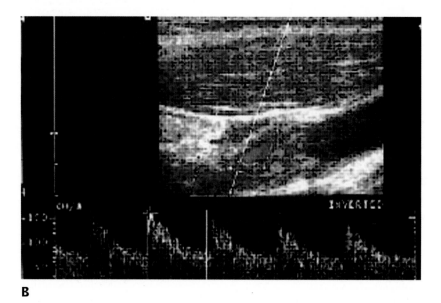

B

Fig 13-1. Carotid US modes (displays). **A.** *B (Brightness) mode*: Echoes are displayed in various levels of gray, depending on the intensity of reflected signals. **B.** *C+D (Color + Doppler) mode*: Doppler signal of blood flow is displayed in color and echo shifts are displayed as a Doppler spectrum. *continues*

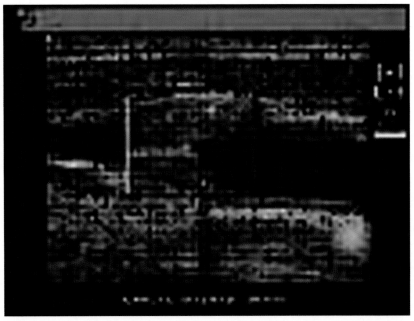

C

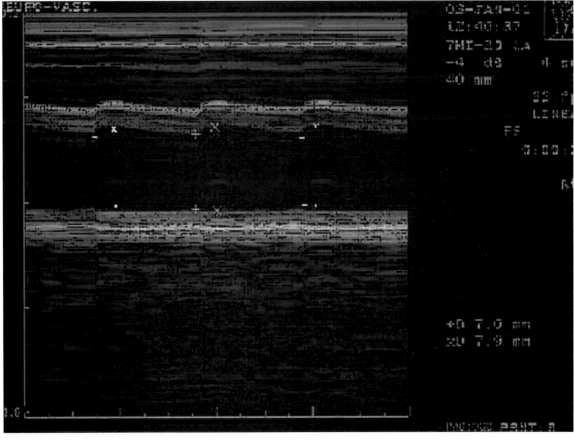

D

Fig 13–1. *continued* **C.** *P (Power) mode*: Doppler signal of blood flow is displayed independent of the angle of insonation and magnified. **D.** *M (Motion) mode*: Perpendicular movement of an image spot in motion is displayed in B-mode.

D (Doppler) mode: where shift in echoes is obtained from the moving blood particles and displayed as a Doppler spectrum, representing the blood flow velocity waveforms.

M (Motion) mode: where perpendicular movement of an image spot in motion is displayed from B-mode.

P (Power) mode: where Doppler signal of blood flow is displayed independent of the angle of insonation and therefore magnified.

An ultrasound system that combines B and D mode is called duplex US. Ultrasound systems that combine B, C, and D mode are called "triplex" systems, or more commonly, color Doppler. Color Doppler provides two-dimensional real-time color-coded flow image superimposed over a real-time gray-scale B-mode image. This permits the synchronous visualization of stationary structures and blood flow over a relatively large plane of section. Newer color Doppler ultrasound systems usually include power mode as well.

Extracranial Doppler

Carotid Artery Anatomy

The carotid arteries are the largest supplying arteries of the brain. The left common carotid artery (CCA) arises from the arch of the aorta, whereas the right common carotid artery branches from the brachio-cephalic trunk (innominate artery) that arises from the aortic arch (Fig 13–2). The left and right common carotid arteries ascend in the neck to approximately the level of the third cervical vertebra at which point they bifurcate into the internal carotid artery (ICA), which supplies the anterior part of the brain, and the external carotid artery (ECA) which supplies the face and neck. The ICA proceeds superiorly and enters the skull through the carotid canal. There are no branches of the ICA in the neck. Inside the cranium, the ICA follows a straight path through the petrous bone and the lateral aspect of the sphe-

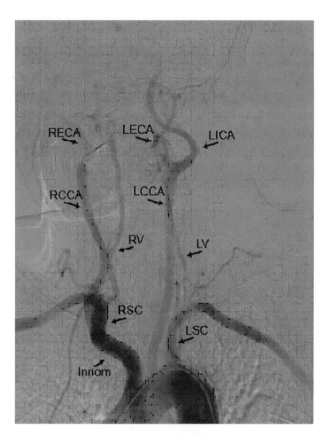

Fig 13–2. Anatomy of extracranial portion of the carotid and vertebral arteries (digital substraction angiography). LSCA = left subclavian artery, RSCA = right subclavian artery, Innom = innominate artery, LVA = left vertebral artery, RVA = right vertebral artery, LCCA = left common carotid artery, RCCA = right common carotid artery, LICA = left internal carotid artery, LECA = left external carotid artery, RECA = right external carotid artery.

noid bone, and ascends into the cavernous portion, forming the carotid siphon where it gives off the ophthalmic artery. On exiting the cavernous sinus, the ICA gives rise to the posterior communicating artery, which joins with the posterior cerebral artery, and then to the anterior choroidal artery. Its terminal portion bifurcates into the anterior and middle cerebral arteries.

The ECA usually does not supply the brain. In the case of occlusion of the carotid or vertebral artery however, several branches of the external carotid artery can become important collateral compensatory pathways. The branches of the extracranial ECA are the ascending pharyngeal, the superior thyroid, the lingual, the external maxillary, the occipital, the facial, the posterior auricular, the internal maxillary, the transverse facial, and the superficial temporal artery. The branches of the external carotid arteries that are most important to collateral circulation are those in communication with the ophthalmic artery from the ICA.

Carotid Artery Hemodynamics

The CCA and the ICA are both low-resistance vessels, but the ICA exhibits greater diastolic flow compared to the CCA. The ECA is a high-resistance vessel so that the diastolic flow is almost zero. The normal range of Doppler blood flow velocities in the carotid arteries may vary with physiologic differences among individuals. The reported peak systolic velocities in the ICA for normal adults range from 55 to 90 cm per sec.[1] Peak systolic velocities exceeding 100 cm per sec in the ICA must be viewed as potentially abnormal. Most of the atherosclerotic plaques in the carotid system are located in the area of carotid bifurcation where turbulent flow occurs. In severe stenosis or occlusion of the internal carotid artery, flow in the CCA is reduced and becomes more resistant with peaky waveforms due to diminished diastolic flow. Flow in the ICA can become more resistant if there is stenosis of the distal portion of ICA, such as in the petrous or cavernous portions. In these situations, collateral pathways become available to compensate for the effect of the restricted flow. When the ECA contributes to the collateral flow, usually via the ophthalmic artery, blood flow in the ECA becomes low resistant and "internalized," resembling the ICA flow waveform. The contralateral ICA may also provide collateral as evident by increased flow velocities. The utilization of the collateral pathways and the direction of the collateral flow depend entirely on the altered pressure gradients and the flow resistance in the collateral system. This is of particular importance in ultrasound examinations of the extracranial carotid and vertebral arteries, and intracranial cerebral arteries.

Carotid Duplex and Color/Power Doppler

Carotid Ultrasound Examination

Carotid ultrasound examination includes longitudinal and transverse scanning of the carotid arteries to visualize anatomy, lesion pathology and perform measurements of flow velocities and vessel diameters. The correct identification of the ICA and the ECA is very important to avoid diagnostic error by their misidentification. Anatomy, size, and the presence of the branches are important distinguishing features, but flow waveform patterns are of the greatest importance for correct vessel identification. The flow characteristics from the ICA and the ECA look and sound different. Tapping on the temporal artery, a branch of the ECA, will cause deflections in the observed spectrum for the ECA but not the ICA, and may therefore be used to distinguish the two vessels.

Diagnostic assessment of the carotid and the vertebral arteries consists of artery identification, description, and measurements of the lesions (eg, atherosclerotic plaque), and hemodynamic measurements. Hemodynamic parameters used for the interpretation of an ultrasound examination include peak systolic and end-diastolic velocity, mean flow velocity (MFV), peak systolic and end-diastolic ICA/CCA velocity ratios, resistance index (difference between peak systolic and end-diastolic velocity over end-diastolic velocity, pulsatility index (difference between peak systolic and end-diastolic velocity over mean velocity), and spectral broadening (Fig 13–3). Flow velocities are measured in the proximal, middle, and distal (just before the bifurcation) portion of the CCA; in the proximal, middle (immediately after the bulb), and distal portion of the ICA; and in the proximal portion of the ECA.

Carotid and Vertebral Artery Scanning Examination

A standard examination of the carotid and vertebral arteries includes longitudinal and transverse examinations, ensuring optimal assessment of the vessel

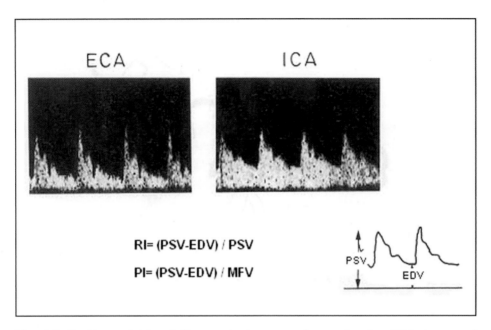

Fig 13–3. Normal blood flow velocity waveforms in the ECA (external carotid artery) and in the ICA (internal carotid artery). RI (resistance index), PI (pulsatility index), PSV (peak systolic velocity), EDV (end-diastolic velocity), MFV (mean flow velocity).

wall, the atherosclerotic plaque, and any luminal narrowing.

- The examination begins with an image survey of the carotid system from the proximal CCA. The transducer is then moved distally to identify the internal and external carotid arteries. This procedure is performed in the anterolateral and posterolateral positions.
- A representative gray-scale (B-mode) image is obtained from a segment of the common carotid artery, documenting any abnormalities. Representative spectral analyses are taken from the proximal, middle, and distal CCA portions, with the spectral cursor adjusted by the examiner so that it is placed in the vessel parallel to the walls and in the center of the flow stream. Color Doppler may be useful for guiding the placement of the spectral cursor in areas with increased turbulence.
- Examination then proceeds distally into the carotid bifurcation, and to the internal carotid artery. The same procedure applies, with detailed documentation of any abnormality. It is important to adjust for the angle of insonation, as the ICA often curves.
- The examination of the external carotid artery is performed using the same scanning procedure. Typically, the ECA is smaller than the ICA and has branches.
- In order to examine the vertebral artery, the transducer is directed posterior, seeking the artery within the vertebral canal of the vertebral bodies. The primary purpose of the vertebral artery examination is to assess vessel patency and flow direction. In the presence of flow abnormalities, the subclavian artery is also examined.
- In the presence of atherosclerotic plaque, its location, surface regularity, and core composition are documented. The severity of luminal narrowing, and the size of the residual lumen are reported. Areas of stenosis are evaluated in the region proximal to the stenosis, at the level of maximal stenosis, and distal to the stenosis.

Indications for Carotid Ultrasound Imaging

The American Institute of Ultrasound in Medicine, in conjunction with the American College of Radiology, has devised standards for the performance and indications for ultrasound examination of the extracranial carotid and vertebral arteries.[2]

Indications include, but are not limited to:

- Evaluation of patients with neurologic symptoms suggesting cerebral ischemia or amaurosis fugax
- Evaluation of patients with a cervical bruit
- Evaluation of a pulsatile mass in the neck
- Evaluation of blunt neck trauma
- Preoperative evaluation of patients undergoing major cardiovascular or other major surgical procedures, including cardiac, liver, and kidney transplant
- Evaluation of unexplained neurologic symptoms
- Follow-up of patients with known carotid artery disease
- Evaluation of postoperative patients following carotid endarterectomy or carotid stenting
- Evaluation of suspected subclavian steal syndrome
- Evaluation of suspected carotid or vertebral artery dissection.

Additional indications pertinent to the head and neck surgeon include evaluation of patients with head and neck neoplasms for carotid involvement or for carotid artery flow that might be suitable for use in microvascular reconstructive surgery.

Evaluation of Carotid Artery Stenosis

Carotid ultrasonography is the most useful imaging modality in the evaluation of patients with symptomatic and asymptomatic carotid artery stenosis. According to the distribution of abnormal blood flow patterns within, proximal to, or distal to a narrowed arterial segment, carotid ultrasound provides data on the extent, site, and degree of lesions of more than 40% lumen narrowing. Ultrasound assessment of the degree of carotid stenosis is a very reliable technique comparable to other noninvasive and invasive imaging methods including MRI and conventional angiography. The sensitivity (92–100%) and specificity (93–100%) of various carotid Doppler techniques have been shown to be similar to those of arteriography.[1,3,4]

Carotid Stenosis and Risk of Stroke and TIA

The atherosclerotic carotid plaque may cause cerebral ischemia by one or more mechanisms: (a) artery-to-artery embolization from the carotid plaque to the intracerebral vessels; (b) occlusion of the ICA with propagation of thrombus to intracranial branches; and (c) hemodynamic compromise, with low flow state downstream causing cerebral perfusion failure.

Artery-to-artery embolization mechanism of stroke largely has been based on inference as scant clinical and pathologic studies are available to precisely document such a mechanism. In the absence of a cardioembolic source, however, it is the most likely underlying pathophysiologic mechanism of infarction in patients with carotid artery stenosis.

The association between degree of carotid stenosis and ischemic risk is well documented in symptomatic patients,[5-9] but remains controversial in asymptomatic patients. The reasons for this discrepancy are not entirely clear, but a lack of standardization of ultrasonographic criteria for the degree of carotid stenosis may be one of the many possible explanations.

An annual risk of stroke or TIA is 8 to 21% in asymptomatic patients with carotid stenosis of 80 to 99%, and 2 to 5% in patients with carotid stenosis less than 80%.[10-13] Besides the degree of carotid stenosis, the rate of progression of carotid stenosis is also an important predictor of stroke and TIA. Asymptomatic patients whose carotid stenosis progressed to stenosis of 80% or more from the baseline examination have a three times greater risk of stroke or TIA compared to those without carotid stenosis progression.[14,15] Progression of asymptomatic carotid stenosis to occlusion can occur in up to 20% of patients and is associated with an additional annual 2 to 6% increased risk of stroke.[16] The majority of neurologic events occur within 6 months of diagnosis of a significant progression of carotid stenosis.[15] It remains controversial whether progression of carotid stenosis precedes or occurs in parallel with neurologic events.[10,11]

Ultrasonographic Criteria for Carotid Artery Stenosis

An international consensus meeting, in conjunction with other professional associations on standardization of performance of carotid ultrasound, has established diagnostic criteria for the quantification of internal carotid artery stenosis.[4,17,18] These criteria, however, are not universally accepted. Major studies do not agree on velocity criteria for defining degree of carotid stenosis. Wide ranges of velocities are used to identify ICA stenosis in clinical practice. Major reasons for such variability in velocity criteria for the degree of carotid stenosis include differences in clinical characteristics of the populations under study, marked variability in collateral circulatory anatomy, differences in level of expertise among sonographers, and variability in instrumentation. The sensitivity and specificity of carotid ultrasonography for detection of severe carotid stenosis reaches 90% in accredited ultrasound laboratories.[19] Accredited ultrasound laboratories maintain rigorous quality control of ultrasound measurements, equipment, and sonographer performance. Conversely, sensitivity and specificity in detecting carotid stenosis by nonaccredited ultrasound laboratories is less than 70%.[19] Each carotid ultrasound laboratory must, therefore, develop its own criteria for defining each level of carotid stenosis. These parameters must be validated with other imaging modalities and/or surgical findings. Furthermore, ongoing quality control programs must be in place. These standards are mandated by ICAVL (Intersocietal Commission for Accreditation of Vascular Laboratories) and other ultrasound accreditation agencies.

The ultrasound hemodynamic parameters for assessment of the degree of stenosis must be eval-

uated in the prestenotic, stenotic, and poststenotic regions. Determination of the degree of carotid stenosis obtained by Doppler parameters can also be confirmed visually on the gray-scale or color ultrasound images. In addition, gray scale (B-mode) will provide information regarding anatomy and presence of lesions. In the case of atherosclerotic plaque, B-mode will provide information regarding plaque size, location, surface characteristics, and composition.

Grading Extracranial Carotid Artery Stenosis

- **Minimal Carotid Stenosis (<40%)** is characterized by a presence of small atherosclerotic plaque and systolic peak velocities below 120 cm per sec (Fig 13-4 and Videos 13A and 13B).
- **Mild Carotid Stenosis (40–59%)** is characterized by a local increase of peak and mean flow velocities. Systolic peak velocities range above 120 cm per sec (Fig 13-5).
- **Moderate Carotid Stenosis (60–79%)** shows a distortion of normal pulsatile flow in addition to a local increase of peak and mean velocities. Typically, systolic flow decelerations are found in the poststenotic segment. The systolic peak velocity ranges from 120 to 250 cm per sec (Fig 13-6 and Video 13C).
- **Severe Carotid Stenosis (80–99%)** produces markedly increased peak flow velocities exceeding 250 cm per sec and occasionally reaching 500 cm per sec (Fig 13-7). In addition, pre- and poststenotic blood flow velocity is significantly reduced compared with the contralateral unaffected carotid artery. Retrograde flow of the ophthalmic artery may occur. *Subtotal stenosis* (close to total occlusion) is characterized by variable, usually low peak flow velocities, which decrease once a stenosis becomes pseudo-occlusive. This condition is difficult to separate from complete occlusion and may be misdiagnosed.

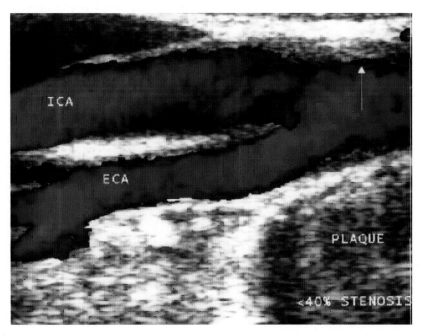

Fig 13–4. Minimal stenosis (<40%) of the internal carotid artery.

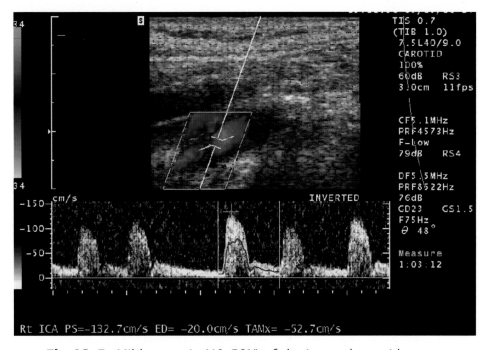

Fig 13–5. Mild stenosis (40–59%) of the internal carotid artery.

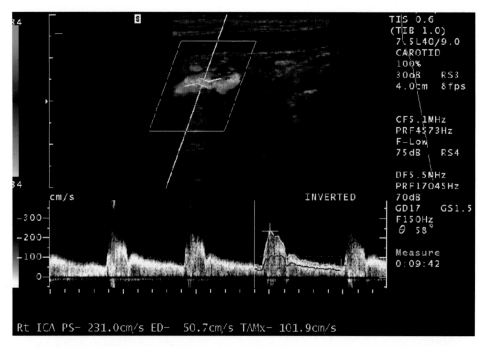

Fig 13–6. Moderate stenosis (60–79%) of the internal carotid artery.

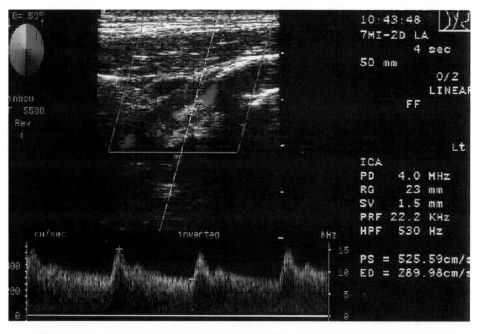

Fig 13–7. Severe stenosis (80–99%) of the internal carotid artery.

■ **ICA Occlusion (100%)** is characterized by the absence of any signal along the cervical course of the ICA (Fig 13-8).

Frequently, a low velocity signal with a predominant reversed signal component and absent diastolic flow can be recorded

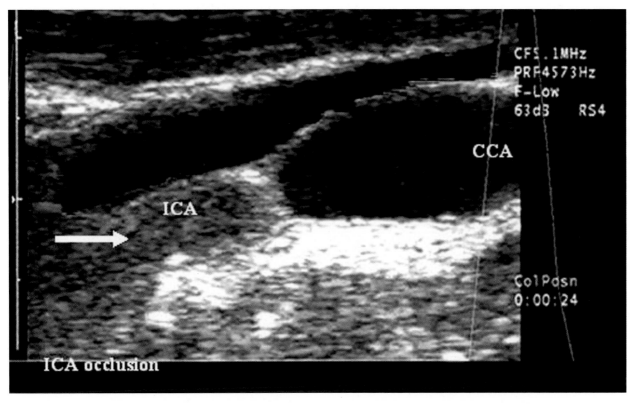

Fig 13–8. Occlusion of the internal carotid artery immediately beyond the carotid bifurcation

at the presumed origin of the ICA (stump flow). Flow velocity in the CCA is reduced, and frequently retrograde perfusion of the ophthalmic artery occurs. Frequently, there is an accompanying marked reduction of the systolic and diastolic flow velocity in the CCA, and an internalized ECA with elevated diastolic flow velocity indicating collateral supply via the ophthalmic artery. The capacity of modern color and power Doppler instruments to detect very slow blood flow velocities has markedly improved the sensitivity for the diagnosis of a subtotal ICA stenosis and pseudo-occlusion.

■ **CCA Occlusion** is a relatively rare condition. It is important to assess whether the ICA distal to the CCA occlusion is patent, as this is a prerequisite for surgical carotid intervention. Color flow imaging typically displays blue-coded

signals in the ECA due to reversed flow direction as a result of anterograde filling of the ICA above its origin and retrograde filling of the occipital branch of the ECA (Fig 13-9).

Carotid Plaque Size and Morphology

Plaque size has a direct correlation with degree of carotid stenosis, but it is also an independent predictor of future cerebral ischemia.[20] Large population-based studies have also shown that carotid plaque size is an independent predictor of future myocardial infarction and vascular mortality, even in individuals with a low degree of carotid stenosis.[21] In patients who present with a carotid plaque without significant hemodynamic stenosis, carotid plaque size measured by any of the ultrasonographic parameters must be evaluated as plaque size is an

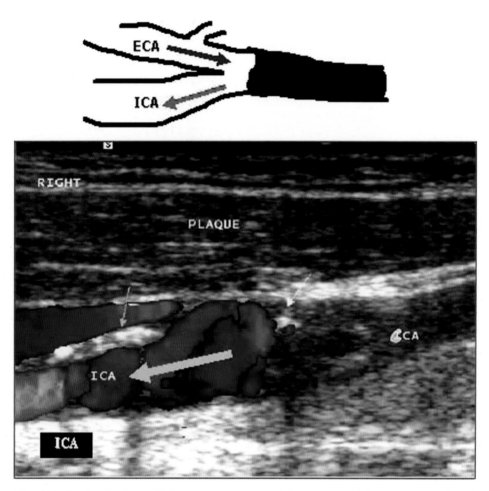

Fig 13–9. Occlusion of the common carotid artery with patent ICA distal to the CCA occlusion.

important marker of subclinical atherosclerosis and a reliable predictor of future vascular events. Ultrasonographic characteristics of carotid plaque may also stratify patients according to level of risk for cerebral ischemia.[22,23]

The main morphologic plaque characteristics include *plaque ulceration* and *plaque echogenicity*. Determinations of such morphologic ultrasonographic features are not always possible in clinical practice. Detection of ulcerated plaques by ultrasound imaging is limited. Sensitivity and specificity of carotid ultrasound for detecting plaque ulceration is moderate at best.[24,25] Plaque *surface irregularity* is another, more reliable parameter that may be useful in vascular risk assessment. In a population-based cohort from the Northern Manhattan Study,

plaque surface irregularity was associated with more than four-fold increased risk of ischemic stroke; and three-fold increase among those with less than 60% carotid stenosis.[26] The cumulative 5-year risk of ischemic stroke among individuals with an irregular plaque was 8% in comparison to less than 3% among those with regular plaque surface (Fig 13–10).

Plaque echogenicity is defined as *hyperechoic* or *echodense* (bright on ultrasound; calcified, Fig 13–11) and *hypoechoic* or *echolucent* (dark on ultrasound; lipid-rich content or blood, Fig 13–12) in comparison to the echodensity of the surrounding soft tissue media or blood (dark on ultrasound, lowest reflection of the ultrasound beam).[27] In the large population-based Cardiovascular Health Study among asymptomatic individuals who were followed for a

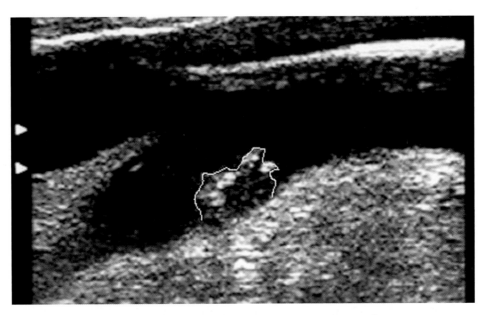

Fig 13–10. Carotid plaque with irregular surface.

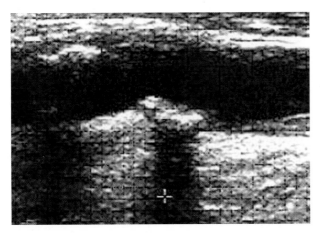

Fig 13–11. Hyperechoic or echodense plaque (bright on ultrasound; calcified) with acoustic shadowing (*white cross*).

mean of 3 years, echolucent carotid plaques were associated with a two-fold increased risk for cerebral infarction, and with a 2.3-fold increased risk of infarction among those who had echolucent plaques in combination with carotid stenosis greater than 50%.[28] In the Tromso study among asymptomatic patients with carotid stenosis, echolucent plaques were associated with a 5 times greater risk of infarction independent of the degree of carotid stenosis

and other cardiovascular risk factors.[29] In contrast, degree of calcium deposition in symptomatic and asymptomatic carotid plaques has been associated with plaque stability. As such, calcification appears to represent the "healing" process following plaque activity during a more dynamic phase. When plaques become less active, they are less prone to rupture, subintimal dissection, and hemorrhage. B-mode ultrasound may be less technically accurate and more operator dependent for the detection of plaque calcification, yet there is histopathologic evidence that echodense plaques contain a greater calcium to lipid ratio content, with the greatest calcium content in homogeneously echodense plaques. Homogeneously calcified plaques have been found to be a good prognostic feature based on the lower rates of cerebral ischemia,[29-32] yet some recent studies have shown quite the opposite results.[33,34] Plaque echodensity and echolucency are descriptive and subjective ultrasonographic morphologic plaque characteristics, and several studies have reported that ultrasonographic plaque morphology evaluation has a low interobserver reliability.[35] Novel, computerized, and standardized ultrasound technologies such as the gray-scale median analyses of plaque echogenicity are more objective methods, and their evaluation is currently underway.[36]

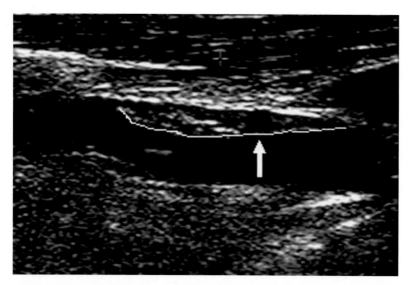

Fig 13–12. Hypoechoic or echolucent plaque (dark on ultrasound; lipid-rich content or blood).

Extracranial Findings in Severe Intracranial Obstructive Disease

Severe intracranial obstructions in the carotid siphon or the middle cerebral artery (MCA) may lead to blunted spectra with elevated resistance pattern in the ipsilateral extracranial ICA. In addition, alterations of flow direction and signal frequency may occur in the ophthalmic artery depending on the site and degree of the lesion. Intracranial arteriovenous malformations (AVM) and shunts may lead to increased flow velocities and a low resistance pattern in the ipsilateral proximal carotid and vertebral segments (indicating feeding AVM arteries). Such findings on extracranial carotid ultrasound examination therefore prompt an appropriate workup for suspected intracranial AVM.

Carotid Artery Dissection

Various flow patterns can be observed in carotid dissection. Color imaging can show marked flow reversal at the origin of the ICA in systole and absent or minimal flow in diastole, corresponding to a bidirectional spectral signal with elevated resistance pattern (Fig 13–13). B-mode scans can demonstrate a tapered lumen and occasionally a floating intimal flap. Narrowing of the true lumen by the false lumen thrombus can occur, and the direction of flow in a patent false lumen can vary from being forward, reversed, or bidirectional. The flow dynamics in carotid dissections are complex and are primarily dependent on the presence of thrombus within the false lumen, the entry and exit flaps if the false lumen is patent, the motion of the flap wall, and the extent of the dissection. In some instances the location of the dissection may lie distal to the insonation site, and if the dissection is not flow limiting normal waveforms may be found.

Follow-up examinations of carotid dissections may demonstrate gradual normalization, indicating recanalization of the ICA within a few weeks to months. The improvement of these findings may occur in more than two-thirds of patients. Carotid aneurysms may result as a complication of ICA dissection. Follow-up with another imaging modality such as MRI/MRA can be complementary.

Carotid Intima-Media Thickness

Carotid intima-media thickness (IMT) assessed by B-mode ultrasound is a validated surrogate marker for atherosclerosis that can efficiently identify and describe populations at cardiovascular risk, and can

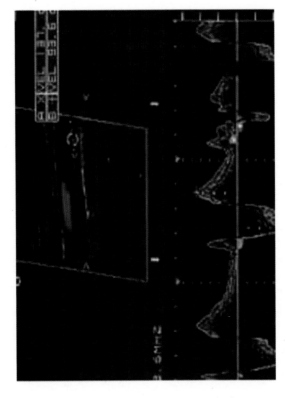

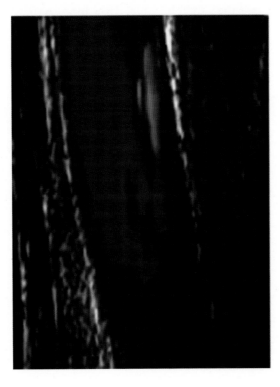

Fig 13–13. Common carotid artery dissection.

determine the therapeutic effect of various drugs. Carotid IMT is also an important surrogate endpoint of vascular events[37] as it is sensitive, easy to evaluate, and more readily available than the clinical endpoint. Also, the causal relationship between carotid IMT and the clinical endpoint has been established on the basis of pathophysiologic, epidemiologic, and clinical studies.[38] In interventional studies, anticipated clinical benefits were deducible from the observed changes in the carotid IMT. Moreover, the strength of carotid IMT as a surrogate marker is enhanced by the fact that it may yield pathophysiologic information at an early stage of the disease process. Carotid IMT measurements are increasingly being performed by clinicians, such as endocrinologists, who utilize ultrasonography in their office practices.

Carotid IMT provides useful information on the early stages of arterial wall thickening prior to lesion formation and is useful in assessing initial arterial wall remodeling in the course of atherosclerosis progression in light of the Glagov effect.[39] B-mode ultrasound imaging technology has evolved to such an extent that the walls of superficial arteries can be imaged noninvasively, in real time and at high resolution. Studies that evaluated the origin of the lumen-intima and the media-adventitia ultrasound interfaces in relation to carotid wall arterial histology demonstrated that the distance between these interfaces reflects the intima-media complex, and consequently this distance is referred to as intima-media thickness or IMT (Fig 13–14).[40,41] As B-mode ultrasound is noninvasive, IMT measurements can be used in observational studies in various populations as well as in atherosclerosis regression trials.[42] Recently, a group of international experts published a consensus document on the assessment of carotid IMT.[43] This document provides the basic guidelines for the use of carotid IMT in the cardiovascular risk stratification, the role of IMT as a surrogate endpoint in the observational studies and clinical trials, and the potential use of IMT in clinical practice.

Carotid IMT and Observational Studies

Carotid IMT measured by B-mode ultrasound has been investigated as a determinant of atherosclerotic disease in the general population. Examples of such large follow-up studies are the Cardiovascular Health Study (CHS), the Rotterdam Study, and the Atherosclerosis Risk in Communities Study (ARIC).[44-50]

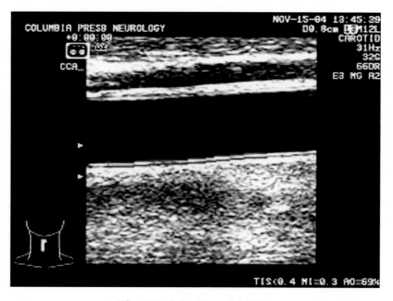

Fig 13–14. Carotid IMT.

- In CHS, among 4,476 participants over 65 years of age without clinical cardiovascular disease, carotid IMT was associated with incident cardiovascular events over a median follow-up time of 6 years.[44] The age/sex-adjusted relative risk of myocardial infarction or stroke for the highest quintile of carotid artery IMT was 3.87 compared with the lowest quintile.[48]
- In the Rotterdam Study, a single-center prospective follow-up study of 8,000 individuals over the age of 55, the associations between carotid IMT and stroke, angina pectoris, myocardial infarction, intermittent claudication and essential hypertension was found during a mean follow-up duration of 2.7 years.[49]
- In ARIC, a study of 15,800 participants, a seemingly small increase of 0.20 mm in mean carotid IMT was associated with a significantly increase in the relative risk of myocardial infarction (33%) and stroke (28%).[50]

Carotid IMT and Interventional Studies

B-mode ultrasound measurements of carotid IMT have been used extensively in clinical trials aimed to demonstrate the "anti-atherosclerotic effect" of various classes of drugs, predominately lipid and blood pressure-lowering medications.

Lipid-Lowering Studies

- The 4-year Cholesterol Lowering Atherosclerosis Study (CLAS) assessed the effects of colestipol-niacin therapy in men with previous coronary bypass surgery and showed statistically significant treatment effects after 2 and 4 years of therapy.[51]
- In the Asymptomatic Carotid Artery Progression Study (ACAPS), a 3-year clinical trial of lovastatin in asymptomatic individuals between 40 and 79 years of age

with early carotid atherosclerosis, it was found that lovastatin, compared to placebo, modified IMT.[52]
- The Kuopio Atherosclerosis Prevention Study (KAPS) investigated the 3-year efficacy of pravastatin in hypercholesterolemic men between 44 and 65 years of age. The primary outcome measure, combined IMT of four carotid arterial wall segments, showed near significance and a highly significant effect on common carotid IMT.[53]
- In the Regression Growth Evaluation Statin Study (REGRESS), the 2-year atherosclerosis regression trial, the efficacy of 40 mg pravastatin was demonstrated by B-mode ultrasound of the peripheral arteries, which was not obtained in any of the coronary angiographic parameters of the REGRESS cohort.[54]
- In the 2-year study of aggressive versus conventional lipid lowering on atherosclerosis progression (ASAP), the effects of atorvastatin 80 mg and 40 mg simvastatin were investigated in 325 patients with familial hypercholesterolemia (FH).[55] In this trial, aggressive cholesterol lowering with statins was more effective than conventional statin treatment. Decrease in carotid IMT was observed in the most aggressively treated group ($\pm$ 51% LDL-cholesterol lowering) whereas the less aggressive treatment ($\pm$ 41% LDL-C lowering) showed inhibition of atherosclerosis progression.
- The outcome of the 1-year ARBITER, a secondary prevention study among 161 patients with cardiovascular disease and LDL-C of 100 mg/dL, was in line with the ASAP findings.[56] In the pravastatin group IMT stabilized whereas in the atorvastatin group the IMT decreased.

Blood Pressure Lowering Studies

- The SECURE trial (Study to Evaluate Carotid Ultrasound changes in patients treated with Ramipril and vitamin E), a substudy of the HOPE (Heart Outcomes Prevention Evaluation) trial, evaluated the effects of long-term treatment (4.5 years) with the angiotensin-converting enzyme (ACE) inhibitor ramipril, and vitamin E on atherosclerosis progression among 732 high-risk patients over the age of 55.[57] The SECURE study demonstrated a significant reduction in IMT progression with ramipril (36%), which could not be explained by the effect of the blood pressure lowering alone. The progression slope of the mean maximum carotid IMT was 0.0217 mm per year in the placebo group, and 0.0137 mm per year in the ramipril 10 mg/dL group ($p = 0.033$). Vitamin E (400 IU/day) had a neutral effect on the carotid IMT.

■ The recently completed β-Blocker Cholesterol-Lowering Asymptomatic Study (BCAPS) showed a significant reduction in progression of IMT in the carotid bulb for those on the ß -blocker metoprolol versus those on placebo that was apparent after 1 year and was sustained after 3 years of treatment.[58]

■ The European Lacidipine Study on Atherosclerosis (ELSA), a randomized, double-blind trial in 2,334 patients with hypertension, the effects of a 4-year treatment based on either lacidipine (a calcium antagonist) or atenolol (a β-blocker) on carotid IMT was compared.[59] A greater efficacy was found of lacidipine on carotid IMT progression and number of plaques per patient, despite a smaller ambulatory blood pressure reduction, indicating an antiatherosclerotic action of lacidipine independent of its antihypertensive action.

■ In the Prospective Randomized Evaluation of the Vascular Effects of Norvasc Trial (PREVENT), a randomized placebo-controlled clinical trial, amlodipine (a calcium-channel blocker) had a significant effect in slowing the 36-month progression of carotid IMT, whereas it had no demonstrable effect on angiographic progression of coronary atherosclerosis.[60]

Standardized Carotid IMT Protocol

High-resolution B-mode carotid IMT imaging is usually performed according to the standardized ultrasound scanning and reading protocols.[61]

Image Acquisition

Subjects are placed in a supine position with the head rotated 45 degrees to the left using a 45-degree head pillow. The jugular vein and carotid artery are located in the transverse view with the jugular vein visualized above the carotid artery. The transducer is then rotated 90 degrees around the central line of the transverse image of the jugular vein-carotid artery to obtain a longitudinal image while maintaining the vessels in the mound position. In addition to the jugular vein above the carotid artery, all images contain anatomic landmarks for reproducing probe angulations, including visualization of the carotid bulb. For each individual, the depth of field, gain, monitor intensity setting, and all other initial instrumentation settings used at baseline examination are maintained and recorded for the future follow-up examinations. A hard copy of each individual's baseline image is used as a guide to match the repeat image to the baseline image. This direct visual aid method for reproducing probe angulations has resulted in a significant reduction of measurement variability between scans.[61] Some protocols use a "mask," an outline of the carotid arteries in to ensure a reliable follow-up IMT examination.

Carotid segments that comprise the IMT measure are defined as (Fig 13–15):

1. the near and the far wall of the carotid segment extending from 10 to 20 mm proximal to the tip of the flow divider into the common carotid artery (CCA);
2. the near and the far wall of the carotid bifurcation beginning at the tip of the flow divider and extending 10 mm proximal to the flow divider tip; and
3. the near and the far wall of the proximal 10 mm of the internal carotid artery (ICA).

Total carotid IMT is calculated as a composite measure (mean of the 12 sites) that combines the near and the far wall IMT of the CCA, carotid bifurcation, and ICA of both sides of the neck (see Fig 13-15) IMT.

Carotid IMT is measured out of the area of plaque. Atherosclerotic plaque is defined as an area of focal wall protrusion or focal thickening more than 50% greater than surrounding wall thickness. If atherosclerotic plaque is present, the measurement of maximal carotid plaque thickness (MCPT) in mm is performed at the highest plaque prominence in any of the three carotid artery segments assessed from the multiangled images.

Carotid IMT and Automatic Computerized Edge Detection (ACED)

The method of computerized edge tracking-multiframe processing of B-mode ultrasound images represents a technologic advance for determining arterial lumen and wall dimensions with direct applicability to noninvasive imaging of atherosclerosis (Fig 13-16).[62,63] ACED processing of B-mode ultrasound images is a highly reproducible, readily available improved method for evaluating arterial diameter, carotid IMT, and plaque size.[62-64]

Carotid IMT: A Surrogate Endpoint of Vascular Outcome

Atherosclerosis is a protracted disease process of the arterial wall with onset decades prior to its clinical manifestations. To understand the determinants of the process and develop therapeutic approaches requires a lifelong follow-up if clinical endpoint data are used. This approach needs extensive time and resources. Therefore, validated surrogate markers for atherosclerosis, such as carotid IMT, that can efficiently identify and describe populations at cardiovascular risk and investigate therapeutic regimens

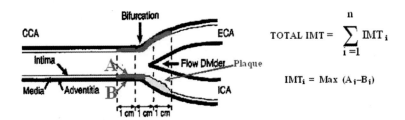

$$\text{TOTAL IMT} = \sum_{i=1}^{n} \text{IMT}_i$$

$$\text{IMT}_i = \text{Max} (A_i - B_i)$$

Fig 13-15. Carotid IMT segments and measurements.

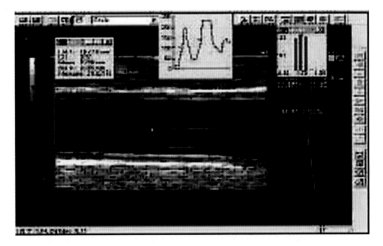

Fig 13-16. ACED of carotid IMT.

are needed. Currently, other imaging modalities such as MRI and soluble surrogate markers such as CRP are strong competitors to ultrasound measurement of carotid IMT. Although a strong association between increased IMT and risk of vascular events has already been established, and that various classes of medication may significantly reduce IMT, the confirmation whether the reduction in IMT translates into the reduction of the risk of vascular events is yet to come. Therefore, the use of IMT in clinical practice is still not standard. Furthermore, the normal IMT values for various populations are lacking. At the moment, carotid IMT may be a useful tool in reassessment of vascular risk among individuals with moderate to high risk for vascular events (eg, among those with 10–20% 10-year CVD risk assessed by the Framingham risk score). The advantage of B-mode ultrasound measurement of IMT is in its user-friendliness and cost-effectiveness. Therefore, in the near future, B-mode ultrasound intima-media thickness measurement will be an important risk assessment and monitoring tool of the arterial wall changes and will complement other, at present competing technologies.

Vertebral Duplex and Color Doppler

Vertebral Artery Anatomy and Hemodynamics

The vertebral arteries (VA) supply the structures of the posterior cerebral fossa, the occipital lobes, and the medial temporal lobes. The VAs are the first branches of the subclavian artery, and ascend to enter the costotransverse foramen of the sixth or the fifth cervical vertebra (V1). From there, the VAs run vertically upward and into the transverse foramina of the cervical vertebrae up until the second cervical vertebra (V2). After leaving the foramen of the second cervical vertebra, the vertebral arteries turn behind the atlas (V3), pierce the dura mater, and enter the skull via the foramen magnum. After leaving the atlas, the VAs give off muscular branches which anastomose with branches of the occipital

artery (occipital-vertebral anastomosis). The last portion of the vertebral artery (V4) is intracranial where it gives off the posterior and anterior spinal artery branches, penetrating branches to the medulla, and the large posterior inferior cerebellar artery. At the level of the pontomedullary junction, both vertebral arteries unite to form the basilar artery.

The vertebral artery waveform, like that of the internal carotid artery, shows little pulsatility. Flow velocities are usually lower in comparison to the CCA or the ICA. Normal peak systolic velocities in the vertebral arteries range from 20 to 40 cm per sec. Systolic velocities below 10 cm per sec are potentially abnormal. Greater velocities may be normal in the potentially dominant vertebral artery or in occlusion of the contralateral vertebral artery. Potentially abnormal ultrasound findings of the vertebral arteries include nonvisualization, very small caliber, absence of flow, considerably increased or decreased flow, and reversal or alternate flow direction.

Ultrasound Examination of the Vertebral Arteries

The technique of ultrasonographic evaluation of the vertebral arteries is similar to that of the carotid arteries. Examination of the vertebral artery is, however, limited by its anatomy. The vertebral artery, unlike the carotid, cannot be traced continuously due to its course within the transverse processes of the cervical vertebrae. Therefore, sonographic examination of the extracranial vertebral artery is reliable only in the origin, intervertebral segments, and at the atlas-loop portion. Color Doppler and power Doppler are particularly useful in the assessment of the calibers of the vertebral arteries. Differences in the caliber of the vertebral arteries is common, and the left vertebral artery is usually larger (dominant). If the difference is substantial, the thinner artery is considered hypoplastic. Tortuosity of the vertebral arteries is also a common finding.

Vertebral Artery Hypoplasia

Vertebral artery (VA) hypoplasia can be found in up to 10% of the normal population. It is defined by a decrease in vascular lumen diameter below 2 mm in pathoanatomic studies. Moderate asymmetry in the caliber of the vertebral arteries does not lead to substantial differences in the transmitted signal. In pronounced hypoplasia, flow velocities are significantly reduced and flow resistance increased. Typical ultrasound findings of VA hypoplasia include substantial differences in lumen caliber between left and right VAs, low-flow velocity (especially in diastole), and an absence of cervical collaterals. The VA on the opposite side is usually easy to image due to its larger caliber, and flow velocities are often in the upper range of normal or elevated.

Vertebral Artery Stenosis

Stenosis and occlusion of the VAs most commonly occurs at the origin, and less frequently in the distal parts of the cervical course (Fig 13–17). Detection of VA stenosis or occlusion is more difficult than for the carotid arteries, due to the difficulty insonating the vessel at its origin, and due to its course within bony foramina. Indirect findings that suggest VA stenosis include a change of the direction of the flow or the presence of a cervical collateral circulation. Proximal stenosis of the VA may produce a distal waveform with decreased pulsatility, and may produce a systolic notch (deceleration). In the presence of a functional collateral circulation, however, a systolic notch or change in the direction of the flow may not occur. Assessment of the collateral circulation is particularly important if a proximal stenosis of the VA is found, if the signals from the distal and proximal portion of the VA are discrepant, and if numerous "hard-to-classify" neck vessels or signals are detected in the region of muscular and cervical brunches of the VA and occipital artery.

Extracranial Findings in Severe Intracranial Vertebrobasilar Stenosis

Mild to moderate asymmetries in VA flow velocities frequently do not have clinical significance. Asymmetry of flow signals from the VAs in the neck is not a reliable criterion for an intracranial stenosis of the VA. Similarly, stenosis of the basilar artery cannot be detected from the findings in the extracranial portion of the VAs. Intracranial stenosis of the vertebrobasilar system is detected directly by the use of transcranial ultrasound. Only the occlusion of the normal-sized VA in the intracranial part or the occlusion of the basilar artery may be detected by extracranial examination of the VAs. Hemodynamically significant obstruction of the intracranial vertebrobasilar system produces a pulsatile VA waveform without diastolic flow, and flow in the VA is usually maintained by small segmental muscular collateral branches.

Vertebral Artery Dissection

There is no pathognomonic ultrasound finding for VA dissection if the lesion affects the cervical segments. Examination of the atlas loop can show absent, low bidirectional, or low poststenotic flow signals. In dissections of the proximal segment, the stenotic segment can sometimes be visualized, whereas absent flow in the intertransverse segments indirectly raises the possibility of VA dissection. Further findings can include a localized increase in the diameter of the artery with hemodynamic signs of stenosis or occlusion at the same level, decreased pulsatility, and the presence of intravascular echogenicity in the enlarged segment. Transcranial ultrasound can be helpful in determining the length of dissection, and in particular in determining whether

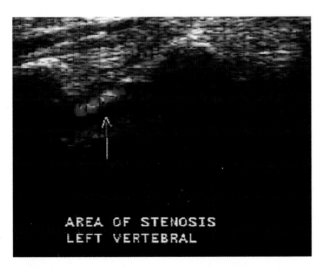

AREA OF STENOSIS
LEFT VERTEBRAL

Fig 13–17. Stenosis of the vertebral artery. Compare to normal vertebral artery flow in **Video 13D**.

the dissection extends intracranially. The combined use of extracranial and transcranial ultrasound along with color/power Doppler increases the diagnostic yield to detect VA dissection. Detection of abnormal but nonspecific flow patterns in the VA in cases of suspected dissection may guide further diagnostic imaging procedures and therapeutic measures. However, as unremarkable ultrasound findings do not exclude the diagnosis of VA dissection, further workup in suspected cases is still mandatory.

Transcranial Ultrasound

Transcranial Doppler (TCD) is a noninvasive ultrasonic technique that monitors blood flow velocity and blood flow direction in large intracranial arteries.[65] In 1982, Aaslid and colleagues introduced TCD to clinical practice by monitoring blood flow in the basal cerebral arteries.[66] Transcranial Doppler assesses flow characteristics in the large proximal cerebral vessels. A low-frequency ultrasound signal capable of penetrating bone is used to insonate the intracranial vessels at various accessible skull regions and cranial foramina. Unlike cervical ultrasound, transcranial ultrasound is for the most part, performed without visual guidance from gray-scale imaging of tissues or color-coded imaging of arteries and veins.

Consequently, transcranial ultrasound is unable to correct for the angle of insonation, but this problem has been somewhat overcome by newer devices capable of B-mode and color-Doppler imaging.

Transcranial ultrasound provides valuable physiologic information about both static (eg, atherosclerotic) and dynamic (eg, vasospasm) conditions, allows for the measurement of cerebrovascular hemodynamic reserve, enables detection of intravascular particles (microemboli), and permits noninvasive analysis of the cranial arterial and venous systems in a multitude of disease states. This section reviews current status of transcranial ultrasound use in cerebrovascular disease.

Anatomy of the Cerebral Vessels

Combined, the two terminal internal carotid arteries (ICA), two anterior cerebral arteries (ACA), one anterior communicating artery (AComm), two posterior communicating arteries (PComm) and the two proximal posterior cerebral arteries (PCA), constitute *the circle of Willis,* the major intracranial collateral system (Fig 13–18). Common anatomic variations pertinent to transcranial insonation include hypoplasia or aplasia of the A1 ACA segment, AComm artery, P1 PCA segment, and PComm vessels.

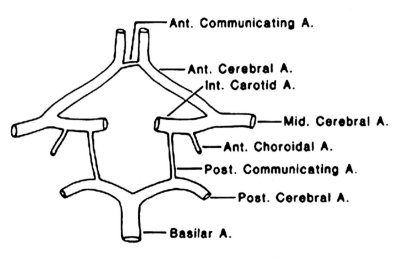

Fig 13–18. The circle of Willis.

TCD Examination Approaches

The intracranial vessels are insonated via temporal, orbital, suboccipital (foramen magnum), and submandibular "windows." The *temporal approach* examines the ICA, MCA, ACA, and PCA, and to some extent the AComm and PComm arteries. The *orbital approach* examines the ophthalmic arteries and ICA siphons, the *suboccipital approach* (via foramen magnum) identifies both vertebral arteries and the basilar artery, and the *submandibular approach* examines the distal extracranial ICA. Parameters used in identifying and assessing the intracranial vessels include distance from the probe, the direction of flow (toward or away from the probe), flow velocities, waveform morphology (numerically represented by pulsatility indexes), and acoustic qualities (Table 13-1).

Anatomy and Hemodynamics of the Cerebral Vessels

Internal Carotid Artery and Ophthalmic Artery

As the internal carotid artery (ICA) ascends intracranially, it gives off three branches—the ophthalmic, posterior communicating artery (PComm), and ante-

rior choroidal arteries—prior to bifurcating into the ACA and MCA. The sigmoidal ICA segment that traverses the cavernous sinus, the ICA "siphon," can be insonated via the orbital window at the distance of 65 to 70 mm. The direction of flow assists in determining which segment of the siphon is being insonated, as under normal conditions flow direction is toward the probe in the inferior portion, away from the probe in the superior portion, and bidirectional in the curved genu. The ICA can also be insonated via the temporal window at distances ranging from 60 to 65 mm, with direction of flow normally toward the probe. The ophthalmic artery is usually insonated at a distance of 30–50 mm, with flow moving toward the probe, and with a low resistance profile. Flow direction in the ophthalmic artery (OA) can quantitate the degree of ipsilateral proximal ICA stenosis, given that the OA anastomoses with facial and orbital arteries originate from the ECA. In severe ICA stenosis collateral flow may be provided from the ECA tributaries to the ACA and MCA by way of retrograde OA filling.

Middle Cerebral Artery

The MCA is the most consistently and reliably identified intracranial vessel, and is frequently insonated not only to diagnose or exclude intrinsic disease, but also for monitoring during vasoreactive testing

Table 13-1. Normal Insonation Distances, Blood Flow Velocities, and Flow Direction Used for the Interpretation of Transcranial Doppler Studies.

Arteries	Insonation Distance (mm)	Mean Velocity (cm/sec)	Flow Direction
MCA	40–60	40–80	Toward
ACA	60–75	40–60	Away
PCA	60–70	30–50	Bidirectional
VA	50–80	30–50	Away
Basilar	80–100+	30–50	Away
OA	30–50	20–30	Toward
ICA (temporal/orbital)	60–65/65–70	30–40/40–50	Away/Bidirectional

and microembolus detection. From its origin, the MCA proceeds laterally along the wing of the sphenoid bone (M1 segment), curves superiorly (M2 portion), bifurcates or trifurcates (M3 portion), and then distributes branches over the superficial cortical regions (M4 vessels). The MCA is optimally insonated at a distance of 40 to 60 mm via the temporal window. Severe proximal stenosis or occlusion of the ipsilateral ICA results in low velocity and low pulsatility waveforms (Fig 13–19). Distal stenosis of the MCA will also show a low-velocity waveform but with elevated pulsatility. Recently, transcranial Doppler has also been utilized as a therapeutic modality to aid in thrombolytic dissolution of thrombus and recanalization of acute MCA occlusion.

Anterior Cerebral Artery and Anterior Communicating Artery

From its origin, the ACA proceeds anteromedially (A1 segment), then superiorly and posteriorly. The A1 segment may be insonated at a distance of 60 to 75 mm also by the temporal window, and the AComm is insonated at 70 to 75 mm (after which the A2 segment of the ACA begins). As the ACA has many variants and often has a curving course, insonation and interpretation of results is often challenging. Direction of flow in the AComm may be toward or away from the probe. The AComm is the first major collateral pathway recruited in instances of severe stenosis or occlusion of the ICA. In such cases, AComm flow is toward the deficient side,

and flow in the ipsilateral A1 segment is reversed to compensate for the hemodynamic compromise (Fig 13–20). A *compression test* of the contralateral ICA may be performed to confirm this cross-filling. While insonating the ipsilateral MCA, compression results in a substantial flow velocity drop if most of the collateral flow comes from the contralateral ICA/ACA. A minor drop in flow velocity confirms that collateral flow predominately comes from other anastomoses.

Posterior Cerebral Artery and Posterior Communicating Artery

Distally the basilar artery bifurcates to form the PCAs, which are typically insonated at a distance of 60 to 70 mm via the temporal window. Flow in the proximal P1 segment is directed toward the probe, whereas flow in the distal P2 segment is away from the probe. The superior cerebellar artery, which lies just inferior, may at times be mistaken for the PCA, but can be distinguished by substantially lower flow velocities. The PComm, originating from the ICA (demarcating the boundary between P1 and P2 segments) is difficult to insonate because of low flow. The P1 to PComm collateral channel is the second major collateral anastomosis to compensate for hemodynamic compromise due to severe stenosis or occlusion of the ICA. Accelerated flow velocities are noted when the collateral anastomosis is functional (Fig 13–21). Up to 20% of the population has an aplastic P1 portion, and a "fetal" PCA composed of the PComm and P2 segment.

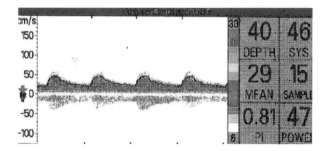

Fig 13–19. Low velocity (blunted waveform) and low pulsatility in the MCA due to severe proximal stenosis of the ipsilateral ICA.

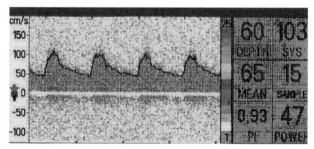

Fig 13–20. Severe stenosis of ICA.

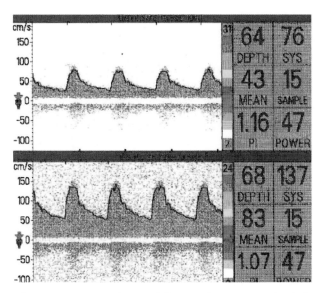

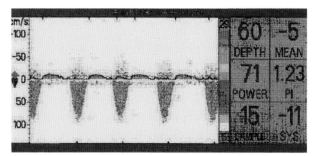

Fig 13–22. Subclavian steal.

Fig 13–21. Accelerated flow velocities in the left PCA ipsilateral to left ICA occlusion.

Vertebral and Basilar Arteries

Intracranially, the bilateral VAs merge to form the solitary basilar artery (BA). By the suboccipital window, the VAs can be insonated from a distance of 50 to 80 mm, whereas the BA usually can be insonated from 80 to 100 mm (sometimes even deeper). Waveform intensity and velocity values obtained during insonation of the VAs will depend on the degree of hypoplasia present, as the caliber of these vessels is frequently asymmetric ("dominant" and "nondominant" vessels). At times, the origin of the BA may be identified by an increase in flow intensity during stepwise insonation of a VA. Insonation of the VAs is essential in diagnosing subclavian steal syndrome, whereby flow in a VA is compromised and diverted to the ipsilateral subclavian artery. Subclavian steal syndrome occurs as a result of subclavian artery stenosis proximal to the origin of the VA, and typically is precipitated by exercise of the ipsilateral arm (Fig 13-22). Physiologically, the arm use causes increased perfusion demand which cannot be met by the stenosed subclavian artery, resulting in competition for perfusion with the vertebral VA, and "steal" of flow from the vertebral to the subclavian. In subclavian steal, flow in the VA may be decreased, retrograde in diastole,

or entirely retrograde. It is usually asymptomatic although it can cause posterior fossa symptoms, including syncope.

Indications for Transcranial Ultrasound

Indications for ultrasound examination of the basal cerebral vessels include:

- Evaluation of patients with acute or longstanding steno-occlusive extracranial or intracranial cerebrovascular disease
- Evaluation and follow-up of patients with sickle cell disease to determine risk for cerebral ischemia and need for transfusions
- Evaluation of patients with spontaneous subarachnoid hemorrhage (SAH) for detection and monitoring of vasospasm
- Identification of microemboli from thromboembolic and cardiogenic sources, with quantification of risk for cerebral infarction and assessment of treatment efficacy
- Testing of vasomotor reactivity in patients with severe intracranial or extracranial arterial stenosis and occlusion
- Testing for cardiac patent foramen ovale (PFO)
- Perioperative monitoring for perfusion adequacy/compromise and embolization
- Evaluation and follow-up of patients with AVM

- Evaluation for venous sinus or cortical vein thrombosis
- Determining cerebral circulatory arrest
- Amplification of intravenous thrombolysis in cases of acute MCA thrombosis
- Assessment of cerebral crossflow in head and neck cancer cases where carotid artery resection is contemplated.

Assessment of TCD Uses by the American Academy of Neurology

In 2004, the American Academy of Neurology Subcommittee on Therapeutics and Technology submitted an assessment for use of TCD.[67] The following are the excerpts of their assessment:

1. TCD is of established value in the screening of children aged 2 to 16 years with sickle cell disease for risk of cerebral ischemia/infarction (Type A, Class I), and for the detection and monitoring of angiographic vasospasm after spontaneous subarachnoid hemorrhage (Type A, Class I to II).
2. TCD provides important information and may have value for the detection of intracranial steno-occlusive disease (Type B, Class II to III), vasospasm after traumatic SAH (Type B, Class III), vasomotor reactivity testing (Type B, Class II to III), cerebral microembolism detection (Type B, Class II to IV), monitoring during carotid surgery (Type B, Class II to III), monitoring during coronary artery bypass surgery (Type B to C, Class II to III), monitoring of cerebral thrombolysis (Type B, Class II to III), and diagnosis of cerebral circulatory arrest (Type A, Class II).
3. Contrast-enhanced studies can provide useful information on cardiac/extracardiac shunts (Type A, Class II), intracranial occlusive disease (Type B, Class II to IV), and aneurismal SAH (Type B, Class II to IV). However, other imaging techniques may be preferable in these settings.

Intracranial Stenosis and Occlusion

Hemodynamically significant narrowing of intracranial arteries may result in focal increases in mean and peak flow velocities, turbulent flow (evident visually and acoustically), and increased waveform pulsatility at the level of stenosis (Fig 13-23). Proximal and distal to the stenosis, reductions in flow velocities may be observed, with corresponding variations in pulsatility indexes. Compensatory collateral flow from uncompromised vessels to deprived

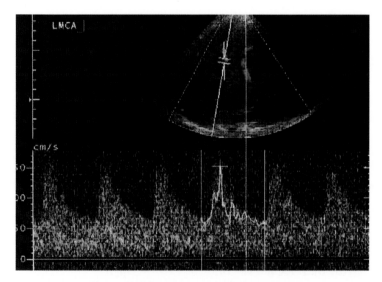

Fig 13-23. Stenosis of the MCA.

areas may result in flow reversal and augmentation of flow. Stenosis of greater than 50% lumen narrowing can reliably be detected in arterial segments with anatomically favorable insonation angles, particularly the M1 segment of the middle cerebral artery. As some patients will have suboptimal temporal windows, failure to obtain a waveform reading does not imply vessel occlusion unless a prior study had demonstrated vessel patency. For such patients, an attempt can be made to insonate the entire anterior circulation from one temporal window. Recently, transcranial ultrasound has even been proposed as an adjunct therapy to intravenous thrombolysis in patients with acute MCA occlusion.[68]

Sickle Cell Disease

Among the various etiologies for cerebrovascular disease, sickle cell anemia affects the youngest patient population, and carries one of the greatest risks for infarction. Patients with sickle cell anemia may experience cerebral ischemia from several mechanisms relating to the deformed erythrocytes, including hyperviscosity at the level of the microarterioles and progressive stenosis at the level of the large basal arteries. Based on the results of two major studies that used transcranial ultrasound as the prime nonclinical measure of disease activity, regular red cell transfusions were shown to decrease the incidence of infarction by a factor of 10,[69] and to maintain a protective effect for as long as transfusions were continued.[70] Parameters that defined patients at risk for cerebral ischemia included mean time-averaged maximum MCA or ICA velocities between 170 to 200 cm per sec, whereas those benefiting from (and thus requiring) regular transfusions were found to have velocities greater than 200 cm per sec.[69,70]

Vasospasm in Subarachnoid Hemorrhage

Transcranial ultrasound has become a standard examination procedure for the detection and quantification of basal artery vasospasm after subarachnoid hemorrhage (SAH), and has also been used to identify and monitor vasospasm following head trauma. Despite limitations in identifying distal vasospasm, most clinically significant spasm occurs in the proximal cerebral vessels which are generally accessible to the insonation beam.[71] Analogous to intracranial steno-occlusive disease, velocity elevations, increased pulsatility, and turbulent flow may be seen at the level of spasm.

As elevated flow velocities can also occur with hyperemia due to postischemic luxury perfusion or loss of autoregulatory mechanisms in the distal resistance arterioles, velocity ratios have been proposed to increase the specificity of ultrasound for identifying vasospasm. For the MCA, ratio measurements are performed by dividing the ipsilateral maximum mean MCA velocity by the maximum mean submandibular extracranial ICA velocity, commonly called "Lindegaard Index."[72] MCA velocities ≥120 cm per sec with MCA/ICA ratios of 3 to 4 are indicative of mild vasospasm, whereas those with ratios of 5 to 6 indicate moderate spasm. Severe spasm is generally defined by velocities ≥200 cm per sec and ratios ≥6.[67] For the BA, maximum BA velocity is divided by the sum of the maximum velocities of each extracranial VA.[73] Flow velocities of ≥80 cm per sec with BA/VA ratios ≥2 are sensitive and specific for detecting vasospasm, and ratios ≥3 reliably identify severe spasm.[73]

Detection of Arteriovenous Malformations

Arteriovenous malformations represent direct communications between the arterial and venous systems, without an intervening capillary bed. As such, no resistance vessels exist to impede or regulate flow, and thus flow measurements from feeding vessels typically demonstrate elevated velocities and low resistance waveforms.[74] Due to the large volume of flow that traverses AVMs, flow patterns may also be altered in vessels not directly connected to the AVM, resulting in alterations of waveform recordings. TCD is very sensitive for the detection of medium to large sized AVMs,[74] yet color Doppler imaging may provide greater yield with regard to anatomic characteristics of AVMs.[75]

Embolus Detection

TCD has been utilized to detect microemboli during carotid endarterectomy, cardiac surgery, stroke associated with atrial fibrillation, in patients with prosthetic heart valves, and carotid artery stenosis.[65-67] Microembolic signals (MES) may be detected by TCD monitoring of an intracranial vessel that may be receiving microemboli from a proximal arterial or cardiac source (Fig 13-24).

Cerebral embolism accounts for up to 70% of all ischemic strokes. The majority of these emboli originate from carotid occlusive disease. Other sources of cerebral emboli include diseases of the heart, aortic arch atheroma, and plaques in vertebral and intracranial arteries. Cerebral microemboli detected by TCD are defined as high-intensity transient signals (HITS) of duration less than 300 msec, exceeding the background signal by at least 3 dB; and are unidirectional within the Doppler velocity spectrum. Automated computer-assisted HITS detection systems are in development and further studies are needed to confirm their reliability before their use becomes widespread in clinical practice. Multigated instruments capable of insonating multiple segments of individual or adjacent vessels may provide greater yield.[76] MES must be differentiated from artifact caused by mechanical interference at the level of the probe, and from patient factors such as jaw tremors. Using multifrequency instruments, MES may be characterized as gaseous or solid, and may provide precise information regarding origin of the

microembolic particles.[75] Gaseous particles have been associated with cardiac sources, whereas solid particles have been connected to arterial thrombo-embolization from proximal atherosclerotic lesions.[77] MES detection may be particularly useful during surgical procedures with potential for cerebral embolization, such as cardiac revascularization or carotid endarterectomy.[78]

TCD-detected microemboli can serve as a clinical marker for stroke and can reliably predict stroke in high-risk populations. Clinical trials of various medical therapies and interventional procedures aimed to demonstrate a reduction of stroke incidence after a reduction of the number of TCD-detected microemboli are currently underway. To ensure better reliability of the MES detection, the International Consensus Group on Microembolus Detection has published MES definitions for spectral Doppler, and subsequent detailed recommendations for reporting MES studies.[79] The future development of automated systems to obtain and process Doppler data and determine MES will best facilitate standardization and routine use in clinical practice.

Detection of "Right-To-Left" Cardiac Shunts

Cardiac patent foramen ovale (PFO) represents the incomplete closure of a fetal intra-atrial communication that persists in approximately 25% of the population. Paradoxic embolism via a patent foramen ovale is often a suspected mechanism of cerebral ischemia in patients with an otherwise uncertain cause. Transcranial ultrasound monitoring of the basal intracranial vessels during intravenous injection of agitated saline or contrast media can be used for the detection of such shunts by documenting MES several seconds following the start of an infusion.[80] Valsalva maneuver, which increases intrathoracic pressure and impedes prepulmonary cardiac output, may assist in this process by enhancing flow across the septal defect.[81] The degree of shunt may also be quantitatively assessed by measuring the number of MES detected, and may correlate to PFO size and degree of shunt.[82] Other less common communications between the venous and arterial systems

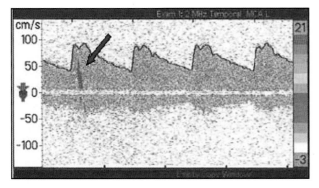

Fig 13–24. Cerebral microembolic signals (MES) or high-intensity transient signals (HITS).

include non-PFO atrial septal defects, ventricular septal defects, patent ductus arteriosus, and pulmonary arteriovenous malformations as occurs with hereditary hemorrhagic telangiectasia.

Cerebral Vasoreactivity (CVR) Testing

Transcranial ultrasound can be used to assess cerebral hemodynamic reserve. When arterial perfusion in compromised, distal regulating arterioles dilate to allow greater flow and prevent cerebral ischemia. Conversely, when excessive perfusion exists, the resistance arterioles constrict to prevent the development of cerebral edema and hemorrhage. Under normal conditions, administration of a pharmacologic vasodilator results in vasodilation of these arterioles. However, when perfusion is severely impaired the arterioles are maximally dilated and the cerebral vasodilatory capacity (CVC) decreases or disappears, indicating a state of exhausted cerebrovascular reserve and "misery" perfusion.[83] Severely impaired

CVC may predict impending ischemia or infarction in patients with extracranial or intracranial artery stenosis or occlusion.[84]

Testing of CVR by the CO_2 Inhalation Test

Several methods of CVR testing exist including breath holding index, blood pressure changes, or the CO_2 inhalation test. The CO_2 inhalation test is reliable, validated, and most commonly used. It is performed by continuous bilateral TCD insonation of the MCAs. End-tidal partial pressure of carbon dioxide (PCO_2) is measured continuously with an in-line capnometer connected via an oral mouthpiece. Continuous tracings of MCA flow velocity, heart rate, respiratory rate, and expiratory PCO_2 are recorded. After 2 minutes of baseline measurements, patients inhale a mixture of 5% CO_2 and air (Carbigene) for 2 minutes. CVC is calculated as the percent rise in MCA mean flow velocity (MFV) per 1 mm Hg PCO_2 increase on the MFV curve plateau (Fig 13–25). Normal CVC is defined as a rise in MCA MFV of >2.0% per mm Hg PCO_2.[84]

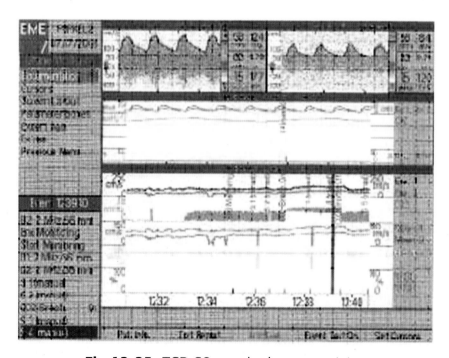

Fig 13–25. TCD-CO_2 cerebral vasoreactivity.

Insonation of the Venous Vessels

Insonation of cerebral veins may provide useful information pertaining to sinus thrombosis. Using the temporal route the basal cerebral vein may be identified,[85] whereas the straight sinus may be identified by the suboccipital route.[86] Evidence exists to suggest utility for TCD in detecting superior sagittal sinus thrombosis.[85] Absence of signal in the basal cerebral vein or straight sinus may indicate thrombosis of these structures, especially if previously imaged and found patent.

Cerebral Circulatory Arrest

Transcranial ultrasound may be used as an adjunct to the clinical exam for assessing and verifying cerebral circulatory arrest. In such cases, systolic spikes (indicating pulsatile flow impacting on an occluded intracerebral circulation) or complete absence of flow may be found.[87] During worsening elevation of intracranial pressure (ICP), flow waveforms progress from normal morphology to waves with low diastolic velocities, systolic peaks with no anterograde diastolic flow, to systolic peaks with retrograde diastolic flow, and finally isolated systolic spikes and complete absence of flow.[65,88]

Cerebral Cross-Flow Assessment

TCD has been used in head and neck cancer patients with suspected carotid artery involvement by neck metastases in their preoperative assessment.[89] Adequate cerebral cross-flow from the contralateral carotid artery and vertebral systems can be reliably determined by TCD when contemplating unilateral carotid resection.

Sonothrombolysis

TCD has recently even been proposed as an adjunct therapy to intravenous thrombolysis in patients with acute MCA occlusion.[68] Augmentation of TPA-associated thrombolysis with 2-MHz TCD was shown to be safe, and may be further enhanced with addition of gaseous microbubbles.[90] Early complete MCA recanalization rate on TCD can be achieved in up to 55% when TPA is given with 2-MHz TCD and microbubbles. This novel approach has currently been tested in a controlled international randomized clinical trial of perflutren-containing microbubbles.[91]

Summary

Transcranial Doppler provides a safe noninvasive method for assessing the anatomy and physiology of the cerebral vessels, and is a reliable technique for detecting, quantifying, and monitoring a multitude of cerebrovascular conditions. Ongoing developments in transcranial ultrasound, such as the use and validation of color/power Doppler, and contrast-enhanced imaging techniques will certainly advance the role and utility of transcranial ultrasonography for the assessment of the intracranial vasculature. Furthermore, novel therapeutic use of TCD ("sonothrombolysis") will expand the role of TCD from a diagnostic and monitoring technique to a powerful therapeutic tool. Recent advances in the field of neurosonology lead to level 1, type A evidence that TCD and carotid duplex are recommended essential components of a comprehensive stroke center.[67,92]

Videos in This Chapter

Video 13A. Normal color Doppler blood flow in the carotid arteries.

Video 13B. Normal color Doppler blood flow in the internal carotid artery.

Video 13C. Normal color Doppler blood flow in the vertebral artery.

Video 13D. Carotid artery stenosis 60 to 79% (systolic BFV >170 cm/sec and diastolic >40 cm/sec).

References

1. Zwiebel WJ, Pellerito JS. *Cerebral vessels: Introduction to Vascular Ultrasonography*, 5th ed. Philadelphia, Pa: Elsevier-Saunders; 2005;Sec II: 107-225.

2. AIUM Standards for the Performance of Ultrasound Examination for the Extracranial Cerebrovascular System. From http://www.acr.org/SecondaryMainMenuCategories/quality_safety/guidelines/us/us_extracranial_cerebrovascular.aspx. Retrieved December 1, 2002.

3. Johnston DC, Goldstein LB. Clinical carotid endarterectomy decision making: noninvasive vascular imaging versus angiography. *Neurology*. 2001;56:1009-1015.

4. De Bray JM, Glatt B. Quantification of atheromatous stenosis in the extracranial internal carotid artery. *Cerebrovasc Dis*. 1995;5:414-426.

5. North American Symptomatic Carotid Endarterectomy Trial collaborators. Beneficial effect of carotid endarterectomy in symptomatic patients with high grade stenosis. *N Engl J Med*. 1991; 325:445-453.

6. European Carotid Surgery Triallists Collaborative Group. MRC European Carotid Surgery Trial: Interim results for symptomatic patients with severe (70-99%) or mild (0-29%) carotid stenosis. *Lancet*. 1991;337:1235-1243.

7. Carra G, Visona A, Bonanome A, et al. Carotid plaque morphology and cerebrovascular events. *Int Angiol*. 2003;22:284-289.

8. Rothwell PM. Risk modeling to identify patients with symptomatic carotid stenosis most at risk of stroke. *Neurol Res*. 2005; 27 (suppl 1):S18-S28.

9. Halliday A, Mansfield A, Marro J, et al. MRC Asymptomatic Carotid Surgery Trial (ACST) collaborative group. Prevention of disabling and fatal strokes by successful carotid endarterectomy in patients without recent neurological symptoms: randomized controlled trial. *Lancet*. 2004;363(9420):1491-1502.

10. Bock RW, Gray-Weale AC, Mock PA, et al. The natural history of asymptomatic carotid artery disease. *J Vasc Surg*. 1993;17(1):160-169.

11. Mackey AE, Abrahamowicz M, Langlois Y, et al. Outcome of asymptomatic patients with carotid disease. *Neurology*. 1997;48:896-903.

12. Nicolaides AN, Kakkos SK, Griffin M, et al. for the Asymptomatic Carotid Stenosis and Risk of Stroke (ACSRS) Study Group. Severity of asymptomatic carotid stenosis and risk of ipsilateral hemispheric ischaemic events: results from the ACSRS study. *Eur J Vasc Endovasc Surg*. 2005;30:275-284.

13. Chambers BR, Norris JW. Outcome in patients with asymptomatic neck bruits. *N Eng J Med*. 1986;315:860-865.

14. Lewis RF, Abrahamowicz M, Cote R, Battista RN. Predictive power of duplex ultrasonography in asymptomatic carotid disease. *Ann Intern Med*. 1997;127:13-20.

15. Roederer GO, Langlois YE, Jager KA, et al. The natural history of carotid arterial disease in asymptomatic patients with cervical bruits. *Stroke*. 1984;15:605-613.

16. Sabeti S, Exner M, Mlekusch W, et al. Prognostic impact of fibrinogen in carotid atherosclerosis: nonspecific indicator of inflammation or independent predictor of disease progression? *Stroke*. 2005;36(7):1400-1404.

17. Meairs S, Steinke W, Mohr JP, Hennerici M. Ultrasound imaging and Doppler sonography. In: Barnett HJM, Mohr JP, Stein BM, Yatsu F, eds. *Stroke: Pathophysiology, Diagnosis and Management*. New York, NY: Churchhill Livingstone; 1998:207-326.

18. Bluth EI, Wetzner SM, Stavros AT, et al: Carotid duplex sonography: a multicenter recommendation for standardized imaging and Doppler criteria. *Radiographics*. 1988;8:487-506.

19. Corriveau MM, Johnston KW. Interobserver variability of carotid Doppler peak velocity measurements among technologists in an ICAVL-accredited vascular laboratory. *J Vasc Surgery*. 2004;39(4):735-741.

20. Dempsey RJ, Diana AL, Moore RW. Thickness of carotid artery atherosclerotic plaque and ischemic risk. *Neurosurgery*. 1990;27(3):343-348.

21. Manolio TA, Burke GL, O`Leary DH, et al. Relationships of cerebral MRI findings to ultrasonographic carotid atherosclerosis in older adults: the Cardiovascular Health Study. CHS Collaborative Research Group. *Arterioscler Thromb Vasc Biol*. 1999;19:356-365.

22. Iemolo F, Martiniuk A, Steinman DA, Spence D. Sex differences in carotid plaque and stenosis. *Stroke*. 2004;35:477-481.

23. Liapis CD, Kakisis JD, Kostakis AG. Carotid stenosis; factors affecting symptomatology. *Stroke* 2001; 32:2782-2786.

24. Streifler JY, Eliasziw M, Fox AJ, et al. Angiographic detection of carotid plaque ulceration. Comparison with surgical observations in a multicenter study. North American Symptomatic Carotid Endarterectomy Trial. *Stroke*. 1994;25(6):1130-1132.

25. Sztajzel R. Ultrasonographic assessment of the morphological characteristics of the carotid plaque. *Swiss Med Wkly*. 2005;135:635-643.

26. Prabhakaran S, Rundek T, Ramas R, et al. Carotid plaque surface irregularity predicts ischemic stroke. The Northern Manhattan Study. *Stroke*. 2006;37(11):2696-2701.

27. De Bray JM, Baud JM, Dauzat M. Consensus concerning the morphology and the risk of carotid plaques. *Cerebrovasc Dis*. 1996;7:289-296.

28. Polak JF, Shemanski L, O`Leary DH, et al. Hypoechoic plaque at US of the carotid artery: an independent risk factor for incident stroke in adults aged 65 years or older. *Radiology*. 1998;208:649-654.

29. Mathiesen EB, Bonaa KH, Joakimsen O. Echolucent plaques are associated with high risk of ischemic cerebrovascular events in carotid stenosis: the Tromso study. *Circulation*. 2001;103:2171-2175.

30. Reilly LM, Lusby RJ, Hugues L, et al. Carotid plaque histology using real-time ultrasonography: clinical and therapeutic implications. *Am J Surg*. 1997;113:1352-1358.

31. Gronholdt ML, Nordestgaard BG, Schroeder TV, et al. Ultrasonic echolucent carotid plaques predict future strokes. *Circulation*. 2001;104:68-73.

32. European Carotid Plaque Study Group. Carotid artery plaque composition and relationship to clinical presentation and ultrasound B-mode imaging. *Eur J Vasc Surg*. 1995;10:23-30.

33. Fanning NF, Walters TD, Fox AJ, Symons SP Association between calcification of the cervical carotid artery bifurcation and white matter ischemia. *AJNR Am J Neuroradiol*. 2006;27(2):378-383.

34. Nandalur KR, Baskurt E, Hagspiel KD, et al. Carotid artery calcification on CT may independently predict stroke risk. *AJR Am J Roentgenol*. 2006;186(2):547-552.

35. Hartmann A, Mohr JP, Thompson JL, Ramos O, Mast H. Interrater reliability of plaque morphology classification in patients with severe carotid artery stenosis. *Acta Neurol Scand*. 1999;99:61-64.

36. Biasi GM, Sampaolo A, Mingazzini P, et al. Computer analysis of ultrasonic plaque echolucency in identifying high risk carotid bifurcation lesions. *Eur J Vasc Endovasc Surg*. 1999;17:476-479.

37. Boissel J-P, Collet J-P, Moleur P, Haugh M. Surrogate endpoints: a basis for a rational approach. *Eur J Clin Pharm*. 1992;43:235-244.

38. Demol P, Weihrauch TR. Surrogate endpoints: their utility for evaluating therapeutic efficacy in clinical trials. *Appl Clin Trials*. 1998;7:45-56.

39. Glagov S, Weisenberg E, Zarins CK, Stankunavicius R, Kolettis GJ. Compensatory enlargement of human atherosclerotic coronary arteries. *N Engl J Med*. 1987;316:1371-1375.

40. Pignoli P, Tremoli E, Poli A, Oreste P, Paoletti R. Intimal plus medial thickness of the arterial wall: a direct measurement with ultrasound imaging. *Circulation*. 1986;74(6):1399-1406.

41. Poli A, Tremoli E, Colombo A, Sirtori M, Pignoli P, Paoletti R. Ultrasonographic measurement of the common carotid artery wall thickness in hypercholesterolemic patients. A new model for the quantitation and follow-up of preclinical atherosclerosis in living human subjects. *Atherosclerosis*. 1988;70(3):253-261.

42. Sidhu PS, Desai SR. A simple and reproducible method for assessing intimal-medial thickness of the common carotid artery. *Br J Radiol*. 1997;70:85-89.

43. Touboul PJ, Hennerici MG, Meairs S. Mannheim intima-media thickness consensus. On behalf of the Advisory board of the 3rd Watching the Risk Symposium 2004, 13th European Stroke Conference, Mannheim, Germany, May 14, 2004. *Cerebrovasc Dis*. 2004;18(4):346-934.

44. O'Leary DH, Polak JF, Kronmal RA, et al. Carotid-artery intima and media thickness as a risk factor for myocardial infarction and stroke in older adults. *N Engl J Med*. 1999;340:14-22.

45. Kuller L, Borhani N, Furberg C, et al. Prevalence of subclinical atherosclerosis and cardiovascular disease and association with risk factors in the Cardiovascular Health Study. *Am J Epidemiol*. 1994;139(12):1164-1179.

46. Bots ML, Hoes AW, Koudstaal PJ, Hofman A, Grobbee DE. Common carotid intima-media thickness and risk of stroke and myocardial infarction: the Rotterdam Study. *Circulation*. 1997;96(5):1432-1437.

47. Chambless LE, Heiss G, Folsom AR, et al. Association of coronary heart disease incidence with carotid arterial wall thickness and major risk factors: the Atherosclerosis Risk in Communities (ARIC) Study, 1987-1993. *Am J Epidemiol*. 1997;146(6):483-494.

48. Touboul PJ, Labreuche J, Vicaut E, Amarenco P; GENIC Investigators. Carotid intima-media thickness, plaques, and Framingham risk score as independent determinants of stroke risk. *Stroke*. 2005;36(8):1741-1745.

49. Bots ML, Hoes AW, Koudstaal PJ, Hofman A, Grobbee DE. Common carotid intima-media thick-

ness and risk of stroke and myocardial infarction: the Rotterdam Study. *Circulation.* 1997;96(5): 1432-1437.

50. Chambless LE, Heiss G, Folsom AR, et al. Association of coronary heart disease incidence with carotid arterial wall thickness and major risk factors: the Atherosclerosis Risk in Communities (ARIC) Study, 1987-1993. *Am J Epidemiol.* 1997;146(6):483-494.

51. Blankenhorn DH, Selzer RH, Crawford DW, et al. Beneficial effects of colestipol-niacin therapy on the common carotid artery. Two- and four-year reduction of intima-media thickness measured by ultrasound. *Circulation.* 1993;88(1):20-28.

52. Furberg CD, Adams HP Jr, Applegate WB, et al. Effect of lovastatin on early carotid atherosclerosis and cardiovascular events. Asymptomatic Carotid Artery Progression Study (ACAPS) Research Group. *Circulation.* 1994;90(4):1679-1687.

53. Salonen R, Nyyssonen K, Porkkala E, et al. Kuopio Atherosclerosis Prevention Study (KAPS). A population-based primary preventive trial of the effect of LDL lowering on atherosclerotic progression in carotid and femoral arteries. *Circulation.* 1995; 92(7):1758-1764.

54. Jukema JW, Bruschke AV, van Boven AJ, et al. Effects of lipid lowering by pravastatin on progression and regression of coronary artery disease in symptomatic men with normal to moderately elevated serum cholesterol levels. The Regression Growth Evaluation Statin Study (REGRESS). *Circulation.* 1995; 91(10):2528-2540.

55. Smilde TJ, van Wissen S, Wollersheim H, Trip MD, Kastelein JJ, Stalenhoef AF. Effect of aggressive versus conventional lipid lowering on atherosclerosis progression in familial hypercholesterolaemia (ASAP): a prospective, randomised, double-blind trial. *Lancet.* 2001;357(9256):577-581.

56. Taylor AJ, Kent SM, Flaherty PJ, Coyle LC, Markwood TT, Vernalis MN. ARBITER: Arterial Biology for the Investigation of the Treatment Effects of Reducing Cholesterol: a randomized trial comparing the effects of atorvastatin and pravastatin on carotid intima medial thickness. *Circulation.* 2002;106(16):2055-2060.

57. Lonn E, Yusuf S, Dzavik V, et al. Effects of ramipril and vitamin E on atherosclerosis: the study to evaluate carotid ultrasound changes in patients treated with ramipril and vitamin E (SECURE). *Circulation.* 2001;103(7):919-925.

58. Wiklund O, Hulthe J, Wikstrand J, Schmidt C, Olofsson SO, Bondjers G. Effect of controlled release/extended release metoprolol on carotid intima-

media thickness in patients with hypercholesterolemia: a 3-year randomized study. *Stroke.* 2002; 33(2):572-577.

59. Zanchetti A, Bond MG, Hennig M, et al. Calcium antagonist lacidipine slows down progression of asymptomatic carotid atherosclerosis: principal results of the European Lacidipine Study on Atherosclerosis (ELSA), a randomized, double-blind, long-term trial. *Circulation.* 2002;106(19): 2422-2427.

60. Pitt B, Byington RP, Furberg CD, Hunninghake DB, Mancini GB, Miller ME et al. Effect of amlodipine on the progression of atherosclerosis and the occurrence of clinical events. PREVENT Investigators. *Circulation.* 2000;102(13):1503-1510.

61. Rundek T, Elkind MS, Pittman J, et al. Carotid intima-media thickness is associated with allelic variants of stromelysin-1, interleukin-6, and hepatic lipase genes: the Northern Manhattan Prospective Cohort Study. *Stroke.* 2002;33(5):1420-1423.

62. Selzer RH, Hodis HN, Kwong-Fu H, et al. Evaluation of computerized edge tracking for quantifying intima-media thickness of the common carotid artery from B-mode ultrasound images. *Atherosclerosis.* 1994;111(1):1-11.

63. Touboul PJ, Prati P, Scarabin PY, Adrai V, Thibout E, Ducimetiere P. Use of monitoring software to improve the measurement of carotid wall thickness by B-mode imaging. *J Hypertens Suppl.* 1992; 10(5):S37-S41.

64. Baldassarre D, Werba JP, Tremoli E, Poli A, Pazzucconi F, Sirtori CR. Common carotid intima-media thickness measurement. A method to improve accuracy and precision. *Stroke.* 1994;25(8):1588-1592.

65. Babikian VL, Feldmann E, Wechsler LR, et al. Transcranial Doppler ultrasonography: year 2000 update. *J Neuroimaging.* 2000;10(2):101-115.

66. Aaslid R, Markwalder TM, Nornes H. Noninvasive transcranial Doppler ultrasound recording of flow velocity in basal cerebral arteries. *J Neurosurg.* 1982;57(6):769-774.

67. Sloan MA, Alexandrov AV, Tegeler CH, et al. *Assessment.* Transcranial Doppler Ultrasonography: Report of the Therapeutics and Technology Assessment Subcommittee of the American Academy of Neurology. *Neurology.* 2004;62:1468-1481.

68. Alexandrov AV, Molina CA, Grotta JC, et al. CLOTBUST investigators. Ultrasound-enhanced systemic thrombolysis for acute ischemic stroke. *N Engl J Med.* 2004;351(21):2170-2178.

69. Adams RJ, McKie VC, Hsu L, et al. Prevention of a first stroke by transfusions in children with sickle

cell anemia and abnormal results on transcranial Doppler ultrasonography. *N Engl J Med*. 1998; 339(1):5–11.

70. Adams RJ, Brambilla D. Optimizing Primary Stroke Prevention in Sickle Cell Anemia (STOP 2) Trial investigators. *N Engl J Med*. 2005;353:2769–2778.

71. Newell DW, Winn HR. Transcranial Doppler in cerebral vasospasm. *Neurosurg Clin North Am*. 1990;1(2):319–328.

72. Lindegaard KF, Nornes H, Bakke SJ, Sorteberg W, Nakstad P. Cerebral vasospasm diagnosis by means of angiography and blood velocity measurements. *Acta Neurochir (Wien)*. 1989;100(1–2):12–24.

73. Soustiel JF, Shik V, Shreiber R, Tavor Y, Goldsher D. Basilar vasospasm diagnosis: investigation of a modified "Lindegaard Index" based on imaging studies and blood velocity measurements of the basilar artery. *Stroke*. 2002;33(1):72–77.

74. Mast H, Mohr JP, Thompson JL, et al. Transcranial Doppler ultrasonography in cerebral arteriovenous malformations. Diagnostic sensitivity and association of flow velocity with spontaneous hemorrhage and focal neurological deficit. *Stroke*. 1995;26:1024–1027.

75. Klotzsch C, Nahser HC, Henkes H, Kuhne D, Berlit P. Detection of microemboli distal to cerebral aneurysms before and after therapeutic embolization. *AJNR Am J Neuroradiol*. 1998;19(7): 1315–1318.

76. Droste DW, Dittrich R, Hermes S, et al. Four-gated transcranial Doppler ultrasound in the detection of circulating microemboli. *Eur J Ultrasound*. 1999;9(2):117–125.

77. Markus HS, MacKinnon A. Asymptomatic embolization detected by Doppler ultrasound predicts stroke risk in symptomatic carotid artery stenosis. *Stroke*. 2005;36(5):971–975.

78. Russell D. Cerebral microemboli and cognitive impairment. *J Neurol Sci*. 2002;203–204:211–214.

79. Ringelstein EB, Droste DW, Babikian VL, et al. Consensus on microembolus detection by TCD. International Consensus Group on Microembolus Detection. *Stroke*. 1998;29:725–729.

80. Jauss M, Kaps M, Keberle M, Haberbosch W, Dorndorf W. A comparison of transesophageal echocardiography and transcranial Doppler sonography with contrast medium for detection of patent foramen ovale. *Stroke*. 1994;25(6):1265–1267.

81. Zanette EM, Mancini G, De Castro S, Solaro M, Cartoni D, Chiarotti F. Patent foramen ovale and transcranial Doppler. Comparison of different procedures. *Stroke*. 1996;27(12):2251–2255.

82. Spencer MP, Moehring MA, Jesurum J, Gray WA, Olsen JV, Reisman M. Power M-mode transcranial Doppler for diagnosis of patent foramen ovale and assessing transcatheter closure. *J Neuroimaging*. 2004;14(4):342–349.

83. Derdeyn CP, Yundt KD, Videen TO, Carpenter DA, Grubb RL Jr, Powers WJ. Increased oxygen extraction fraction is associated with prior ischemic events in patients with carotid occlusion. *Stroke*. 1998;29(4):754–758.

84. Marshall RS, Rundek T, Sproule D, et al. Monitoring of cerebral vasodilatory capacity with transcranial Doppler carbon dioxide inhalation in patients with severe carotid disease. *Stroke*. 2003;34:945–949.

85. Valdueza JM, Schultz M, Harms L, Einhaupl KM. Venous transcranial Doppler ultrasound monitoring in acute dural sinus thrombosis. Report of two cases. *Stroke*. 1995;26(7):1196–1199.

86. Baumgartner RW, Nirkko AC, Muri RM, Gonner F. Transoccipital power-based color-coded duplex sonography of cerebral sinuses and veins. *Stroke*. 1997;28(7):1319–1323.

87. Hassler W, Steinmetz H, Pirschel J. Transcranial Doppler study of intracranial circulatory arrest. *J Neurosurg*. 1989;71(2):195–201.

88. Aaslid R, Lindegaard KF. *Cerebral Hemodynamics. Transcranial Doppler Sonography*. New York, NY: Springer-Verlag; 1986.

89. Mann WJ, Beck A, Schreiber J, Maurer J, Amedee RG, Gluckmann JL. Ultrasonography for evaluation of the carotid artery in head and neck cancer. *Laryngoscope*. 1994;104(7):885–888.

90. Molina CA, Ribo, M, Rubiera, M, et al. Microbubble administration accelerates clot lysis during continuous 2-MHz ultrasound monitoring in stroke patients treated with intravenous tissue plasminogen activator. *Stroke*. 2006;37:425–429.

91. Alexandrov AV, Bornstein NM. Advances in neurosonology 2005. *Stroke*. 2006;37:299–300.

92. Alberts MJ, Latchaw RE, Selman WR, et al. for the Brain Attack Coalition. Recommendations for comprehensive stroke centers: a consensus statement from the Brain Attack Coalition. *Stroke*. 2005;36: 1597–1618.

Chapter 14

DYNAMIC IMAGING OF THE TONGUE, LARYNX, AND PHARYNX DURING SWALLOWING

Jeri L. Miller
Barbara C. Sonies

Advancements in ultrasound imaging technologies have provided clinicians a wide range of qualitative and quantitative imaging techniques to examine the dynamic and functional aspects of the lingual, laryngeal, and pharyngeal mechanisms. Because ultrasound is uniquely suited for observation of dynamic, real-time movements of soft tissue structures, several methods have been developed to evaluate oral–motor functions, swallowing, laryngeal movements, and lateral pharyngeal wall movements. Dynamic sonography is an imaging modality that is relatively low cost in comparison to radiographic and MRI techniques and offers the ability to obtain quantitative data (eg, temporal-spatial displacement, vascular flow) simultaneously with high-resolution images of targeted aerodigestive structures. Portability, the ability to acquire moving images, and the lack of bioeffects make ultrasound extremely suitable for evaluation of swallowing and laryngeal function in patients with pathology, trauma, and surgical complications. Ultrasound imaging techniques can be easily adapted for use in pediatric to geriatric populations and unlike radiographic imaging, can be conducted across repeated or extended assessments. Because no contrast agents are needed, a variety of bolus types can be tested to identify the effects of therapeutic interventions, surgeries or pharmacologic agents on lingual, laryngeal, or pharyngeal functions. Recorded static images or real-time movies provide clinicians with archival records to chart the progression of pathology, the results of medical-surgical interventions, changes to swallowing physiology, or to demonstrate treatment efficacy. Picture archiving formats allow for repeated viewing and measurements at central workstations. These advantages underscore the value of ultrasound as an imaging modality uniquely suited for examination of aerodigestive function (Table 14–1).

This chapter focuses on the basic procedures for conducting dynamic evaluations of swallowing function in adult and pediatric populations within lingual, laryngeal, and pharyngeal structures. Whereas previous chapters provide information on normal anatomy, this chapter stresses techniques to identify tissue changes across physiologic tasks and clinical methods to measure swallowing, sucking or vocal function. Descriptions of normal and abnormal swallowing patterns are highlighted from various clinical studies and special approaches with pediatric populations provided. The necessary sonographic system

Table 14–1. Benefits and Limitations of Ultrasound Imaging in Functional Evaluation of Swallowing

Benefits	Limitations
Dynamic, real-time imaging of oral sequences	Partial views of aerodigestive region due to transducer aperture.
Multiple plane views of oral anatomy; Potential for 3D volumetric data (dynamic and static)	Echo-free or acoustic shadow regions caused by bones in scanning field.
Tracks hyoid motion and bolus flow in real time	Reduced visualization of hard palate, tongue tip, and hypopharynx depending on task, age, and size of oral cavity
Noninvasive, no bioeffects, comfortable procedure	
Regular foods and liquids visualized	
Use of typical furniture without special seating for feeding	Limited detection of aspiration
Determine duration of chewing and bolus preparation during typical tasks.	Manual analysis; Limited normative data
Determine duration of oropharyngeal swallow from tracking hyoid movement.	
Portability	
Minimal patient preparation required	
Suited for pediatric population	
Acquire multiple trials without scan time restriction	
Multiple recording format (still images, movie clips, Video-CD-DVD formats)	
Biofeedback during therapeutic trials	
Low cost	

requirements, transducer placements, and scanning techniques for clinical examinations of aerodigestive function are emphasized with images and video clips of dynamic motion studies during swallowing and lingual activity provided to assist beginning clinicians.

Functional Examination of Oral Musculature and Lingual-Hyoid Activity During Swallowing

Transducer Selection and Equipment Requirements

Sonographic examination of lingual function during swallowing requires the selection of appropriate transducer arrays, image settings, and transducer placements (Table 14–2). Most real-time B-mode ultrasound systems can provide high-resolution images of lingual function during swallowing. Commercially available systems can easily record dynamic swallowing events directly onto computer hard drives in video/movie formats. In order to conduct a functional analysis the study must be recorded onto disk (CD, DVD, optical disk), taped (VHS, SVHS), or saved to the system's or a networked hard drive for review. Selection of the appropriate transducer for functional studies should be guided by patient age, size, and required field of view of the targeted tissue structures. Real-time sector, convex, or curvilinear transducers producing wedge pie-shaped fields-of-view provide suitable image fields of the adult lingual anatomy extending from the anterior tongue tip to the base of tongue and upper pharynx. Large sector probes provide 90- to 120-degree imaging fields for

Table 14–2. Equipment for Functional Swallowing Studies

B-mode real-time ultrasound system

Integrated recording format, monitor display, and device (videotape, CD/DVD, optical disk)

3.5- to 7.5-MHz transducer frequency, abdominal convex/curvilinear probes (adult), pediatric abdominal probes (child); linear probes for pharyngeal-laryngeal imaging (minimum 5-MHz frequency)

Small-parts image preset capability for optimization of image resolution

Additional scanning packages: duplex imaging, M-mode, color Doppler, power Doppler

Selected bolus items in a variety of volumes and viscosities

Feeding utensils and systems (spoons, cups, bottle/nipple, adaptive or therapeutic equipment)

Transducer cleaner, sterile gloves

adults, whereas smaller pediatric abdominal probes or small curvilinear probes can provide appropriate views of the pediatric oral cavity. Transducer frequencies ranging from 3.5 to 7.5 MHz provide sufficient depth penetration to view the oral cavity from the floor-of-the-mouth to the lingual-palatal surface in most adult patients as well as for children. Higher frequency probes greater than 10 MHz provide high resolution of soft tissues particularly along surface margins such as the floor of the mouth or neck and may also be useful for small children or infants. Acoustic coupling gel spread on the patient's skin in the targeted region of insonation ensures appropriate acoustic transmission through the tissues. Rarely are acoustic stand-off pads required; however, abnormal surface deformations due to tumors, cysts, post-surgical malformation, and so forth may benefit from the use of an additional coupling medium. Peng, Jost-Brinkmann, and Miethke[1] have promoted the use of a specialized, noncommercial stand-off pad that reduces the need for hand-held, free-scan imaging; however, clinical scanning often dictates that the clinician perform free-hand scans of targeted regions generally using submental transducer placement.[1]

Procedures for Evaluation of Swallowing

The evaluation of swallowing function can be conducted for a variety of purposes without the use of specialized seating systems or adaptive imaging suites (Table 14–3). Portable units can be taken bedside if necessary. With the patient in a normal upright position, the transducer is placed submentally at approximate midline to obtain a sagittal plane image of the tongue (Table 14–4, Basic Procedures for Sonographic Study of Swallowing). A correct placement of the transducer is essential to maintain clear identification of soft tissue anatomy and reproducible fiducial markers. Slight angling of the probe will ensure visualization of the lingual surface margin and hyoid shadow.

Table 14–3. Ultrasound Applications for Functional Analyses of Swallowing

Evaluate oral and pharyngeal soft tissue anatomy

Evaluate lingual symmetry/asymmetry/surface deformation-contour

Evaluate oral bolus preparation, control, and transport

Evaluate oral phase swallowing timing-duration

Evaluate effects of bolus types, volumes, single-multiple swallows and continuous drinking

Evaluate nutritive and non-nutritive sucking and swallowing patterns in infants

Evaluate response to feeding device, utensils, nipple systems

Evaluate tongue-hyoid interactions

Evaluate effects of reduced saliva

Evaluate effects of medication

Monitor therapeutic interventions

Evaluate effects of pathologic conditions (neuromuscular, postradiation-surgery, developmental delay)

Evaluate effects of aging

Evaluate vascular effects, lateral pharyngeal wall function, gross vocal fold activity

Table 14–4. Basic Procedures for Sonographic Study of Swallowing.

I. Transducer Placement

  A. Midline sagittal view with transducer placed in submental region

  B. Move transducer as needed slightly left-right (parasagittal) to obtain clear view of anatomy and curved surface margins of tongue.

  C. Rotation-angling of transducer to observe acoustic shadow of hyoid bone and mandible

  D. Maintain this positioning to view swallow duration.

  E. Command dry (saliva) swallows. Observe response and repeat three times to identify patient variations and effect of reduced moisture.

  F. Trial boluses using water, liquids, puree. Repeat command. Obtain single and multiple swallows.

  G. Vary utensil (straw, cup, and spoon).

  H. Observe response to therapeutic maneuvers.

  I. Rotate transducer 90 degrees at midline to obtain coronal view. Repeat dry, liquid, and bolus trials.

II. Anatomic Landmarks

  A. Lingual surface at midline (coronal and sagittal)

  B. Lingual central groove (coronal) and symmetry

  C. Genioglossus muscle

  D. Floor of mouth musculature (mylohyoid, geniohyoid, anterior belly digastricus)

  E. Palate (coronal or sagittal—may not be visible)

  F. Hyoid (sagittal) and mandibular (sagittal and coronal) shadows

  G. Muscular attachment at hyoid (sagittal)

  H. Oropharynx (sagittal)

  I. Vallecula shadow, upper border of epiglottis

  J. Palate, tonsils, cervical vertebrae in infants and children

  K. Adenoids, upper oropharynx in children

III. Measurement of Swallowing Duration

  A. Made from sagittal view from movement of hyoid bone

  B. Measurement should be made from stop-frame-by-frame analysis with video editor. Measurement begins at the frame when hyoid bone begins to move forward/upward.

  C. The measurement at the end of the swallow is the frame when the hyoid returns to resting position.

  D. The total time is then measured by subtracting the starting time from the ending time. Time at end of movement minus time of initial movement of hyoid bone is equal to the total time of the swallowing event.

IV. Abnormalities

  A. Delayed initiation of swallow

  B. Excessive preparatory gestures of tongue and floor of mouth

  C. Multiple forward-upward motions of the hyoid

  D. Hyoid held at maximum anterior position for extended duration

  E. Multiple swallows to transport bolus

  F. Slow, irregular, jerking motions of hyoid or tongue

  G. Density changes (echogenicity) of musculature

  H. Adipose deposits—connective tissue wasting

  I. Asymmetry of musculature during bolus transport or at rest

  J. Rapid lingual anterior-posterior motion (pumping) or bunching

Table 14–4. *continued*

K. Lingual rigidity or spasms

L. Mid-tongue contractions ("dipping") patterns

M. Lingual dystonia

N. Extraneous lingual-hyoid movements that do not result in swallow

O. Pooling of secretions in the oropharynx

P. Abnormal mastication or bolus lateralization patterns

Q. Multiple swallows for small boluses (3–5 cc)

V. Biofeedback for Swallowing Therapy

A. Tracking bolus transport

B. Tracking and imitation of proper temporal sequences

C. Feedback on effectiveness (safety) of swallow techniques of maneuvers such as laryngeal elevation, effortful swallows, and breath holding.

D. Feedback on increased strength-force of swallow

E. Feedback on lingual-hyoid activity

F. Feedback on bolus viscosity or volume

G. Feedback on positioning effect

H. Feedback on adaptive utensil—feeding system use

Source: From A. L. Perlman (ref. 45) *Dysphagia: A Continuum of Care* (pp. 168–169), B. C. Sonies, ed., 1997, Gaithersburg, Md: Aspen Publishers, Inc. Copyright 1997 by Pro-Ed, Inc. Adapted with permission.

Requesting that the subject hold a small bolus of water or preswallow a bolus of carbonated soda may serve to better differentiate surface margins prior to functional analysis.[2-3] B-mode gain, time compensation gain, and adjustments to depth/focal zone settings may also be modified to ensure clear identification of a hyperechoic lingual surface, homogeneous gray-scale speckle display of the lingual musculature, and connective tissue boundaries.

The lingual surface and mucosal covering should be clearly identified as a broad hyperechoic band which usually appears 4 to 6 cm from the floor of the mouth (Fig 14–1). Posterior angling of the transducer will permit visualization of the acoustic shadow created from the attenuation of the ultrasound signal at the hyoid bone whereas anterior angling visualizes the mandible. The acoustic shadow of the hyoid appears posteriorly as an inverted triangle from the lingual surface margin approximately 45 degrees from midline. The mandibular shadow has a similar acoustic shadow appearance in the anterior region of the image field in the sagittal plane. These landmarks should be used as fiducial markers to track displacements of the tongue and bolus during repeated swallowing tasks.

In this plane the musculature of the tongue is easily distinguished in both resting (Figs 14–1A and 14–1B) and contraction states (Figs 14–1C and 14–1D). These include the intrinsic verticalis and transversus musculature, the genioglossus, geniohyoid, and mylohyoid (see Fig 14–1). Connective tissue such as the fibrous septum can also be seen. Rotation of the transducer 90 degrees from the sagittal placement provides views of the tongue in a longitudinal coronal plane (or also referred as a transverse plane) (Fig 14–2). In this plane, target anatomic markers for tracking function include the lingual surface, the genioglossus, the geniohyoid-mylohyoid complex, the fascia and paramedian septum, and the acoustic shadow of the mandible flanking the ventral margins of the image.[4] Functional observation of bolus holding, lingual propulsion, lingual-palatal contact, tongue tip and dorsum motion, bolus clearance, and hyoid excursion can be evaluated in the sagittal plane (Video 14A). The addition of color-flow or power-flow Doppler

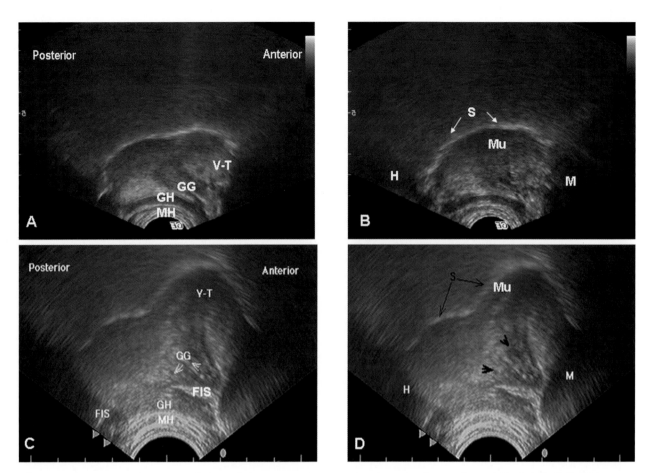

Fig 14–1. Two image sets of the adult tongue in a sagittal scan plane. **A** and **B.** Adult 7.5-MHz sector scans of tongue at rest. Transducer contact is at the bottom of the screen. **C** and **D.** Adult tongue with tongue blade elevated to contact hard palate. 7.0-MHz convex sector scans. Anatomy: V-T (verticalis, transversus), GG (genioglossus), GH (geniohyoid), MH (mylohyoid), FIS (fibrous intermuscular septum). In B and D, the lingual surface (*S* and *arrows*) and mucosal covering should be clearly identified as a broad hyperechoic band which usually appears 4 to 6 cm from the floor of the mouth. The musculature (*Mu*) appears in a darker gray-scale color. The attenuated shadow of the hyoid bone (*H*) and mandible (*M*) are seen as dark triangular regions.

(Fig 14–3) within a gated volume of interest may also allow the clinician to identify lingual vascularization or changes in lingual hemodynamics due to pathology or radiation effects.[5-6]

In the coronal plane, the tongue has a trapezoidal shape with the triangular genioglossus muscle clearly demarcated in the center of the tongue body. The intramuscular septum will appear as a hyperechoic boundary separating the tongue body from the geniohyoid, mylohyoid, and anterior digastric muscles located along the floor of the mouth.[4] This scan plane permits identification of changes to lingual surface deformations during alteration of various bolus volumes and viscosities, the identification of the depth of the central lingual groove during bolus holding and transport, the symmetry and motion of the lateral lingual margins needed to elevate and hold the bolus, and various contraction patterns of the musculature of the floor of the mouth and tongue body (Videos 14B and 14C).

The capability of ultrasound to use non-barium-based foodstuffs provides clinicians the opportunity to evaluate oral phase deglutition skills of actual patient diets throughout an unlimited number of

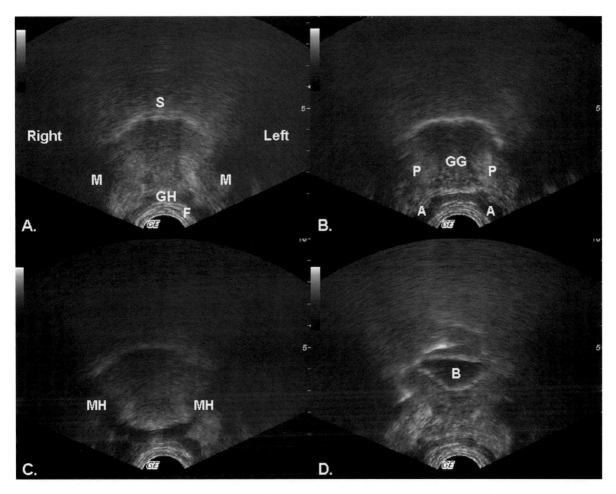

Fig 14–2. Rotation of the transducer 90 degrees from the sagittal placement provides views of the tongue in a longitudinal coronal plane. **A.** Tongue at rest with transducer placement at bottom of image. Anatomy: mandibular acoustic shadows (*M*), dermal layers and fascia (*F*), tongue surface (*S*), geniohyoid (*GH*). **B.** Scaning plane is slightly more posterior than **A.** Anatomy: genioglossus (*GG*), anterior belly digastricus (*A*), paramedian septum (*P*). **C.** Scan plane now shows the sling-shape mylohyoid (*MH*). **D.** Coronal plane with tongue holding a bolus (*B*). Note the contractions of the lateral muscular margins, the change in the configuration of the musculature and the cupping of the bolus along the tongue surface.

swallowing trials (see Table 14–3). The type of bolus, however, may influence sound transmission. Thus added carbonation or thickening agents may permit better visualization of fluid boluses.[2] During each bolus trial, the displacement patterns of the lingual musculature and the timing of swallows can be reviewed through the use of real-time playback of recorded swallowing trials whereas more sophisticated procedures to extract quantitative data on kinematic patterns during swallowing events require the use of image extraction, image processing, and

motion analysis software packages.[7-8] Qualitative information regarding the oral preparatory and oral phases of swallowing, however, can be derived from observations of lingual tissue configurations and hyoid shadow displacements.[9-12] For example, at rest, prior to swallow activity, the acoustic shadow of the hyoid bone created by the attenuated ultrasound signal can be seen as an inverted triangular region in the posterior section of the image plane (Video 14D). The lingual tissues of the tongue body at rest may appear in a forward, flattened posture, or

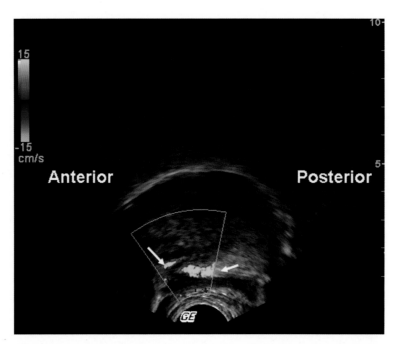

Fig 14–3. The addition of color-flow or power-flow Doppler allows the clinician to identify lingual vascularization or changes in lingual hemodynamics. Adult tongue in sagittal plane with gated volume (*box region*). Color Doppler flow in these regions depicts vascular flow (*arrows*) within the lingual tissues.

in a curved configuration with the posterior dorsum of the tongue body appearing relaxed against the backdrop of an open oropharynx (Fig 14–4). During bolus intake or loading, the anterior lingual structures will cup the bolus into a medial channel created by contractions of the lateral intrinsic musculature. Initial bolus propulsion will begin with a superior and posterior elevation of the anterior lingual segment and simultaneous anterior-posterior excursions by the hyoid shadow. Continued propulsion of the bolus toward the oropharynx is identified by the sequential wavelike deformations of the tongue surface. A maximum anterior-superior displacement of the hyoid shadow occurs at the peak of the swallow as the posterior tongue contacts the palate to propel the bolus into the oropharynx. This displacement represents the important function of laryngeal elevation to assist in airway protection and drive the bolus from the oropharynx into the hypopharynx. The epiglottis may be seen momentarily during the

swallow as an echo-free region posterior to the hyoid shadow. With completion of the oropharyngeal swallow, the tongue body and hyoid shadow descend to original resting postures (see Fig 14–4).

Knowledge of the sonographic changes to lingual tissue configurations and movement patterns of the hyoid shadow during a bolus swallow provides a baseline reference from which to address abnormal or compensatory movements as a result of pathology, structural alteration, or aging. Although some intrasubject variability is expected in both healthy and impaired patient populations,[13] key areas of differentiation between normal and abnormal swallowing patterns can be identified using sonographic imaging. These features include incomplete anterior–superior excursion of the hyoid, spasmodic-dissynchronous and extraneous movements, or a lack of movement as indices of abnormal function. For example, patients with neuromuscular disorders such as postpolio may exhibit slowed, asymmetric

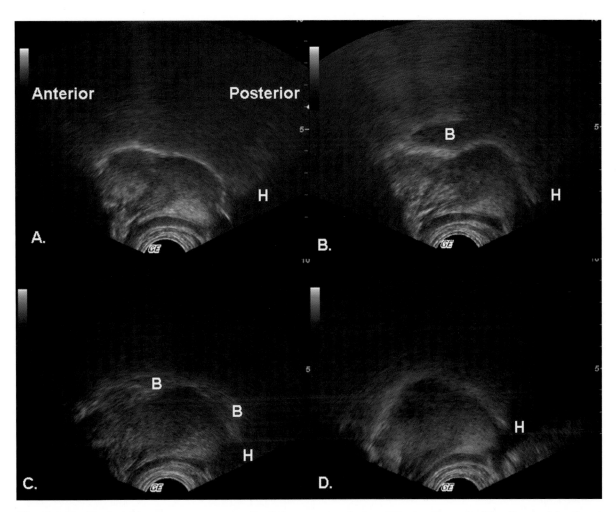

Fig 14–4. Sagittal image sequence of a 10-cc water bolus (*B*) swallow. **A.** The lingual body at rest may appear in forward, flattened posture or curved with the posterior dorsum relaxed against the backdrop of an open oropharynx. **B.** During bolus intake or "loading," the anterior lingual structures will cup the bolus into the medial channel created by contractions of the lateral muscular margins (see 14–20). **C.** Initial bolus propulsion begins with a superior and posterior elevation of the anterior lingual segment. This movement causes a simultaneous anterior and superior excursion by the hyoid shadow (*H*). Continued propulsion of the bolus toward the oropharynx can be seen as sequential wavelike deformations of the tongue surface. **D.** A maximum anterior-superior displacement of the hyoid shadow occurs at the peak of the swallow as the posterior tongue-palate contacts to propel the bolus into the oropharynx. This displacement represents the important function of laryngeal elevation to assist in airway protection and drive the bolus from the oropharynx into the hypopharynx. The epiglottis may be seen momentarily during the swallow as an echo-free region posterior to the hyoid shadow. With completion of the oropharyngeal swallow, the tongue body and hyoid shadow descend to original resting postures.

or compensatory movement patterns in an attempt to initiate lingual movements during a swallow.[14-15] Sustained posterior elevation or bunching of the tongue is typical of Parkinsonian patients, whereas patients with progressive supranuclear palsy exhibit fewer continuous swallows, longer durations to complete swallows, and dystonic movements associated with tremors and fasciculations of the lingual tip, body or base.[16-17] Changes in salivary gland fluid secretion as part of normal aging or as a result of primary Sjögren's syndrome may influence the timing, duration, and degree of hyoid-lingual gestures despite maintenance of the temporal aspects of overall swallowing ability.[18-19] Multiple hyoid gestures and lingual gestures occur prior to completion of a swallow in normal aging populations.[20-21]

Pediatric Applications

B-mode imaging by virtue of its safety and noninvasiveness is well suited for observation of pediatric lingual-hyoid patterns during sucking on the breast or bottle, and during bolus feeding and swallowing.[22-24] The first dynamic applications of ultrasound in pediatrics focused on descriptions of the surface configurations created by the tongue pressing against nipple systems during breast or bottle feeding.[25-26] These studies, conducted with early B-mode imaging systems, identified the key contractions of the lingual musculature required to create the posterior wave of superior-inferior and medial lingual surface displacements during compression of the nipple and the movements of the tongue to propel expressed boluses toward the oropharynx. The lateral margins of the lingual musculature have also been identified sonographically to provide important movements to enclose and channel the bolus.

Today, several ultrasound applications can be used to examine structures of the oral cavity during sucking and swallowing evaluations. The transducer can be placed along the child's cheek to obtain images of lateral compression and elongation of nipple systems by the posterior and vertical motions of the tongue. Submental placement of the transducer provides an image field of the mid-dorsal region of the tongue to observe lingual compression of the nipple against the palate, lingual movements during breast- or bottle-feeding, oral adaptive or compensatory responses to changing feeding systems, and the functionality of lateral margin elevation important for channeling fluids to the oropharynx.

Clinical testing of feeding and swallowing skills can be conducted in both nutritive and non-nutritive sucking contexts. In some instances, the air interface created by pacifier or nipple systems may alter image resolution. However, image adjustment should allow identification of integrated movements of the oropharynx and are optimized through use of pediatric transducers that are of dimensions appropriate to submental placement in infants and small children. These transducers will provide a complete view of the oral cavity from the anterior tongue tip to the superior laryngeal and pharyngeal margins. Velopharyngeal closure necessary to prevent nasal reflux and laryngeal elevation to prevent tracheal penetration are easily observed in these populations. The peristaltic actions of the cervical esophagus also may be viewed in small infants.

To conduct a pediatric evaluation of swallowing, the clinician should identify an appropriate feeding position with input from the caregiver. Submental transducer placement is effective when the child is cradled in the caregiver's arms or when the child is seated in a portable car seat. The clinician, when possible, should be seated in front of the child in order to observe transducer placement and feeding responses. For infants, prepared formula, expressed breast milk, juices, purees, and soft solids can all be tested when the infant is alert and cooperative. Imaging of many swallow trials throughout the entire meal is important to observe the effects of satiation or fatigue on sucking and swallowing patterns. Trials of different foodstuffs, bolus volumes, or adaptive feeding equipment can also be documented for evaluation of clinical effect. In addition, the handling of natural salivary secretions or non-nutritive sucking patterns can be tested with a pacifier when the infant is sleeping provided the clinician's placement of the transducer does not disrupt the child. Similar approaches can be used for young children and toddlers.

Several authors have provided sonographic descriptions of normal versus impaired swallowing skills in specific pediatric populations. Yang, Loveday, Metreweli, and Sullivan reported that malnourished children with oral motor dysfunction due to neurologic impairment demonstrated altered oral and pharyngeal bolus transport across the tongue and through the hypopharyngeal region.[27] Lingual surface patterns during swallowing in children with open-bite demonstrated a tongue thrust motion forming a regional depression in the posterior region. This differed from the central groove produced during normal swallow patterns.[28]

Developmental patterns of tongue movement have been examined in normal children[29] and in children with spastic cerebral palsy.[30-33] These experimental studies showed that children with cerebral palsy demonstrate high variability across swallows. Liquid boluses are often the most difficult to control, due to posterior elevation of the lingual musculature. The timing of the swallow may be abnormal as it may take longer to achieve maximum anterior displacement of the hyoid. In addition, short-latency apnea may be observed during salivary swallows, whereas long-latency apnea may be observed during semisolid or liquid swallows.[33]

Laryngeal Function

Glottic function can be examined using a 5.0- to 7.5-MHz linear-array transducer. The transducer is placed at the level of the thyroid notch and angled slightly until clear depiction of laryngeal anatomy is achieved (Fig 14–5).[34] The general status of the laryngeal region and symmetry patterns during glottic adduction-abduction can be visualized while the patient phonates or hums. Trials during a patient

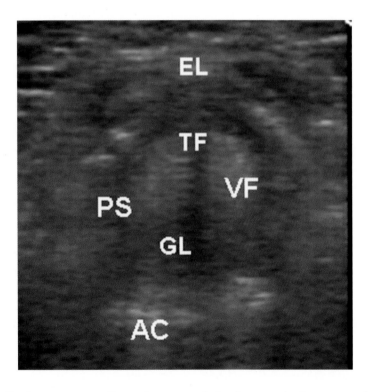

Fig 14–5. A transverse B-mode scan of the larynx during normal breathing using a 5.0- to 7.5-MHz linear-array transducer. The transducer is placed at the level of the thyroid notch and angled slightly until clear depiction of laryngeal anatomy is achieved. The ventricular folds (*VF*), true folds (*TF*), epiglottic ligament (*EL*), piriform sinus (*PS*), glottis (*GL*), and arytenoid cartilage (*AC*) are seen.

cough, throat clear, or production of repeated /k/ consonants provides visual confirmation of vocal fold adductor strength and the patient's ability to protect the airway from entrance of foreign material into the subglottic space (Video 14E). The degree of laryngeal elevation can be measured on the system monitor via the electronic calipers or measured off-line based on the thyrohyoid distance, namely, the distance between the hyoid shadow and the superior margin of the thyroid cartilage.[35] Vocal fold paralysis, asymmetry, laryngeal tumors, and masses should be observed during phonatory and swallowing functional tasks to ascertain degree of impairment, effectiveness of airway protection, and impact on swallowing-phonatory efficiency. Any residue pooled in the laryngeal vestibule detected on the vocal folds or in the valleculae should be noted and patient response recorded. Although material penetrating into the trachea cannot be visualized, inferences can be made regarding the potential threat of aspiration. In addition, laryngeal responses to various therapeutic measures (eg, supraglottic swallow, Mendelsohn maneuver) can be evaluated and the visual information used during patient biofeedback or laryngeal exercise programs.

Duplex B/M-Mode Imaging of Lateral Pharyngeal Wall and Lingual Function

The sequential contraction of the pharyngeal constrictors propels the bolus through the pharynx. Evaluation of these movements can be addressed through a combination of B-mode imaging of the lateral pharyngeal wall tissues and M-M-mode (motion-mode) displays of temporal-spatial displacement patterns of the tissue interfaces during swallowing activity.[36-37] The use of duplex B/M-mode ultrasound permits real-time gray-scale imaging of the anatomy of the pharyngeal wall with simultaneous split-screen images depicting the motion of tissue margins during physiologic movement. In this ultrasound technique an echo reflector along a single line of site is selected within a B-mode gray-scale image. Any tissue movements along this line will be depicted on the M-mode image as concomitant echo traces

from hyperechoic tissue margins within the structure. The vertical axis of the M-mode trace provides a moving representation of soft tissue displacement whereas the horizontal margin represents movement at tissue margins over time (Fig 14-6). Convex sector or linear transducers can be used within a frequency range of 5 to 10 MHz.

Appropriate gain and focus should be selected to allow identification of necessary tissue interface echoes. The sweep speed should be set at minimum to allow sufficient display of contiguous movements. Transducer placements can occur with the subject seated upright. The transducer can be placed at two preferred viewing sites. The first placement provides a beam directed orthogonally to the center of the transducer vertically oriented at the side of the neck. The upper edge of the transducer field should correspond to approximately 1.0 cm below the external auditory canal in an adult patient. The sampling region with this orientation will provide an image display at the level of the superior aspect of the ramus of the mandible and functionally corresponds to the mid-oropharynx. The transducer can then be angled manually a few degrees to obtain images of the base of the tongue in the mid-oropharyngeal region. In this plane of view, the transducer should be slightly angled until clear echoes from the lateral pharyngeal wall are obtained (Fig 14-7). Repetition by the subject of the phonemes /a/ and /i/ can substantiate the adequacy of the lateral wall traces and appropriate transducer orientation.

The displacements of the lateral pharyngeal wall provide information on the integrity of mesial and lateral motions of the pharynx during swallows of various boluses, volumes, or during various postural maneuvers.[36-37] Images recorded in real time to video, disk or hard drive provide the clinician the opportunity for playback review and frame-by-frame analysis of temporal-spatial kinematic patterns of movements within the target region. A similar application of Duplex B/M-mode imaging has been used to identify temporal-spatial patterns of lingual movements during oral bolus swallows.[1] A line of sight can be placed vertically through a selected point of the tongue body and the soft tissue displacements recorded during functional tasks. Several research studies have used this approach to identify complex lingual movement patterns[38] and gender differences.[39]

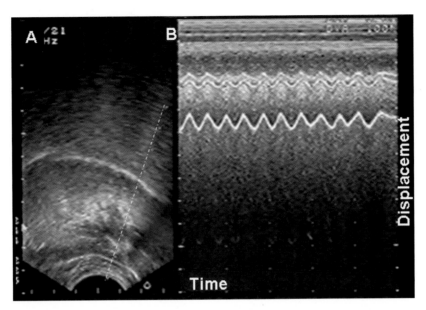

Fig 14–6. B/M-mode image example of tongue movements during rapid movements of the tongue tip. **A.** B-mode image of tongue in sagittal plane. An echo reflector from a single line of sight (*white dashed line*) is selected within the gray-scale image. **B.** Movements along this line are shown as concomitant echo traces (hyperechoic boundaries of tissue margins) within the structure. The vertical axis of the M-mode trace provides a moving representation of soft tissue displacement whereas the horizontal margin represents movement at tissue margins over time.

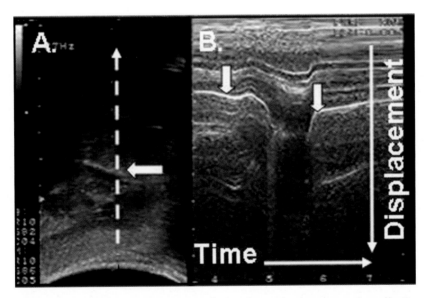

Fig 14–7. B/M-mode image of the lateral pharyngeal wall. **A.** Shows the B-mode image of the lateral wall (*white arrow*) and line of sight (*dashed line*) where motion is depicted in M-mode. **B.** The M-mode trace of movements of tissues along the line of sight. The white echo (*arrows*) indicates the lateral wall displacement (in centimeters) over time (*seconds*).

Real-Time Visualization of Fetal Aerodigestive Tract

The upper aerodigestive tract can also be examined in the fetus using clinical obstetric sonographic systems.[40] Using standard obstetric probes, two-dimensional B-mode ultrasound images from a variety of scan planes can be used to view the fetal face, oral cavity, pharynx, and larynx. More recent three-dimensional imaging systems also provide surface renderings of the fetal facial area (Fig 14–8). In the two-dimensional B-mode plane, specific bony and soft tissue fiducial markers serve as anatomic landmarks for repeated scanning. The fetal face can be observed from a frontal image taken in an axis containing the soft tissues of the nasum and mentum (Fig 14–9A). The transducer is oriented by the sonographer to identify the nose, mouth, and lower facial anatomy. With power Doppler or color Doppler flow imaging superimposed on the nares, fetal ingestive and oral-nasal respiratory-related activity can be observed as the influx or efflux of amniotic fluid.

Rotating the transducer 90 degrees provides a second long-axis view of the oral cavity. The transducer is angled to obtain an image of the level inferior (caudal) to the maxilla producing cross-sectional images of the oral cavity, mandibular rami, tongue, and oropharynx (Fig 14–9B). The presence of distinctive circular hyperechoic signals representing the vertebral bodies confirms the level of the imaging plane and provides views of the buccal (sucking) fat pads and masseter musculature within the buccal mucosa. The emerging tooth buds may be detected as small circular objects seen within the alveolar ridge. The tongue is visualized lying medially within the alveolar ridge and, depending on gestational age, may be observed in real time to thrust forward, cup, or produce anterior-posterior sucking motions.[41–42] A hypoechoic midline region represents the median raphe whereas the uvula may be seen in cross-section as a circular object adjacent to the posterior aspect of the tongue. A "D"-shaped anechoic region posterior to the tongue represents the upper pharynx in transverse view. The use of a transaxial image plane of the oropharynx has been useful in studying lingual movements and oropharyngeal contraction patterns.[40,42] A longitudinal coronal imaging plane (Fig 14–9C) along the posterior aspect of the neck will identify the central loca-

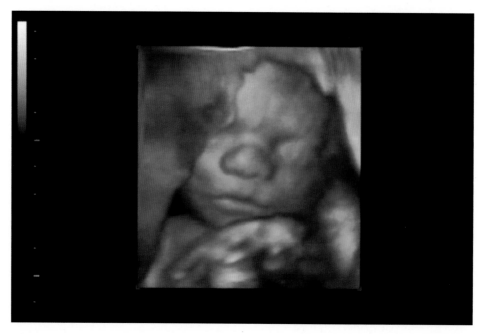

Fig 14–8. Example of a three-dimensional surface rendering of the fetal facial area.

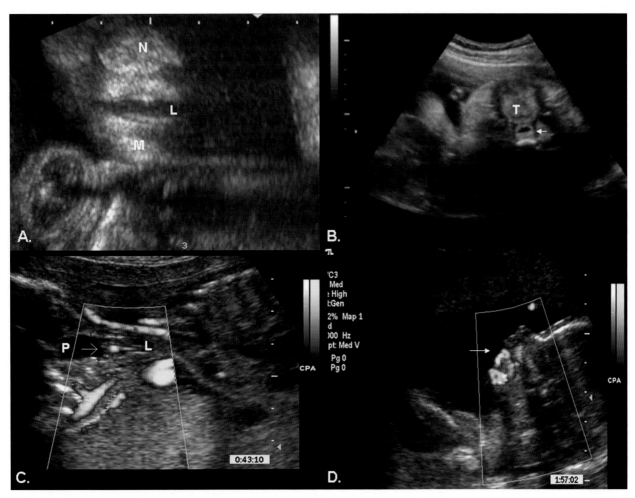

Fig 14–9. A. The fetal face can be observed from a frontal image taken in an axis containing the soft tissues of the nasum and mentum. The transducer is oriented by the sonographer to identify the nose (N), mouth (M), lips (L), and lower facial anatomy. **B.** Rotating the transducer 90 degrees provides long-axis cross-sectional images of the oral cavity, mandibular rami, tongue, and oropharynx. The tongue (T) is visualized lying medially within the alveolar ridge. A hypoechoic midline region represents the upper oropharynx (arrows) in transverse view. **C.** The transducer is angled to obtain an image of the level inferior (caudal) to the maxilla along the posterior aspect of the neck will identify the central location of the pharynx (P) and larynx (L) within soft tissues adjacent to the anterior aspect of the cervical spine. The thin white arrow depicts Power Doppler detected amniotic fluid within the pharyngeal space. Carotid artery flow identified by power-flow Doppler is seen lateral to the activity in the pharyngeal/laryngeal area. **D.** A parasagittal view of the fetal profile allows observation of amniotic fluid flow (*arrow*) in and out of the oral cavity during ingestion.

tion of the pharynx and larynx within soft tissues adjacent to the anterior aspect of the cervical spine. This plane is acquired by centering the transducer transversely on the third cervical vertebra, then rotating the transducer ninety degrees. Activating color flow or power Doppler assists in locating the pulsing coplanar carotid arteries ventral to the

medial pharynx and larynx. In this plane, the epiglottis can be seen extending into the pharyngeal lumen as a small arcuate projection at the base of the tongue, whereas bilateral piriform recesses can be seen at the inferior ventral aspects of the pharynx. The larynx is delimited by the presence of amniotic fluid extending into the cervical trachea.

The laryngeal additus is seen as an echogenic structure central to the piriform recesses. The thin echoic interfaces of the inner margins of the lateral pharyngeal walls in this plane are well defined in fetuses prior to 32 weeks when the pharynx is relaxed and therefore fluid-filled. This permits real-time observation of pharyngeal contraction patterns and changes to pharyngeal dimensions when in distended fluid-filled states.[40-42] A final transducer orientation is obtained by bringing the transducer forward and translating an additional 90 degrees to permit a parasagittal view of the fetal profile (Fig 14-9D). This plane allows observations of amniotic fluid flow during ingestion or respiration.

Ultrasound Use During Evaluation of Sleep Apnea

Ultrasound has been used to monitor oral behaviors during sleep in persons suffering from obstructive sleep apnea.[43] When paired with polysomnography to record sleep waves, ultrasound imaging allowed visualization of lingual activity during sleep and wakefulness. This pilot study demonstrated that shortly after an apneic episode the tongue elevated and moved posteriorly to produce a swallowlike gesture which ended the apnea possibly by opening the airway. Thus, it appears that ultrasound can be used to monitor oropharyngeal activity during sleep as well as during wakefulness.

Summary

Ultrasound is easy to use to image the oropharynx during swallowing and oral motor maneuvers, and can also be applied to the study of tongue motions in speech and to viewing the larynx during swallowing and phonation.[44-45] It is a technique that can be applied to subjects of all ages, from fetus to infant to adult, for evaluation of a wide variety of neuromuscular conditions and oral and pharyngeal tumors, and to obtain noninvasive, real-time dynamic views of the many functions of the upper aerodigestive system.

Videos in This Chapter

Video 14A. Sagittal plane anatomic markers for tracking function include the lingual surface, the genioglossus, the geniohyoid-mylohyoid complex, the fascia and paramedian septum, and the acoustic shadow of the mandible flanking the ventral margins of the image. Functional observation of bolus holding, lingual propulsion, lingual-palatal contact, tongue tip and dorsum motion, bolus clearance, and hyoid excursion can be evaluated in the sagittal plane.

Videos 14B and 14C. B. B-mode scanning through the tongue body. In the coronal plane, the tongue has a trapezoidal shape with the triangular genioglossus muscle clearly demarcated in the center of the tongue body. The intramuscular septum will appear as a hyperechoic boundary separating the tongue body from the geniohyoid, mylohyoid, and anterior digastric muscles located along the floor of the mouth. **C.** This scan plane permits identification of changes to lingual surface deformations during alteration of various bolus volumes and viscosities (as a round echoic region on the mid-surface of tongue), the identification of the depth of the central lingual groove during bolus holding and transport, the symmetry and motion of the lateral lingual margins needed to elevate and hold the bolus, and various contraction patterns of the musculature of the floor of the mouth and tongue body as the bolus is swallowed.

Video 14D. Lingual tissue configurations and hyoid shadow displacements during swallow activity. The acoustic shadow of the hyoid bone created by the attenuated ultrasound signal can be seen as an inverted triangular region in the posterior section of the image plane. The patterns of displacement and propulsion can thus be observed during various swallow trials. During bolus intake or loading, the anterior lingual structures will cup the bolus into a medial channel created by contractions of the lateral intrinsic musculature. Initial bolus propulsion will begin with a superior and posterior elevation of the anterior lingual segment and simultaneous anterior-posterior excursions by the hyoid shadow. Continued propulsion of the bolus toward the oropharynx is identified by the sequential wavelike deformations of the tongue surface. A maximum anterior-superior displacement of the hyoid shadow occurs at the peak of the swallow as the posterior tongue contacts the palate to propel the bolus into the oropharynx. This displacement represents the important function of laryngeal elevation to assist in airway protection and drive the bolus from the oropharynx into the hypopharynx.

Video 14E. Video demonstration of laryngeal imaging. The general status of the laryngeal region and symmetry patterns during glottic adduction-abduction can be visualized while the patient phonates or produces repeated /k/ consonants. Additional observations of coughs or throat clears provide visual confirmation of vocal fold adductor strength and the patient's ability to protect the airway from entrance of foreign material into the subglottic space.

References

1. Peng CL, Jost-Brinkmann PG, Miethke RR. The cushion scanning technique: a method of dynamic tongue sonography and its comparison with the transducer–skin coupling scanning technique during swallowing. *Acad Radiol.* 1996;3:239–244.

2. Casas MJ, Seo AH, Kenny DJ. Sonographic examination of the oral phase of swallowing: bolus image enhancement. *J Clin Ultrasound.* 2002;30(2): 83–87.

3. Epstein MA, Stone M. The tongue stops here: ultrasound imaging of the palate (Letter). *JASA.* 2005; 118(4):2128–2131.

4. Shawker TH, Sonies BC, Stone M. Soft tissue anatomy of the tongue and floor of the mouth: an ultrasound demonstration. *Brain Lang.* 1984;21: 335–350.

5. Miller JL, Watkin KL. Color flow Doppler US of lingual vascularization in postoperative oral cancer subjects. *Dysphagia.* 1997;2:114.

6. Miller JL, Watkin KL. Color flow Doppler ultrasound of lingual hemodynamics: a preliminary study. *Dysphagia.* 1996;11:158.

7. Chi-Fishman G, Sonies BC. Effects of systematic bolus viscosity and volume changes on hyoid movement kinematics. *Dysphagia.* 2002A;17:278–287.

8. Chi-Fishman G, Sonies BC. Kinematic strategies for hyoid movement in rapid sequential swallowing. *J Speech Lang Hearing Res.* 2002B;45:457–468.

9. Stone M, Shawker T. An ultrasound examination of tongue movement during swallowing. *Dysphagia.* 1986;1:78–83.

10. Sonies BC, Parent L, Morrish K, Baum BJ. Durational aspects of the oral-pharyngeal swallow in normal adults. *Dysphagia.* 1998;3:1–10.

11. Sonies BC, Wang C, Sapper DJ. Evaluation of normal and abnormal hyoid bone movement during swallowing by use of ultrasound duplex-Doppler imaging. *Ultrasound Med Biol.* 1996;22:1169–1175.

12. Chi-Fishman G, Stone M, & McCall GN. Lingual action in normal sequential swallowing. *J Speech Lang Hear Res,* 1998;41:771–785.

13. Soder N, Miller N. Using ultrasound to investigate intrapersonal variability in durational aspects of tongue movement during swallowing. *Dysphagia.* 2002;17(4):288–297.

14. Sonies BC, Dalakas MC. Dysphagia in patients with post-polio syndrome. *N Engl J Med.* 1991;324: 1162–1167.

15. Sonies BC, Dalakas MC. Progression of oral-motor and swallowing symptoms in post-polio syndrome. *Ann NY Acad Sci.* 1995;753:87–95.

16. Sonies BC. Speech and swallowing disturbances. In Litvan I, Agid Y, eds. *Progressive Supranuclear Palsy.* New York, NY: Oxford University Press; 1992:240–253.

17. Litvan I, Sastry N, Sonies BC. Characterizing swallowing abnormalities in progressive supranuclear palsy. *Neurology.* 48(6):1654–1662.

18. Caruso AJ, Sonies BC, Atkinson JS, Fox PC. Objective measures of swallowing in patients with primary Sjögren's syndrome. *Dysphagia.* 1989;4:101–105.

19. Sonies BC, Ship JA, Baum J. Relationship between saliva production and oropharyngeal swallow in healthy, different-aged adults. *Dysphagia.* 1989; 4(2):85–89.

20. Sonies BC, Parent L, Morrish K, Baum BJ. Durational aspects of the oropharyngeal swallow in normal adults. *Dysphagia.* 1998;31–40.

21. Sonies BC, Stone M, Shawker T. Speech and swallowing in the elderly. *J Gerontol.* 1984;3:115–123.

22. Bosma JF, Hepburn LG, Josell SD, Baker K. Ultrasound demonstration of tongue motions during suckle feeding. *Dev Med Child Neurol.* 1990;32:223–229.

23. Bullock F, Woolridge MW, Baum J D. Development of co-ordination of sucking, swallowing and breathing: ultrasound study of term and preterm infants. *Dev Med Child Neurol.* 1990;32:669–678.

24. Weber F, Woolridge MW, and Baum J D. An ultrasonographic study of the organization of sucking and swallowing by newborn infants. *Dev Med Child Neurol.* 1986;28:19–24.

25. Nowak AJ, Smith WL, Erenberg A. Imaging evaluation of breast-feeding and bottle-feeding. *J Pediatr.* 1995;126:S130–S134.

26. Smith WL, Erenberg A, Nowak A. Imaging evaluation of the human nipple during breast-feeding. *Am J Dis Child.* 1998;42:76–78.

27. Yang WT, Loveday EJ, Metreweli C, Sullivan PB. Ultrasound assessment of swallowing in malnourished disabled children. *Br J Radiol.* 1997;70(838):992–994.

28. Kikyo T, Saito M, Ishikawa M. (1999). A study comparing ultrasound images of tongue movement between open bite children and normal children in the early mixed dentition period. *J Med Dent Sci.* 1999;46(3):127–137.

29. Ayano R, Tamura F, Ohtsuka Y, Mukai Y. The development of normal feeding and swallowing: Showa University study of the feeding function. *Int J Orofacial Myology.* 2000;(36):24–32.

30. Casas MJ, McPherson KA, Kenny DJ. Durational aspects of oral swallow in neurologically normal children and children with cerebral palsy—an ultrasound investigation. *Dysphagia.* 1995;10:155–159.

31. Casas MJ, Kenny DJ, McPherson K. Swallowing/ventilation interactions during oral swallow in normal children and children with cerebral palsy. *Dysphagia.* 1994;9:140–146.

32. Wein B, Bockler R, Klajman S. Temporal reconstruction of sonographic imaging of disturbed tongue movements. *Dysphagia.* 1991;6:135–139.

33. Kenny DJ, Casas MJ, McPherson KA. Correlation of ultrasound imaging of oral swallow with ventilatory alterations in cerebral palsied and normal children: preliminary observations. *Dysphagia.* 1989;4:112–117.

34. Sonies BC. Instrumental procedures for dysphagia diagnosis. *Sem Speech Lang.* 1991;12(3):185–198.

35. Kuhl V, Eicke BM, Dieterich M, Urban PP. Sonographic analysis of laryngeal elevation during swallowing. *J Neurol.* 2003;250(3):333–337.

36. Miller JL, Watkin KL. Lateral pharyngeal wall motion during swallowing using real time ultrasound. *Dysphagia.* 1997;12:125–132.

37. Watkin KL, Miller JL. Lateral pharyngeal wall motion during swallowing: analysis of B/M-mode ultrasound imaging. *Dysphagia.* 1996;11:161.

38. Peng CL, Jost-Brinkmann PG, Yoshida N, Miethke RR, Lin CT. Differential diagnosis between infantile and mature swallowing with ultrasonography. *Eur J Orthod.* 2003;25(5):451–456.

39. Peng, CL, Lin CT, Jost-Brinkmann PG, Miethke RR. Comparison of tongue functions during swallowing between females and males. *J Dental Res.* 1997;76:1218.

40. Macedonia C, Miller JL, Sonies BC. Power Doppler imaging of the fetal upper aerodigestive tract: a four-point standardized evaluation. *J Ultrasound Med.* 2002;21:869–878.

41. Miller JL, Macedonia C, Sonies BC. A gender-comparison of the developing fetal upper airway and oral-facial systems: are there prenatal differences in emerging oral-motor behaviors? *Dev Med Child Neurol.* In press.

42. Miller JL, Sonies BC, Macedonia C. Emergence of oropharyngeal, laryngeal, and swallowing activity in the developing fetal upper aerodigestive tract: an ultrasound evaluation. *Early Hum Dev.* 2000;71(1):61–87.

43. Siegel H, Sonies BC, Graham B, McCutchen C, et al. Obstructive sleep apnea: a study by simultaneous polysomnography and ultrasonic imaging. *Neurology.* 2000;54(9):1872.

44. Sonies BC, Chi-Fishman G, Miller JL. Ultrasound imaging and swallowing. In: B. Jones, ed. *Normal and Abnormal Swallowing Imaging in Diagnosis and Therapy.* 2nd ed. New York, NY: Springer-Verlag, Inc; 2003:119–138.

45. Perlman AL. Application of instrumental procedures to the evaluation and treatment of dysphagia. In Sonies BC, ed. *Dysphagia: A Continuum of Care.* Gaithersburg, Md: Aspen Publishers, Inc; 1997:168–169.

Chapter 15

ULTRASOUND SURVEILLANCE FOR HEAD AND NECK CANCER

Michiel W. M. van den Brekel

Jonas A. Castelijns

Introduction

Lymphatic metastasis is the most important prognostic indicator for head and neck cancer.[1,2] Not only the presence, but also the number of nodal metastases, the level in the neck, the size of the nodes, and presence of extranodal spread (ENS) are important prognostic features. The incidence of distant metastases, survival, and locoregional tumor control are dependent on the status of the cervical lymph nodes. De Bree et al[3] have shown that in patients with 3 or more nodal metastases, bilateral or low jugular lymph node metastases, large lymph node metastases ($\geq$ 6 cm) or second primary malignancies, a search for distant metastases, based on a high risk, is warranted. In a recent study by Ljumanovic, MRI characteristics of lymph node metastases were evaluated for their predictive value for the development of distant metastases. In the multivariate analysis, ENS as diagnosed on MRI was the only independent predictor for distant metastasis.[4]

Not only in mucosal squamous cell carcinoma, but also in melanoma and nonmelanoma skin cancer as well as in salivary gland cancer do lymph node metastases predict survival.[5-7] On the other hand, whereas neck node metastases increase the risk of locoregional recurrences, in well-differentiated thyroid carcinoma the influence on survival is limited.[8,9] Because of the lower incidence of occult metastases and disputable prognostic impact of elective treatment in these tumors, elective neck dissection is not routine practice in salivary gland, skin and papillary thyroid carcinoma.[10-13] Imaging can thus play a role in detecting occult metastases in an early stage, which might, but is not proven to, be beneficial for survival.

Any patient with a known primary malignancy in the head and neck region without palpable metastases is at risk of harboring occult metastasis. This risk is to a large extent dependent on the size and site and other characteristics of the primary tumor. For many head and neck primary malignancies not only the ipsilateral neck is at risk but the contralateral neck has a significant risk to harbor metastases as well, especially when the primary has grown close to or extends across the midline. In a neck without palpable nodes, imaging can help in detecting occult metastases leading to appropriate treatment or diminishing the risk of delayed metastases. Negative imaging results can be used as an argument to refrain from elective treatment of the neck.[14-19] In many studies, a risk below 20% is considered to be low enough for a wait-and-see policy, although this cutoff point is very arbitrary. In most studies, CT, MRI, and PET have not yielded sufficient accuracies to be used routinely to exclude metastases and refrain from elective neck treatment.[20-23] As a consequence most patients with nonglottic, infiltrating tumors undergo some form of elective neck treatment. Disadvantages of this policy are costs, overtreatment, and morbidity for the majority of the patients.

Ultrasonography (US) of the Neck

In many countries US is widely and routinely used to assess lymph node metastases in the neck for initial evaluation and follow-up of patients with known primary head and neck carcinomas. Improvements in US transducers and processing computers have tremendously increased the quality of the images, the details depicted, and the ease of US scanning. As the US images are not very easy to interpret in retrospect, unlike in CT or MRI, it is crucial that the ultrasonographer is well trained and aware of the clinical questions, known patterns of metastases, and limitations of the examination. Furthermore, the corresponding report should be quite detailed describing not only the level and measurements of the lymph nodes but also other characteristics important for discriminating metastatic from reactively enlarged lymph nodes. This is especially important if US is used during follow-up.

In general, US is reported to be superior to palpation in detecting lymph node metastases.[24,25] Whereas some authors report US to be superior to contrast-enhanced CT and MRI,[26] others have found similar accuracies.[27,28] Advantages of US over other imaging techniques include its low price, lack of radiation, and low patient burden. Furthermore, US is the only available imaging technique that can be used for frequent routine follow-up. It is important to realize that none of the currently available imaging techniques are able to depict small tumor deposits like micrometastases inside lymph nodes. As the incidence of exclusively micrometastases in clinically N0 necks with occult metastases is over 25%, no imaging technique can ever reach a sensitivity over 75% without losing a high specificity.[29] In melanoma, the incidence of micrometastases is even higher (over 60% of all metastases), and the sensitivity of imaging will thus be lower.[30,31]

In the following sections, the criteria for metastases, and the indications and applicability of US are discussed.

US Criteria for Metastases

The accuracy of US for neck node metastases is to a great extent determined by the criteria used.[32,33] Using US, nodal metastases are diagnosed on the basis of size, shape, presence of irregularities within lymph nodes caused by tumor and tumor necrosis, and extranodal tumor spread. The characteristics of metastatic lymph nodes that can be depicted are increased size, a rounder shape, absence of a hilum, widening of the cortex, irregular reflection patterns, high or low echogeneity, unsharp borders, and an irregular shape (Figs 15–1 through 15–4). As a consequence, the US report should describe the exact location (level), size (minimal and maximal diameter),

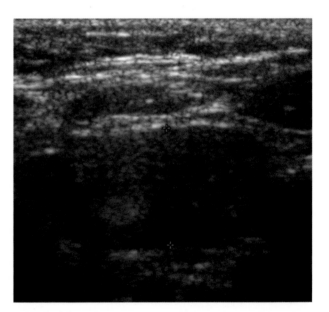

Fig 15–1. US, using a 7.5-MHz transducer. The lymph node clearly has a heterogeneous reflection pattern, suggestive of metastasis. Histopathology confirmed the presence of a metastasis. Unfortunately, this US pattern is rarely seen in small lymph node metastases.

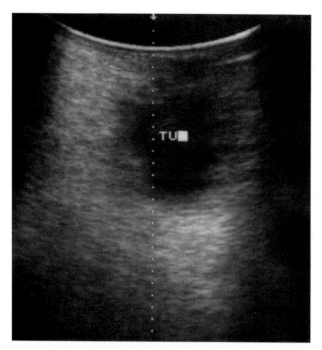

Fig 15–2. Lymph node that is not sharply delineated, suspicious of a metastasis. Indeed this proved to be a metastatic lymph node.

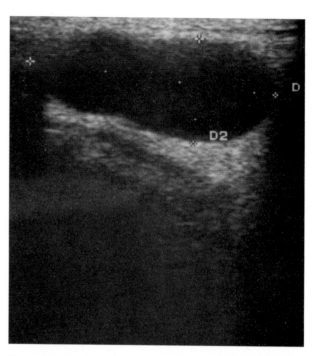

Fig 15–3. Anechogenic lymph node with an oval shape that is clearly demarcated. This is a difficult lymph node to judge. Metastases can be anechogenic and in these cases the size is probably the most useful sign. This proved to be a reactively enlarged lymph node.

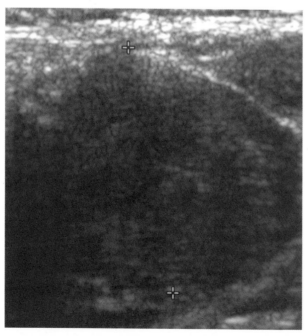

Fig 15–4. Lymph node of 18 mm with slight irregularities in reflection pattern and not very well demarcated toward the surrounding tissue. This most likely is a metastasis.

shape, reflection pattern (anechogenic, irregular, echogenic), presence of cortical widening, presence of a hilum, and sharpness of the borders.

In the literature, there is no consensus on what nodal size should be considered pathologic. Criteria vary from as high as 15 mm down to 8 mm (Table 15-1). Most studies defined and studied the size criteria in patient populations with the majority of patients having large palpable lymph node metastases. As a consequence, in these series a large cutoff point still renders a high sensitivity and the criteria are not valid in clinically N0 populations. A major problem of using the size criterion is that the smaller the cutoff point is defined, the higher the sensitivity, but the lower the specificity (Table 15-2). Wang also reported this and found that using a minimal axial diameter of 8 mm showed the highest accuracy (73%) with 45% sensitivity and 93% specificity.[34]

Several studies have tried to define criteria by evaluating nodal size and shape and the histopathologic outcome in neck dissection specimens.[33,35-37] Friedman et al[37] studied the maximal axial diameter and defined a cutoff point of 1 cm. By comparing three lymph node diameters from three axes we and others found that the minimal axial diameter is a better criterion than the more widely used maximal axial diameter or the longitudinal diameter.[33,34,38]

Table 15–1. Examples of Criteria for Metastases by Several Authors

Author	Criteria
Stern[39]	15 mm all levels
Som[32]	15 mm levels I, II 10 mm levels III–V
Mancuso[40]	15 mm all levels 3 or more 8 to 15 mm
Friedman[41]	10 mm all levels
Steinkamp[42]	8 mm (max. ax.) and L / T <2 or 8 mm (min. ax.)
Vassallo[26]	L / T <2 or absence of hilus or focal cortical widening
van den Brekel[33]	11 mm level II (min. ax.) 10 mm elsewhere (min. ax.) 3 or more 8 to 10 mm (min. ax.)

L/T = longitudinal/transverse diameter

Table 15–2. Comparison of Sensitivity and Specificity for Metastases for Various Lymph Node Size Criteria

Minimal Diameter*	Sensitivity	Specificity
4 mm	90%	33%
5 mm	86%	44%
6 mm	80%	59%
7 mm	61%	76%
8 mm	41%	84%
9 mm	27%	95%

When the size criterion for metastases is larger, the sensitivity drops, whereas the specificity rises. It is very difficult to define an optimal criterion from these figures.

*The cutoff point for lymph nodes in Level II was 1 mm larger than for the other levels of the neck.[43]

Don et al[35] found that 68 of 102 (67%) metastatic nodes had a longitudinal diameter smaller than 1 cm, whereas in our study the number was 48 of 144 (33%). For the minimal or smallest axial diameter we even found that 102 of 144 (71%) are smaller than 1 cm. As a consequence, the current size criterion of 1 cm or larger misinterprets the majority of all metastases.

In a previous study on the size of lymph nodes in different levels, as measured with US in clinically negative neck sides, we found that a criterion of 1 cm rendered a very low sensitivity[43] (see Table 15-2). We also found that the sizes of lymph nodes varied considerably in different lymph node levels. In fact, the size criterion should thus be different in different levels of the neck. In the palpably N0 neck, for level 2 a criterion of 7 mm for the minimal diameter renders the best accuracy, whereas for the rest of the neck, lymph nodes with a minimal diameter of 6 mm should be considered suspicious.

A round nodal shape is considered more suspicious than an oval or flat shape (Figs 15-4 and 15-5).[44] As the minimal diameter is the same as the maximal diameter in round lymph nodes, this explains that the minimal diameter is more reliable than the maximal. In reactively enlarged lymph nodes, the ratio of the longest diameter over the shortest diameter is 2:1 or higher in 86% of cases[45] (Figs 15-5 and 15-6). Perhaps even better is mea-

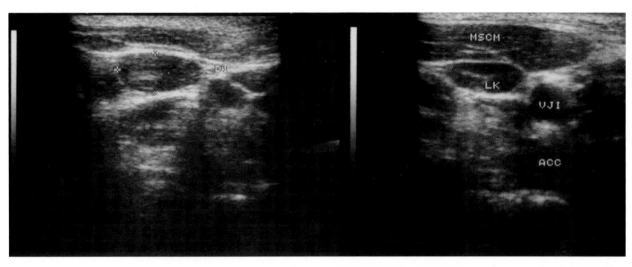

Fig 15–5. Typical reactively enlarged lymph nodes with an oval shape and a hilum of fat depicted.

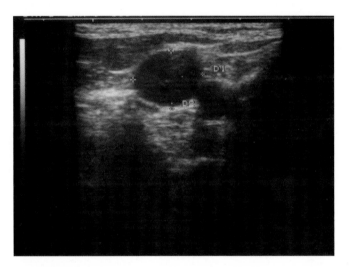

Fig 15–6. A round lymph node of 9 mm, suggestive of a metastasis. However, often lymph nodes smaller than 6 to 7 mm are round rather than oval. This indeed was a metastasis.

suring the axial surface area. In a study by Umeda et al, a surface area of 45 mm^2 correlated better with histopathology than using a minimal or maximal axial diameter.[46]

From these studies, we can conclude that size and shape criteria are always hampered by either a low sensitivity or a low specificity. Thus, apart from size, additional criteria are necessary to increase the accuracy of metastatic node detection. These criteria can be either US characteristics or cytologic features found in US-guided aspiration cytology (US-FNAC). The advantage of cytology is that false positives are extremely rare and the specificity is very high (almost 100%). During follow-up, a very important feature suggestive of metastasis is an increase in size with time. To document such change, US characteristics of lymph nodes should be reported and categorized meticulously.[47]

Apart from size and shape, the US reflection patterns can help in diagnosing metastatic lymph nodes (Figs 15-7 and 15-8). Hypoechogenic (hypoechoic)

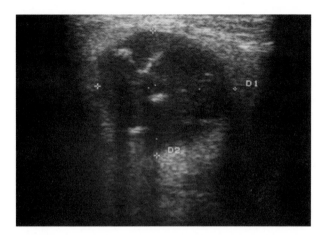

Fig 15–7. Lymph node with irregular reflections suggestive of calcifications. These can be seen sometimes after radiotherapy, in tuberculous lymph nodes or metastases from thyroid cancer.

or anechogenic (anechoic) lymph nodes, lymph nodes without a hilum, or lymph nodes with a very irregular reflection pattern are more suspicious. Morphologic criteria, such as focal cortical widening or depiction of small tumor areas or necrotic areas inside a lymph node, have become more important as the contrast and spatial resolution of imaging techniques has increased, a concept that was predicted even years ago.[48] However, these criteria involving reflection patterns are not always reliable (Figs 15-9 and 15-10). Shin, in a study of axillary lymph nodes, found that using nodal shape, hypoechogenicity, absence of a hilum and focal cortical widening had a reasonable sensitivity (70%) and high specificity (93%) in diagnosing metastases in sentinel lymph nodes.[49] Yusa defined an equation using the minimal diameter, irregular internal echo pattern and absence of a hilum and found very high values for sensitivity (82%) and specificity (91%) in selected lymph nodes, not only from clinically N0 patients.[38] Lee[50] showed that internal echogenicity is more reliable than lymph node size but the two

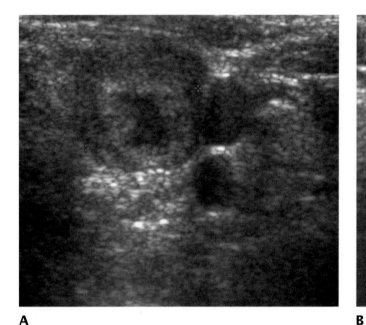

A

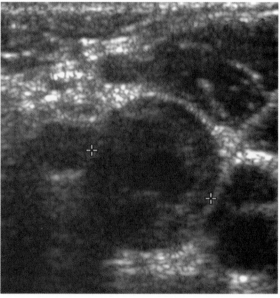

B

Fig 15–8. Although the minimal axial diameter is the most relevant and objective parameter in predicting malignancy in lymph nodes, intranodal reflection patterns can be important as well. In lymph nodes larger than 1 cm the presence of intranodal cystic necrosis, as shown in these two US images, may also be indicative of metastasis. Unfortunately, this feature is rarely seen in lymph nodes under 1 cm.

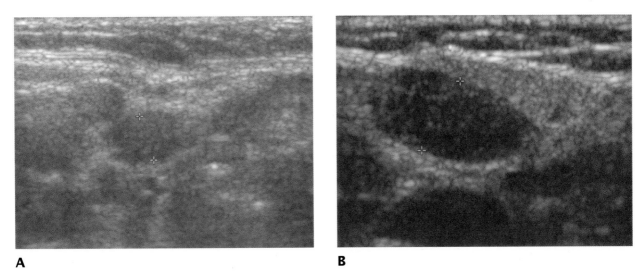

Fig 15–9. Patient with a T2N0 supraglottic carcinoma. **A.** A level 2 lymph node, minimal diameter of 5 mm, homogeneous. At US-FNAC the cytology was negative for malignancy. **B.** A right level 2 lymph node, 6 mm and also homogeneous, somewhat less echogenic that proved to be a metastasis. These figures show how difficult it is to interpret echogenicity reliably.

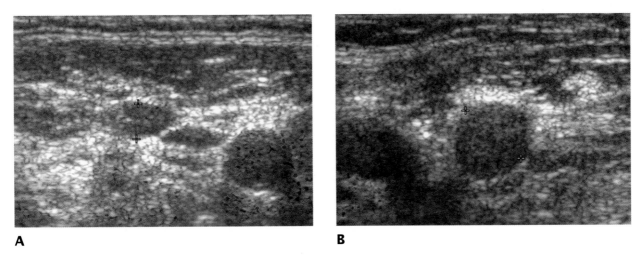

Fig 15–10. Example showing the unreliability of the morphologic US criteria. This patient clinically had a left-sided T3N0 tonsil carcinoma. The lymph node in the figure on the left (**A**) of 6 mm with a hilum within the left neck, level 2, was tumor positive at cytology whereas the lymph node in the figure on the right (**B**) with a round shape, measuring 9 mm in level 3 and without a hilum from the right neck was tumor negative.

criteria should be used in conjunction. In contrast to squamous metastases, hyperechogenicity and punctate calcification are typical features for metastatic nodes from papillary or medullary carcinoma of the thyroid[51] (see Fig 15-7).

An important feature of metastatic lymph nodes is tumor necrosis as this is a very specific criterion for lymph node metastases. Unfortunately, this criterion is quite rare in small lymph node metastases.[36] Therefore, necrosis hardly contributes to the overall accuracy of imaging in studies concerning the clinically negative neck.[52] Curtin[36] and Yousem[53] found that CT is more sensitive and accurate than MRI in depicting nodal necrosis. King[54] studied the accuracy of CT, MRI, and US in detecting necrosis and found that US has a significantly lower sensitivity (77%) than CT (91%) and MRI (89%). None of the modalities studied could detect areas smaller than 3 mm. As a consequence, although specific, it is not very useful in small lymph node metastases. On the other hand, apart from being a criterion, it is also important for prognostication and prediction of treatment response. In general, lymph nodes with major necrosis are less likely to be cured with radiotherapy.[55] Indeed, Dietz has shown that diminished vascularity in lymph nodes as shown with duplex Doppler is a poor predictive sign for patients treated with chemoradiation.[56]

Another technique to increase the accuracy of gray-scale US is to add duplex Doppler and spectral Doppler criteria (Fig 15–11). This technique enables the visualization of irregularities in vascularization.[57-59] Doppler US criteria for lymph node metastases are an avascular pattern, a subcapsular/peripheral vessel pattern, a scattered pattern of vessels (parenchymal), focal defects in vascularity, and absence of hilar vessels. Doppler criteria have been reported to be more accurate than gray-scale criteria.[58] Using spectral Doppler, the metastatic lymph nodes have a higher vascular resistance and a high pulsatility index.[51] Unfortunately, these patterns and spectral changes are seldom visible in lymph nodes smaller than 1 cm where these additional criteria would be most useful. A combination of morphologic, size, and Doppler criteria might be optimal. Wang found that combined criteria of the minimal axial diameter larger than 8 mm together with spotted or peripheral vascular pattern revealed an accuracy of 82%, a sensitivity of 77% and specificity of 86%.[34] Also, Ariji found that combining parenchymal vascular pattern

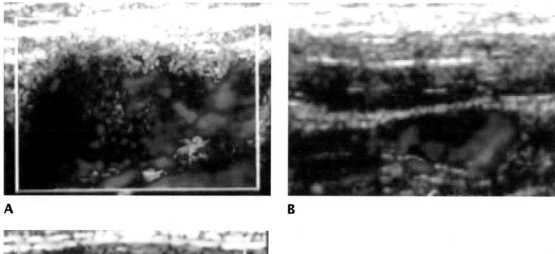

Fig 15–11. Color power Doppler US criteria for detecting metastatic lymph nodes, as suggested in the literature, are a focal perfusion defect (**A**), a scattered pattern (**B**), and a subcapsular or peripheral pattern (**C**).

and transverse to longitudinal size ratio increased the accuracy (sensitivity 92%, specificity 100%).[60] Chikui and Chang, on the other hand, found no advantage in adding color Doppler criteria to minimal axial diameter and hilar absence.[61,62]

The value of contrast-enhanced ultrasound needs to be assessed further. After the administration of Levovist® (galactose-palmitic acid ultrasound contrast agent, Berlex, Canada), lymph nodes reveal more vascular detail than before the administration of Levovist®.

US-Guided FNAC

To overcome the disadvantages of morphologic US criteria, US-guided aspiration cytology can be used (Fig 15–12). Although the technique is not difficult, considerable training is required to aspirate from lymph nodes as small as 4 to 5 mm and still obtain sufficient cells,[63,64] and to select the most suspicious lymph nodes from which to aspirate. The major

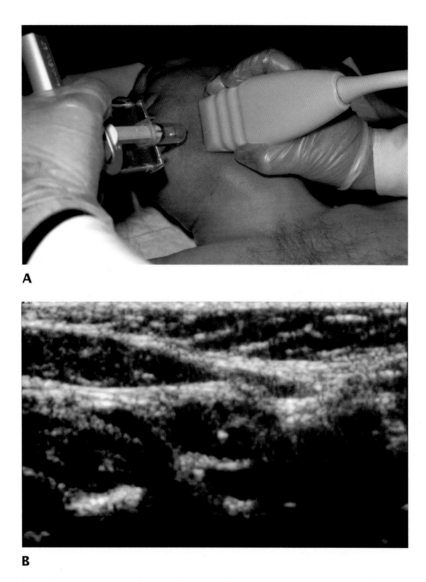

A

B

Fig 15–12. US-FNAC procedure. The needle can be introduced in line with the linear transducer (short-axis technique), or just opposite to it (long-axis technique), as shown in this figure. At US the needle tip can be seen as it moves inside the lymph node. **Video 15A** demonstrates the US-FNAC procedure in real time.

advantage of using cytologic criteria is that false positive cytology of lymph node aspirates is extremely rare. As a consequence, the specificity of US-FNAC is always in the order of 100% in the nonirradiated neck. The disadvantage of using US-FNAC is that the reliability of this modality becomes even more dependent on the ultrasonographer as well as the cytopathologist and it is an invasive modality with potential discomfort to the patient. This is especially the case if repeated examinations are being conducted during follow-up.

The choice of the lymph node to be aspirated is crucial, and so is the aspiration technique. A high sensitivity can only be obtained if the correct lymph node is aspirated. As not all lymph nodes can be aspirated, a selection should be made of the most suspicious ones. The aforementioned criteria play a large role in this selection, as do the known patterns of metastases. To obtain a high sensitivity, in some cases lymph nodes as small as 4 to 5 mm in the first two echelons should be aspirated. Although aspirating smaller nodes will increase the sensitivity, it is difficult to obtain a diagnostic aspirate from nodes of 3 to 4 mm or smaller. In a previous report, we found that with use of US-guided FNAC we obtained a sensitivity of 73% with a specificity of 100% in N0 necks.[27,63] This was significantly better than CT or MRI. Several other studies compared US-FNAC to CT and MRI and found it to be superior as well.[65-67] On the other hand, Takes reported a sensitivity of only 42% for the N0 neck.[68] Righi found a sensitivity of 50%, which was inferior to 60% for CT[69]; however, in Righi's study, most false negatives were found in the beginning of the study, consistent with a learning curve for US-guided FNAC, and some of these were irradiated patients or nonsquamous cell carcinoma patients. In a recent survey in the Netherlands Cancer Institute, we found that the sensitivity is significantly lower in small T1 tumors as compared to T2 carcinomas and that it was lower in oral cavity as compared to oropharyngeal or laryngeal carcinomas. The main reasons are probably that lymph node metastases are smaller in small carcinomas and level 1 nodes are more easily overlooked. Furthermore, as in the small tumors a wait-and-see policy was conducted, another reason for this lower sensitivity could be that small lymph node metastases were overlooked by the pathologist in the larger tumors.

It is well known that routine histopathologic examination, as conducted in the electively treated group, overlooks 5 to 15% of the small metastases.[72] As a consequence, we believe that the reported sensitivities in the literature, always based on the pathology report of the neck dissection specimen, are probably overestimated.

We have conducted several studies to determine the causes of false negative US-FNAC examinations.[70] Using sentinel node scintigraphy and specific aspiration from the sentinel lymph nodes we have tried to increase the sensitivity of US-FNAC.[14] Furthermore, we tried to increase the detection of tumor cells in aspirates using RT-PCR techniques.[71] Patients were clinically N0 and subsequently underwent elective neck dissection for RT-PCR and histopathologic evaluation. From these studies we have learned that the main cause of false negative US-FNAC is not improper lymph node selection, but actual sampling of a wrong part of the correct lymph node. This is mainly caused by small metastases inside lymph nodes, not detectable by imaging or aspiration (micrometastases).[29] An important finding from these studies was that sentinel lymph node aspiration did not increase the sensitivity.

US Assessment of Different Levels of the Neck

Like dictated operative reports, the US report should describe findings in terms of lymph node levels, according to internationally standardized guidelines.[73] With use of US it is quite easy to define the exact levels in the neck. US is ideal to assess lymph nodes in levels 2 through 5. Level 1 nodes on the other hand, especially those around the facial artery, are more easily overlooked unless diligently sought out. Although an N-staging lymph node level is used only in nasopharyngeal carcinomas, several studies have shown the prognostic importance of lymph node level in other primary tumor sites of the head and neck.[74,75] The relevance of staging of the exact number and levels of metastases is becoming increasingly important now that selective neck dissections are being performed more widely, even for limited disease, and radiotherapy is frequently the primary treatment modality and no histopathology will become available.[76,77] Unfortunately, there are no studies on the accuracy of US to assess the number of lymph nodes and levels involved. One can expect the sensitivity per level to be relatively low, as relatively large detectable metastases are very often accompanied by small undetectable micrometastases.[33,72]

A limitation of US is that retropharyngeal lymph nodes are not depicted. The incidence of these lymph nodes has never been studied in detail compared with the other lymph node levels, and the retropharyngeal nodes are not generally incorporated into the typical neck dissection. A recent study from Gross et al showed an incidence of retropharyngeal nodal metastases of over 27% in surgically treated non-nasopharynx head and neck carcinomas, whereas this incidence is even higher in nasopharynx carcinoma.[78,79] Imaging of the retropharynx thus seems to be a clinically significant limitation of US.

Another level of clinical and prognostic relevance is level VI.[80] Unfortunately, it is our experience that US, as well as CT, are not very sensitive in detecting metastases at this level,[81] especially when the thyroid gland is present. This might be due to the small size of metastases in this level. Perhaps endoscopic transesophageal US-FNAC or CT-PET are more appropriate to assess this level in the neck[82-84] (see Chapter 10). Because of the limited accuracy of imaging, elective paratracheal dissection is recommended in aggressive thyroid cancer, laryngeal cancer with subglottic extension, and hypopharyngeal and proximal esophageal cancer.

Tumor Extent and Extranodal Spread

In general, the borders of metastatic lymph nodes, certainly if small, are sharp. Extranodal spread (ENS, also known as extracapsular spread or ECS) is an important prognostic feature and radiologically it is characterized by ablation of fat planes and irregular nodal borders. Close et al have reported that CT can identify extranodal spread in large nodes,[85] and Som has even reported a 100% sensitivity for CT.[32] Yousem on the other hand found an accuracy of CT of 90%, whereas in their study MRI had an accuracy

of 78%.[53] Carvalho also studied the value of CT in detecting extranodal spread and found a sensitivity of 63% and a specificity of 60%.[86] In a study by Woolgar, in 16% of the cases that were N0 at CT, ENS was present at pathology.[87] These figures show that ENS can be present in small lymph node metastases and can be difficult to diagnose radiologically. Recently, King et al have shown that both CT and MRI have an accuracy in the order of 73 to 80% to detect ENS.[88] No studies on US have been done in this field. We have previously looked at the inter- and intraobserver variation in diagnosing ENS histopathologically.[89] From these studies it became clear that even among pathologists there is no consensus on the criteria of ENS and that frequently it is a subtle feature not detectable radiologically. In our opinion, only major macroscopic extranodal spread (infiltration) can be detected with imaging techniques.

Assessment of invasion of vital structures can be both prognostically and therapeutically relevant, as the resectability becomes uncertain and prognosis very poor once vital structures are invaded. In this respect, invasion of the common or internal carotid artery is probably most important,[90] although invasion of the internal jugular veins, the skull base, or thoracic inlet pose similar therapeutic challenges. Initial reports on the accuracy of US in detecting tumor invasion into the carotid artery were quite optimistic.[91,92] A more recent report, on the other hand, found no advantage of US over palpation or CT.[93] However, no correlation with operability has ever been performed. Palpation simultaneous with real-time US ("sonopalpation") can be helpful to detect carotid wall invasion.[94]

Clinical Impact of US in Squamous Cell Carcinomas

As discussed above, a positive finding at palpation or US will guide our therapeutic approach to the neck. There is still debate on the optimal modality and extent of neck treatment, but this discussion is not pursued in this chapter. As US, and especially US-FNAC, are very specific assessment techniques to detect metastases, a positive finding will thus influence management.

The extent of neck disease is more difficult to assess than is the mere presence or absence of any positive findings using US. Exact assessment of the levels involved, assessment of retropharyngeal and paratracheal lymph nodes, as well as infiltration into the carotid artery or other vital structures, remains difficult. As a consequence, US only plays a limited role in the assessment of each level separately and in determining the operability of a lesion when such aggressive features are present.

US-FNAC can play a major role in confirming a neck-side to be tumor negative. In these cases, the potential for US-negative occult disease might be judged to be low enough to refrain from elective neck treatment. In small oral cavity, pharyngeal, and laryngeal carcinomas, several centers in the world have adapted their policy of elective neck treatment in selected patients.[14-16] In selected patients who can be treated with transoral excision for T1 (and T2) oral/oropharyngeal carcinomas, laser excision of T1-2 supraglottic carcinomas, or selected patients who undergo laryngectomy for laryngeal carcinomas, the authors rely on the US-guided FNAC findings and do not routinely treat the neck electively. These patients are followed very meticulously, using US-guided FNAC at 12-week intervals for 1 year. Our experience with this wait-and-see policy has been encouraging. Only about 20% of the patients with oral cancer treated with transoral excision develop a neck node metastasis during follow-up, but over 80% of these can be salvaged by timely treatment.[14,15] This high salvage rate is certainly related to the short delay of diagnosis due to follow-up by US-guided FNAC.

Clinical Impact of US (-FNAC) in Thyroid Carcinomas

Regional lymph nodes metastases are present in 50 to 75% of cases of well-differentiated and medullary carcinomas of the thyroid gland at the time of diagnosis. Because radioactive iodine can cure small metastases after thyroidectomy for well-differentiated thyroid carcinoma, imaging has relatively few implications if no palpable neck nodes are present. However, to detect metastases early, US with guided

FNAC has shown to be a reliable technique, that can be used routinely for follow-up.[95-97] Furthermore, since US of the thyroid is the preferred imaging technique, the opportunity to survey the cervical lymph nodes during preoperative thyroid US should not be wasted. More recently, BRAF mutation and RET/PTC rearrangements have been identified as molecular markers of papillary thyroid carcinoma that can be applied to aspirates in adjunct to traditional cytology.[98] Because of the prognostic significance, in medullary carcinomas elective neck dissection is often recommended but still controversial and imaging can play a pivotal role in decision-making. As imaging of the paratracheal nodes is not very reliable, a routine paratracheal dissection is generally recommended.

Clinical Impact of US (-FNAC) in Salivary Gland Carcinomas

Lymph node metastases are an important prognostic factor in salivary gland carcinomas.[99] A common approach is to perform frozen section of the first echelon nodes in level 2. If these are positive, the parotidectomy will be followed by a neck dissection. However, this policy has the disadvantage that surgery time is difficult to plan. Therefore, preoperative assessment of the neck, using either MRI or US (-FNAC) is a logical approach, although there is no literature on its accuracy.[64] As the treatment of most parotid carcinomas is surgery with postoperative radiotherapy there is a tendency to treat the primary tumor with surgery and postoperative radiotherapy, and to treat the neck with elective radiotherapy if staged N0 preoperatively and at frozen section of level 2 nodes.

Clinical Impact of US (-FNAC) in Skin Cancer

In melanoma and nonmelanoma skin cancer, lymph node metastases are important prognostic features.[5,6] The incidence of lymph node metastases is very low in basal cell carcinomas, it increases in squamous cell carcinomas to 7 to 15% and is even higher in merkel cell carcinomas and infiltrating melanomas.[6] The incidence of lymph node metastases is in the range of 20% for intermediate-thickness melanomas. The patterns of metastases of melanoma are less predictable than in squamous cell carcinomas.[100] Because of this unpredictability, the sentinel node procedure has gained widespread acceptance although it has not yet been clarified with certainty whether early detection of lymph node metastases (and early treatment) has prognostic importance in skin melanoma. For the head and neck area, the accuracy of the sentinel node procedure is less than for other parts of the body, and in over 10% of patients, the SN cannot be identified or renders false negative results.[101-103] To assess the neck nonsurgically, several authors have shown that US or US-FNAC is the modality of first choice, more reliable than palpation or CT, and can be used during follow-up.[104-109] Preoperative US-FNAC can be used to stage advanced skin squamous cancers and melanomas. In case the US-FNAC is negative, a sentinel node procedure should be considered in intermediate-thickness melanomas. Several authors have tried to use US to obviate the need for sentinel lymph node biopsy. However, as the incidence of undetectable micrometastases is very high in melanoma,[31] US can only detect 21 to 71% of the occult metastases and can only spare 5 to 12% patients from a sentinel node procedure.[107,110,111]

Clinical Impact of US-FNAC on Recurrent Disease in the Neck

Detection of recurrences is clinically most relevant if therapeutic options are still present. As many patients have had initial treatment of the neck with neck dissection and postoperative radiotherapy, regional recurrences in these necks can rarely be treated effectively. However, even for these patients the establishment of a diagnosis is important. In patients treated for the primary tumor only (wait and see for the neck), or those treated in the neck exclusively with radiotherapy, chemoradiation, or limited surgery, routine follow-up examinations of the neck using imaging to detect early recurrences

seem warranted. Thus far, CT and MRI have been disappointing in the early detection of recurrent or residual disease in the neck. Radiation therapy and surgery can lead to anatomic changes that may mask the detection of disease by physical examination. Computed tomography, MRI, and US are reported to have a poor specificity to distinguish radiation or postsurgical edema and scarring from recurrent tumor.[112,113] However, based on our experience, we believe that US is very appropriate to evaluate a treated neck. Changes in lymph node appearance on serial exams can be very telling. Suspicious areas may be seen with low echogenicity and irregular borders. US-FNAC of these regions may then be performed and may confirm malignancy in these areas. Cytology, however, is sometimes inaccurate in discriminating necrotic tumor cells from viable tumor. MRI can be helpful in selecting patients for further examination under general anesthesia after chemoradiation.[114] The use of US, US-FNAC, or duplex Doppler for the follow-up of the treated neck has been studied by several authors.[17,115-117] Westhofen showed that US-FNAC was superior to CT in detecting neck recurrences after previous treatment.[17] In our opinion, routine US-FNAC follow-up for at least one year is warranted if the neck was not treated electively (except for T1-2 glottic carcinomas, small skin carcinomas, or noninfiltrating carcinomas). We also use US to assess the N+ neck treated with chemo(radiation), 6 to 8 weeks post-treatment. In these cases however, the cytology is much more difficult to interpret and necrotic tumor cells can be both a sign of good response as well as residual disease. Of course US-FNAC can also be used to confirm findings at post treatment PET scans.[118]

Videos in This Chapter

Video 15A. See legend for Figure 15–12.

References

1. Snow GB, Annyas AA, van Slooten EA, Bartelink H, Hart AAM. Prognostic factors of neck node metastasis. *Clin Otolaryngol.* 1982;7:185–192.

2. Zoller M, Goodman ML, Cummings CW. Guidelines for prognosis in head and neck cancer with nodal metastasis. *Laryngoscope.* 1978;88:135–140.

3. De Bree R, Deurloo EE, Snow GB, Leemans CR. Screening for distant metastases in patients with head and neck cancer. *Laryngoscope.* 2000;110 (3 pt 1):397–401.

4. Ljumenovic R, Langendjk JA, Hoekstra OS, Leemans CR, Castelijns JA. Distant metastases in head and neck carcinoma: identification of prognostic groups with MR imaging. *Eur J Radiol.* 2006;60(1):58–66.

5. Grunhagen DJ, Eggermont AM, van Geel AN, Graveland WJ, deWilt JH. Prognostic factors after cervical lymph node dissection for cutaneous melanoma metastases. *Melanoma Res.* 2005; 15(3):179–184.

6. Moore BA, Weber RS, Prieto V, et al. Lymph node metastases from cutaneous squamous cell carcinoma of the head and neck. *Laryngoscope.* 2005; 115(9):1561–1567.

7. Terhaard CH, Lubsen H, van der Tweel I, et al. Salivary gland carcinoma: independent prognostic factors for locoregional control, distant metastases, and overall survival: results of the Dutch head and neck oncology cooperative group. *Head Neck.* 2004;26(8):681–692.

8. Mazzaferri EL, Jhiang SM. Long-term impact of initial surgical and medical therapy on papillary and follicular thyroid cancer. *Am J Med.* 1994; 97(5):418–428.

9. Sato N, Oyamatsu M, Koyama Y, Emura I, Tamiya Y, Hatakeyama K. Do the level of nodal disease according to the TNM classification and the number of involved cervical nodes reflect prognosis in patients with differentiated carcinoma of the thyroid gland? *J Surg Oncol.* 1998;69(3):151–155.

10. Korkmaz H, Yoo GH, Du W, et al. Predictors of nodal metastasis in salivary gland cancer. *J Surg Oncol.* 2002;80(4):186–189.

11. Zbaren P, Schupbach J, Nuyens M, Stauffer E. Elective neck dissection versus observation in primary parotid carcinoma. *Otolaryngol Head Neck Surg.* 2005;132(3):387–391.

12. Fisher SR. Elective, therapeutic, and delayed lymph node dissection for malignant melanoma of the head and neck: analysis of 1444 patients from 1970 to 1998. *Laryngoscope.* 2002;112(1): 99–110.

13. Shaha AR. Management of the neck in thyroid cancer. *Otolaryngol Clin North Am.* 1998;31(5): 823–831.

14. Nieuwenhuis EJ, Castelijns JA, Pijpers R, et al. Wait-and-see policy for the N0 neck in early-stage oral and oropharyngeal squamous cell carcinoma using ultrasonography-guided cytology: is there a role for identification of the sentinel node? *Head Neck.* 2002;24(3):282–289.

15. van den Brekel MW, Reitsma LC, et al. Sonographically guided aspiration cytology of neck nodes for selection of treatment and follow-up in patients with N0 head and neck cancer. *AJNR Am J Neuroradiol.* 1999;20(9):1727–1731.

16. Quetz JU, Bosse M, Sperlich D, Heissenberg MC. Sonography for detection of late lymph node metastases in the head and neck region: an effective method of follow-up screening? *Br J Cancer.* 1998;77 (suppl 1):15.

17. Westhofen M. Ultrasound b-scans in the follow-up of head and neck tumors. *Head Neck Surg.* 1987;9:272–278.

18. Schipper J, Gellrich NC, Marangos N, Maier W. [Value of B-image ultrasound in patients with carcinomas of the upper aerodigestive tract and N0 lymph node stage]. *Laryngorhinootologie.* 1999; 78(10):561–565.

19. Szmeja Z, Wierzbicka M, Kordylewska M. The value of ultrasound examination in preoperative neck assessment and in early diagnosis of nodal recurrences in the follow-up of patients operated for laryngeal cancer. *Eur Arch Otorhinolaryngol.* 1999;256(8):415–417.

20. Borjesson PK, Jauw YW, Boellaard R, et al. Performance of immuno-positron emission tomography with zirconium-89-labeled chimeric monoclonal antibody U36 in the detection of lymph node metastases in head and neck cancer patients. *Clin Cancer Res.* 2006;12(7):2133–2140.

21. Wagner JD, Schauwecker D, Davidson D, et al. Inefficacy of F-18 fluorodeoxy-D-glucose-positron emission tomography scans for initial evaluation in early-stage cutaneous melanoma. *Cancer.* 2005; 104(3):570–579.

22. Hao SP, Ng SH. Magnetic resonance imaging versus clinical palpation in evaluating cervical metastasis from head and neck cancer. *Otolaryngol Head Neck Surg.* 2000;123(3):324–327.

23. Stuckensen T, Kovacs AF, Adams S, Baum RP. Staging of the neck in patients with oral cavity squamous cell carcinomas: a prospective comparison of PET, ultrasound, CT and MRI. *J Craniomaxillofac Surg.* 2000;28(6):319–324.

24. Ishii J, Amagasa T, Tachibana T, Shinozuka K, Shioda S. US and CT evaluation of cervical lymph

node metastasis from oral cancer. *J Craniomax-illofac Surg.* 1991;3:123-127.

25. Prayer L, Winkelbauer H, Gritzmann N, Winkelbauer F, Helmer M, Pehamberger H. Sonography versus palpation in the detection of regional lymph-node metastases in patients with malignant melanoma. *Eur J Cancer.* 1990;26:827-830.

26. Vassallo P, Edel G, Roos N, Naguib A, Peters PE. In vitro high-resolution ultrasonography of benign and malignant lymph nodes. a sonographic-pathologic correlation. *Invest Radiol.* 1993;28:698-705.

27. van den Brekel MW, Castelijns JA, Stel HV, Golding RP, Meyer CJ, Snow GB. Modern imaging techniques and ultrasound-guided aspiration cytology for the assessment of neck node metastases: a prospective comparative study. *Eur Arch Otorhinolaryngol.* 1993;250:11-17.

28. Giancarlo T, Palmieri A, Giacomarra V, Russolo M. Pre-operative evaluation of cervical adenopathies in tumours of the upper aerodigestive tract. *Anticancer Res.* 1998;18:2805-2809.

29. van den Brekel MWM, van der Waal I, Meyer CJLM, Freeman JL, Castelijns JA, Snow GB. The incidence of micrometastases in neck dissection specimens obtained from elective neck dissections. *Laryngoscope.* 1996;106:987-991.

30. Giese T, Engstner M, Mansmann U, Hartschuh W, Arden B. Quantification of melanoma micrometastases in sentinel lymph nodes using real-time RT-PCR. *J Invest Dermatol.* 2005;124(3):633-637.

31. Spanknebel K, Coit DG, Bieligk SC, Gonen M, Rosai J, Klimstra DS. Characterization of micrometastatic disease in melanoma sentinel lymph nodes by enhanced pathology: recommendations for standardizing pathologic analysis. *Am J Surg Pathol.* 2005;29(3):305-317.

32. Som PM. Detection of metastasis in cervical lymph nodes: ct and mr criteria and differential diagnosis. *Am J Roentgenol.* 1992;158:961-969.

33. van den Brekel MWM, Stel HV, Castelijns JA, et al. Cervical lymph node metastasis: assessment of radiologic criteria. *Radiology.* 1990;177:379-384.

34. Wang Q, Takashima S, Takayama F, et al. Detection of occult metastatic lymph nodes in the neck with gray-scale and power Doppler US. *Acta Radiol.* 2001;42(3):312-319.

35. Don DM, Anzai Y, Lufkin RB, Fu YS, Calcaterra TC. Evaluation of cervical lymph node metastases in squamous cell carcinoma of the head and neck. *Laryngoscope.* 1995;105:669-674.

36. Curtin HD, Ishwaran H, Mancuso AA, Dalley BW, Caudry DJ, McNeil BJ. Comparison of CT and MR imaging in staging of neck metastases. *Radiology.* 1998;207:123-130.

37. Friedman M, Mafee MF, Pacella BL Jr, Strorigl TL, Dew LL, Toriumi DM. Rationale for elective neck dissection in 1990. *Laryngoscope.* 1990;100:54-59.

38. Yusa H, Yoshida H, Ueno E. Ultrasonographic criteria for diagnosis of cervical lymph node metastasis of squamous cell carcinoma in the oral and maxillofacial region. *J Oral Maxillofac Surg.* 1999;57(1):41-48.

39. Stern WBR, Silver CE, Zeifer BA, Persky MS, Heller KS. Computed tomography of the clinically negative neck. *Head Neck.* 1990;12:109-113.

40. Mancuso AA, Maceri D, Rice D, Hanafee W. CT of cervical lymph node cancer. *AJR Am J Roentgenol.* 1981;136:381-385.

41. Friedman M, Roberts N, Kirshenbaum GL, Colombo J. Nodal size of metastatic squamous cell carcinoma of the neck. *Laryngoscope.* 1993;103:854-856.

42. Steinkamp HJ, Cornehl M, Hosten N, Pegios W, Vogl T, Felix R. Cervical lymphadenopathy: ratio of long- to short-axis diameter as a predictor of malignancy. *Br J Radiol.* 1995;68:266-270.

43. van den Brekel MW, Castelijns JA, Snow GB. The size of lymph nodes in the neck on sonograms as a radiologic criterion for metastasis: how reliable is it? [see comments]. *AJNR Am J Neuroradiol.* 1998;19(4):695-700.

44. Steinkamp HJ, Hosten N, Richter C, Schedel H, Felix R. Enlarged cervical lymph nodes at helical *Ct Radiology.* 1994;191:795-798.

45. Bruneton JN, Balu-Maestro C, Marcy PY, Melia P, Mourou MY. Very high frequency (13 Mhz) ultra-sonographic examination of the normal neck: detection of normal lymph nodes and thyroid nodules. *J Ultrasound Med.* 1994;13:87-90.

46. Umeda M, Nishimatsu N, Teranobu O, Shimada K. Criteria for diagnosing lymph node metastasis from squamous cell carcinoma of the oral cavity: a study of the relationship between computed tomographic and histologic findings and outcome. *J Oral Maxillofac Surg.* 1998;56(5):585-593.

47. Yuasa K, Kawazu T, Kunitake N, et al. Sonography for the detection of cervical lymph node metastases among patients with tongue cancer: criteria for early detection and assessment of follow-up examination intervals. *AJNR Am J Neuroradiol.* 2000;21(6):1127-1132.

48. Vassallo P, Wernecke K, Roos N, Peters PE. Differentiation of benign from malignant superficial lymphadenopathy: the role of high-resolution US. *Radiology.* 1992;183:215-220.

49. Shin JH, Choi HY, Moon BI, Sung SH. In vitro sonographic evaluation of sentinel lymph nodes for detecting metastasis in breast cancer: comparison with histopathologic results. *J Ultrasound Med.* 2004;23(7):923-928.

50. Lee N, Inoue K, Yamamoto R, Kinoshita H. Patterns of internal echoes in lymph nodes in the diagnosis of lung cancer metastasis. *World J Surg.* 1992;16(5):986-993.

51. Ahuja A, Ying M. An overview of neck node sonography. *Invest Radiol.* 2002;37(6):333-342.

52. Giancarlo T, Palmieri A, Giacomarra V, Russolo M. Pre-operative evaluation of cervical adenopathies in tumours of the upper aerodigestive tract. *Anticancer Res.* 1998;18(4B):2805-2809.

53. Yousem DM, Som PM, Hackney DB, Schwaibold F, Hendrix RA. Central nodal necrosis and extracapsular neoplastic spread in cervical lymph nodes: MR imaging versus CT. *Radiology.* 1992;182(3):753-759.

54. King AD, Tse GM, Ahuja AT, et al. Necrosis in metastatic neck nodes: diagnostic accuracy of CT, MR imaging, and US. *Radiology.* 2004;230(3):720-726.

55. Grabenbauer GG, Steininger H, Meyer M, et al. Nodal CT density and total tumor volume as prognostic factors after radiation therapy of stage III/IV head and neck cancer. *Radiother Oncol.* 1998;47(2):175-183.

56. Dietz A, Delorme S, Rudat V, et al. Prognostic assessment of sonography and tumor volumetry in advanced cancer of the head and neck by use of doppler ultrasonography. *Otolaryngol Head Neck Surg.* 2000;122(4):596-601.

57. Ahuja A, Ying M, Yuen YH, Metreweli C. Power Doppler sonography to differentiate tuberculous cervical lymphadenopathy from nasopharyngeal carcinoma. *AJNR Am J Neuroradiol.* 2001;22(4):735-740.

58. Moritz JD, Ludwig A, Oestmann JW. Contrast-enhanced color Doppler sonography for evaluation of enlarged cervical lymph nodes in head and neck tumors. *AMJ Am J Roentgenol.* 2000;174(5):1279-1284.

59. Sato N, Kawabe R, Fujita K, Omura S. Differential diagnosis of cervical lymphadenopathy with intranodal color doppler flow signals in patients with oral squamous cell carcinoma. *Oral Surg Oral Med Oral Path Oral Radiol Endod.* 1998;86:482-488.

60. Ariji Y, Kimura Y, Hayashi N, et al. Power Doppler sonography of cervical lymph nodes in patients with head and neck cancer. *AJNR Am J Neuroradiol.* 1998;19(2):303-307.

61. Chikui T, Yonetsu K, Nakamura T. Multivariate feature analysis of sonographic findings of metastatic cervical lymph nodes: contribution of blood flow features revealed by power Doppler sonography for predicting metastasis. *AJNR Am J Neuroradiol.* 2000;21(3):561-567.

62. Chang DB, Yuan A, Yu CJ, Luh KT, Kuo SH, Yang PC. Differentiation of benign and malignant cervical lymph nodes with color doppler sonography. *AJR Am J Roentgenol.* 1994;162:965-968.

63. van den Brekel MW, Castelijns JA, Stel HV, et al. Occult metastatic neck disease: detection with US and US-guided fine-needle aspiration cytology. *Radiology.* 1991;180:457-461.

64. McIvor NP, Freeman JL, Salem S, Elden L, Noyek AM, Bedard YC. Ultrasonography and ultrasound-guided fine-needle aspiration biopsy of head and neck lesions: a surgical perspective. *Laryngoscope.* 1994; 104:669-674.

65. Hodder SC, Evans RM, Patton DW, Silvester KC. Ultrasound and fine needle aspiration cytology in the staging of neck lymph nodes in oral squamous cell carcinoma. *Br J Oral Maxillofac Surg.* 2000;38(5):430-436.

66. Atula TS, Varpula MJ, Kurki TJI, Klemi PJ, Grenman R. Assessment of cervical lymph node status in head and neck cancer patients—palpation, computed tomography and low field magnetic resonance imaging compared with ultrasound-guided fine-needle aspiration cytology. *Euro J Radiol.* 1997;25:152-161.

67. Kau RJ, Alexiou C, Stimmer H, Arnold W. Diagnostic procedures for detection of lymph node metastases in cancer of the larynx. *ORL J Otorhinolaryngol Relat Spec.* 2000;62(4):199-203.

68. Takes RP, Righi P, Meeuwis CA, et al. The value of ultrasound with ultrasound-guided fine-needle aspiration biopsy compared to computed tomography in the detection of regional metastases in the clinically negative neck. *Int J Rad Oncol Biol Physics.* 1998;40:1027-1032.

69. Righi PD, Kopecky KK, Caldemeyer KS, Ball VA, Weisberger EC, Radpour S. Comparison of ultrasound fine needle aspiration and computed tomography in patients undergoing elective neck dissection. *Head Neck Surg.* 1997;19:604-610.

70. Colnot DR, Nieuwenhuis EJ, van den Brekel MW, et al. Head and neck squamous cell carcinoma: US-guided fine-needle aspiration of sentinel lymph nodes for improved staging-initial experience. *Radiology.* 2001;218(1):289-293.

71. Nieuwenhuis EJ, Leemans CR, Kummer JA, Denkers F, Snow GB, Brakenhoff RH. Assessment and clinical significance of micrometastases in lymph nodes of head and neck cancer patients detected by E48 (Ly-6D) quantitative reverse transcription-polymerase chain reaction. *Lab Invest.* 2003;83(8):1233-1240.

72. van den Brekel MW, Stel HV, van der Valk P, van der Waal I, Meyer CJ, Snow GB. Micrometastases from squamous cell carcinoma in neck dissection specimens. *Eur Arch Otorhinolaryngol.* 1992; 249:349-353.

73. Robbins KT, Clayman G, Levine PA, et al. Neck dissection classification update: revisions proposed by the American Head and Neck Society and the American Academy of Otolaryngology-Head and Neck Surgery. *Arch Otolaryngol Head Neck Surg.* 2002;128(7):751-758.

74. Jones AS, Roland NJ, Field JK, Phillips DE. The level of cervical lymph node metastases: their prognostic relevance and relationship with head and neck squamous carcinoma primary sites. *Clin Otolaryngol.* 1994;19:63-69.

75. O'Brien CJ, Smith JW, Soong SJ, Urist MM, Maddox WA. Neck dissection with and without radiotherapy: prognostic factors, patterns of recurrence, and survival. *Am J Surg.* 1986;4:456-463.

76. van den Brekel MW, Bartelink H, Snow GB. The value of staging of neck nodes in patients treated with radiotherapy. *Radiother Oncol.* 1994;32:193-196.

77. Hermans R, Op dB, van den BW, et al. The relation of CT-determined tumor parameters and local and regional outcome of tonsillar cancer after definitive radiation treatment. *Int J Radiat Oncol Biol Physics.* 2001;50(1):37-45.

78. Gross ND, Ellingson TW, Wax MK, Cohen JI, Andersen PE. Impact of retropharyngeal lymph node metastasis in head and neck squamous cell carcinoma. *Arch Otolaryngol Head Neck Surg.* 2004;130(2):169-173.

79. Ng SH, Chang JT, Chan SC, et al. Nodal metastases of nasopharyngeal carcinoma: patterns of disease on MRI and FDG PET. *Eur J Nucl Med Mol Imaging.* 2004;31(8):1073-1080.

80. Plaat RE, De Bree R, Kuik DJ, et al. Prognostic importance of paratracheal lymph node metastases. *Laryngoscope.* 2005;115(5):894-898.

81. Yang CY, Andersen PE, Everts EC, Cohen JI. Nodal disease in purely glottic carcinoma: is elective neck treatment worthwhile? *Laryngoscope.* 1998; 108:1006-1008.

82. Chandawarkar RY, Kakegawa T, Fujita H, Yamana H, Toh Y, Fujitoh H. Endosonography for preoperative staging of specific nodal groups associated with esophageal cancer. *World J Surg.* 1996; 20(6):700-702.

83. Larsen SS, Vilmann P, Krasnik M, et al. Endoscopic ultrasound guided biopsy versus mediastinoscopy for analysis of paratracheal and subcarinal lymph nodes in lung cancer staging. *Lung Cancer.* 2005;48(1):85-92.

84. Shim SS, Lee KS, Kim BT, et al. Non-small cell lung cancer: prospective comparison of integrated FDG PET/CT and CT alone for preoperative staging. *Radiology.* 2005;236(3):1011-1019.

85. Close LG, Merkel M, Vuitch MF, Reisch J, Schaefer SD. Computed tomographic evaluation of regional lymph node involvement in cancer of the oral cavity and oropharynx. *Head Neck.* 1989;11: 309-317.

86. Carvalho P, Baldwin D, Carter R, Parsons C. Accuracy of CT in detecting squamous carcinoma metastases in cervical lymph nodes. *Clin Radiol.* 1991;44:79-81.

87. Woolgar JA, Vaughan ED, Scott J, Brown JS. Pathological findings in clinically false-negative and false-positive neck dissections for oral carcinoma. *Ann R Coll Surg Engl.* 1994;76(4):237-244.

88. King AD, Tse GM, Yuen EH, et al. Comparison of CT and MR imaging for the detection of extranodal neoplastic spread in metastatic neck nodes. *Eur J Radiol.* 2004;52(3):264-270.

89. van den Brekel MWM, van der Waal I, Stel HV, Snow GB. Het histopathologisch onderzoek van halsklierdissectie preparaten en de beoordeling van kapseldoorbraak. *Ned Tijdschr Geneeskd.* 1996;140(6):337.

90. Freeman SB, Hamaker RC, Borrowdale RB, Huntley TC. Management of neck metastasis with carotid artery involvement. *Laryngoscope.* 2004; 114(1):20-24.

91. Mann WJ, Beck A, Schreiber J, Maurer J, Amedee RG, Gluckmann JL. Ultrasonography for evaluation of the carotid artery in head and neck cancer. *Laryngoscope.* 1994;104:885-888.

92. Pradeep VM, Padmanabhan V, Sen P, et al. Sonographic evaluation of operability of malignant cervical lymph nodes. *Am J Clin Oncol.* 1991;14: 438-441.

93. Sarvanan K, Bapuraj JR, Sharma SC, Radotra BD, Khandelwal N, Suri S. Computed tomography and ultrasonographic evaluation of metastatic cervical lymph nodes with surgicoclinicopathologic correlation. *J Laryngol Otol.* 2002;116(3):194-199.

94. Gritzmann N, Grasl MC, Helmer M, Steiner E. Invasion of the carotid artery and jugular vein by lymph node metastases: detection with sonography. *AJR Am J Roentgenol.* 1990;154:411-414.

95. Franceschi M, Kusic Z, Franceschi D, Lukinac L, Roncevic S. Thyroglobulin determination, neck ultrasonography and Iodine-131 whole-body scintigraphy in differentiated thyroid carcinoma. *J Nucl Med.* 1996;37(3):446-451.

96. Frasoldati A, Pesenti M, Gallo M, Caroggio A, Salvo D, Valcavi R. Diagnosis of neck recurrences in patients with differentiated thyroid carcinoma. *Cancer.* 2003;97(1):90-96.

97. Kouvaraki MA, Shapiro SE, Fornage BD, et al. Role of preoperative ultrasonography in the surgical management of patients with thyroid cancer. *Surgery.* 2003;134(6):946-954.

98. Salvatore G, Giannini R, Faviana P, et al. Analysis of BRAF point mutation and RET/PTC rearrangement refines the fine-needle aspiration diagnosis of papillary thyroid carcinoma. *J Clin Endocrinol Metab.* 2004;89(10):5175-5180.

99. VanderPoorten V, Balm AJ, Hilgers FJ, et al. The development of a prognostic score for patients with parotid carcinoma. *Cancer.* 1999;85(9):2057-2067.

100. de Wilt JH, Thompson JF, Uren RF, et al. Correlation between preoperative lymphoscintigraphy and metastatic nodal disease sites in 362 patients with cutaneous melanomas of the head and neck. *Ann Surg.* 2004;239(4):544-552.

101. Jansen L, Koops HS, Nieweg OE, et al. Sentinel node biopsy for melanoma in the head and neck region. *Head Neck.* 2000;22(1):27-33.

102. Maffioli L, Belli F, Gallino G, et al. Sentinel node biopsy in patients with cutaneous melanoma of the head and neck. *Tumori.* 2000;86(4):341-342.

103. Stadelmann WK, Cobbins L, Lentsch EJ. Incidence of nonlocalization of sentinel lymph nodes using preoperative lymphoscintigraphy in 74 consecutive head and neck melanoma and Merkel cell carcinoma patients. *Ann Plast Surg.* 2004;52(6):546-549.

104. Tregnaghi A, Decandia A, Calderone M, et al. Ultrasonographic evaluation of superficial lymph node metastases in melanoma. *Eur J Radiol.* 1997;24:216-221.

105. Blum A, Schlagenhauff B, Stroebel W, Breuninger H, Rassner G, Garbe C. Ultrasound examination of regional lymph nodes significantly improves early detection of locoregional metastases during the follow-up of patients with cutaneous melanoma—Results of a prospective study of 1288 patients. *Cancer.* 2000;88(11):2534-2539.

106. van den Brekel MW, Pameijer FA, Koops W, Hilgers FJ, Kroon BB, Balm AJ. Computed tomography for the detection of neck node metastases in melanoma patients. *Eur J Surg Oncol.* 1998;24:51-54.

107. Voit C, Mayer T, Proebstle TM, et al. Ultrasound-guided fine-needle aspiration cytology in the early detection of melanoma metastases. *Cancer Cytopathol.* 2000;90(3):186-193.

108. Ross GL, Soutar DS, Gordon MD, et al. Sentinel node biopsy in head and neck cancer: preliminary results of a multicenter trial. *Ann Surg Oncol.* 2004;11(7):690-696.

109. Rossi CR, Scagnet B, Vecchiato A, et al. Sentinel node biopsy and ultrasound scanning in cutaneous melanoma: clinical and technical considerations. *Eur J Cancer.* 2000;36(7):895-900.

110. Hocevar M, Bracko M, Pogacnik A, et al. The role of preoperative ultrasonography in reducing the number of sentinel lymph node procedures in melanoma. *Melanoma Res.* 2004;14(6):533-536.

111. Rossi CR, Mocellin S, Scagnet B, et al. The role of preoperative ultrasound scan in detecting lymph node metastasis before sentinel node biopsy in melanoma patients. *J Surg Oncol.* 2003;83(2):80-84.

112. Mukherji SK, Mancuso AA, Kotzur IM, et al. Radiologic appearance of the irradiated larynx. Part II. Primary site response. *Radiology.* 1994;193:149-154.

113. Pameijer FA, Hermans R, Mancuso AA, et al. Pre- and post-radiotherapy computed tomography in laryngeal cancer: imaging-based prediction of local failure. *Int J Radiat Oncol Biol Physics.* 1999;45(2):359-366.

114. van den Broek GB, Rasch CR, Pameijer FA, Peter E, van den Brekel MW, Balm AJ. Response measurement after intraarterial chemoradiation in advanced head and neck carcinoma: magnetic resonance imaging and evaluation under general anesthesia? *Cancer.* 2006;106(8):1722-1729.

115. Ahuja A, Leung SF, Ying M, Metreweli C. Echography of metastatic nodes treated by radiotherapy. *J Laryngol Otol.* 1999;113(11):993-998.

116. Hessling KH, Schmelzeisen R, Reimer P, Milbradt H, Unverfehrt D. Use of sonography in the follow-up of preoperatively irradiated efferent lymphatics of the neck in oropharyngeal tumours. *J Cranio-Max-Fac Surg*. 1991;19:128–130.

117. Steinkamp HJ, Maurer J, Cornehl M, Knobber D, Hettwer H, Felix R. Recurrent cervical lymphadenopathy: differential diagnosis with color-duplex sonography. *Eur Arch Oto-Rhino-Laryngol*. 1994;251:404–409.

118. Yao M, Graham MM, Hoffman HT, et al. The role of post-radiation therapy FDG PET in prediction of necessity for post-radiation therapy neck dissection in locally advanced head-and-neck squamous cell carcinoma. *Int J Radiat Oncol Biol Physics*. 2004;59(4):1001–1010.

INDEX

V